Mayo Clinic
Essential Neurology

Andrea C. Adams, MD

T0386165

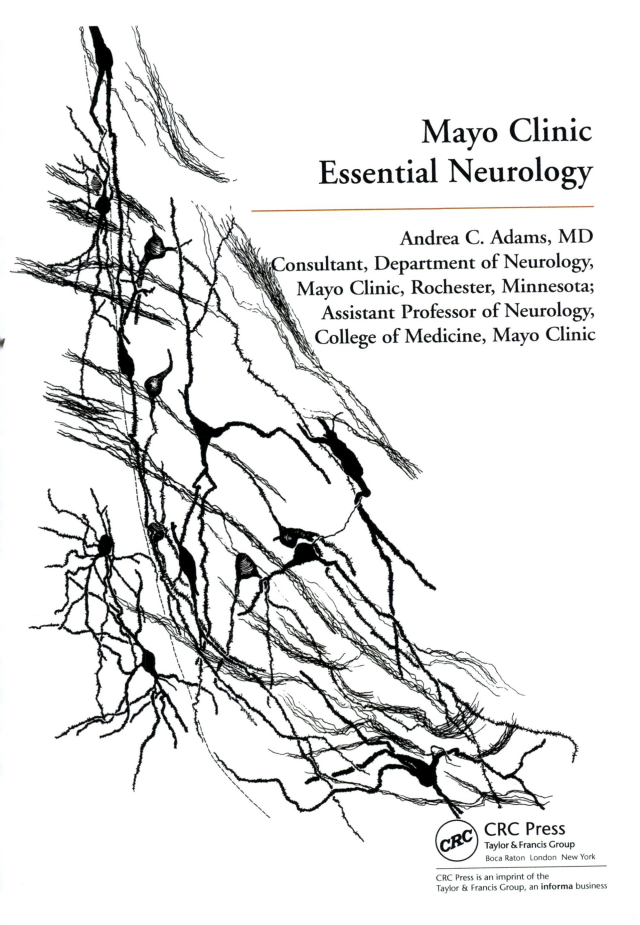

Mayo Clinic
Essential Neurology

Andrea C. Adams, MD
Consultant, Department of Neurology,
Mayo Clinic, Rochester, Minnesota;
Assistant Professor of Neurology,
College of Medicine, Mayo Clinic

CRC Press
Taylor & Francis Group
Boca Raton London New York

CRC Press is an imprint of the
Taylor & Francis Group, an **informa** business

CRC Press
Taylor & Francis Group
6000 Broken Sound Parkway NW, Suite 3000
Boca Raton, FL 33487-2742

First issued in paperback 2020

© 2008 Mayo Foundation for Medical Education and Research.
CRC Press is an imprint of Taylor & Francis Group, an Informa business

No claim to original U.S. Government works

ISBN-13: 978-1-4200-7973-9 (pbk)

This book contains information obtained from authentic and highly regarded sources. While all reasonable efforts have been made to publish reliable data and information, neither the author[s] nor the publisher can accept any legal responsibility or liability for any errors or omissions that may be made. The publishers wish to make clear that any views or opinions expressed in this book by individual editors, authors or contributors are personal to them and do not necessarily reflect the views/opinions of the publishers. The information or guidance contained in this book is intended for use by medical, scientific or health-care professionals and is provided strictly as a supplement to the medical or other professional's own judgement, their knowledge of the patient's medical history, relevant manufacturer's instructions and the appropriate best practice guidelines. Because of the rapid advances in medical science, any information or advice on dosages, procedures or diagnoses should be independently verified. The reader is strongly urged to consult the relevant national drug formulary and the drug companies' and device or material manufacturers' printed instructions, and their websites, before administering or utilizing any of the drugs, devices or materials mentioned in this book. This book does not indicate whether a particular treatment is appropriate or suitable for a particular individual. Ultimately it is the sole responsibility of the medical professional to make his or her own professional judgements, so as to advise and treat patients appropriately. The authors and publishers have also attempted to trace the copyright holders of all material reproduced in this publication and apologize to copyright holders if permission to publish in this form has not been obtained. If any copyright material has not been acknowledged please write and let us know so we may rectify in any future reprint.

Except as permitted under U.S. Copyright Law, no part of this book may be reprinted, reproduced, transmitted, or utilized in any form by any electronic, mechanical, or other means, now known or hereafter invented, including photocopying, microfilming, and recording, or in any information storage or retrieval system, without written permission from the publishers.

For permission to photocopy or use material electronically from this work, please access www. copyright. com (http://www.copyright.com/) or contact the Copyright Clearance Center, Inc. (CCC), 222 Rosewood Drive, Danvers, MA 01923, 978-750-8400. CCC is a not- for-profit organization that provides licenses and registration for a variety of users. For organizations that have been granted a photocopy license by the CCC, a separate system of payment has been arranged.

Trademark Notice: Product or corporate names may be trademarks or registered trademarks, and are used only for identification and explanation without intent to infringe.

Library of Congress Cataloging-in-Publication Data

Mayo Clinic essential neurology / Andrea C. Adams.
      p. ; cm.
  Includes bibliographical references and index.
  ISBN-13: 978-1-4200-7973-9 (pbk. : alk. paper)
  ISBN-10: 1-4200-7973-5 (pbk. : alk. paper) 1. Neurology--Handbooks, manuals, etc. 2. Nervous system--Diseases--Handbooks, manuals, etc. 3. Neurologic examination--Handbooks, manuals, etc. I. Adams, Andrea C., 1955- II. Mayo Clinic. III. Title: Essential neurology.
  [DNLM: 1. Nervous System Diseases--diagnosis--Handbooks. 2. Diagnostic Techniques, Neurological--Handbooks. 3. Nervous System Diseases--physiopathology--Handbooks. 4. Nervous System Diseases--therapy--Handbooks. WL 39 M478 2008]
  RC355.M39 2008
  616.8--dc22

2007049858

Visit the Taylor & Francis Web site at
http://www.taylorandfrancis.com

and the CRC Press Web site at
http://www.crcpress.com

About the Cover

The cover is a camera lucida drawing of a 160-μm–thick section of part of the striatum and adjoining globus pallidus. Brain tissue from a 19-day-old rat was processed according to the rapid Golgi method, which selectively impregnates neuronal cell bodies, dendrites, and axons. The cells on the left of the dashed line are medium spiny neurons typical of the striatum. They are the target of the dopaminergic axons that arise in the substantia nigra. Degeneration of these dopaminergic axons alters the function of the medium spiny neurons, leading to Parkinson disease. The medium spiny neurons send axons to neurons in the globus pallidus (cells on the right). These striopallidal axons form the fiber bundles that cross the section diagonally. The pallidal neurons are larger than the medium spiny neurons and have fewer but longer and thicker dendrites; their axons form the major efferent pathways of the basal ganglia.

Image from Millhouse, OE: Pallidal neurons in the rat. J Comp Neurol 254:209-227, 1986. Used with permission.

About the Cover

To Gene and Maude

Foreword

The field of neurology continues to evolve rapidly. Treatment options are increasing in number and improving in efficacy, diagnostic imaging allows us to see more detail in a noninvasive manner, and there are few areas of the field not affected by the tools of molecular genetics. Despite all this, it is the clinical interaction with the patient—the history and examination—that continues to be the underpinnings of the specialty. It is within this framework that *Mayo Clinic Essential Neurology*, by Dr. Andrea Adams, has a prominent role on the desk or bookshelf.

The book has been written by a most experienced neurology clinician-educator. As a highly regarded educator in a large neurology residency program and medical school basic neuroscience course and as a neurologist involved in the evaluation and management of patients with virtually all symptoms and disease types, she has made use of her wealth of experience in developing this textbook. The text, tables, figures, and images are a concise source of information that will be useful to the neurologist or nonneurologist evaluating patients with a wide array of neurologic conditions and symptoms, as seen in the office or hospital. It also is a superb review text for neurology in-service examinations and the neurology boards. For nonneurologists, *Mayo Clinic Essential Neurology* contains a wealth of information presented in a learner-friendly manner that will demystify many aspects of the evaluation and management of neurologic problems encountered in most any field of medicine.

I congratulate Dr. Adams on the completion of this textbook and thank her for her dedication to the education of those interested in the field of neurology across the spectrum of specialties and levels of experience and for making a major impact on the care of our patients by sharing her knowledge in this manner.

Robert D. Brown, Jr, MD, MPH
Chair, Department of Neurology, Mayo Clinic
Professor of Neurology, College of Medicine, Mayo Clinic
Rochester, MN

Preface

Mayo Clinic Essential Neurology is intended to provide succinct and essential neurologic information. Because time is a rare commodity for physicians, the text, tables, and illustrations have been designed to provide information quickly and concisely. The book is similar to the earlier *Neurology in Primary Care*. The book consists of three sections: the neurologic examination and diagnostic testing, common neurologic symptoms, and common neurologic diseases.

Neurology is a rapidly changing specialty, with an increasing number of therapeutic options available for managing neurologic disease. Neurologic symptoms such as headache, backache, and dizziness are frequent complaints that cause patients to seek medical care. *Mayo Clinic Essential Neurology* is designed to provide clinicians the necessary neurologic information for the diagnosis and management of these common neurologic problems.

This book will be useful to all clinicians who evaluate patients who have neurologic problems. It will be useful for medical students and residents in neurology, internal medicine, and psychiatry. The book also will be helpful to paramedical personnel who need a concise source of information on outpatient neurologic practice.

I want to thank O. Eugene Millhouse, PhD, Roberta J. Schwartz, Virginia Dunt, Traci Post, and Ann Ihrke of the Section of Scientific Publications for their conscientious help in editing and preparing the manuscript for publication. I also want to thank Jonathan Goebel, Karen Barrie, James J. Tidwell, and Jim Postier for their expert help with the illustrations. Thanks also to Doctors Marian McEvoy and Mark Pittelkow and the Department of Dermatology. Special thanks to my colleagues in Neurology, including Doctors Barbara Westmoreland, Kelly Flemming, Brad Boeve, Eliot Dimberg, and Robert D. Brown, Jr, for their help with the illustrations and radiographs. Finally, it is a pleasure to thank all my colleagues in the Department of Neurology at Mayo Clinic for their support and collegiality.

Production Staff

MAYO CLINIC SECTION OF SCIENTIFIC PUBLICATIONS

O. Eugene Millhouse, PhD	Editor
Roberta J. Schwartz	Production editor
Virginia Dunt	Editorial assistant
Traci Post	Scientific publications specialist
Ann Ihrke	Copy editor/proofreader

MAYO CLINIC SECTION OF ILLUSTRATION AND DESIGN

Jonathan Goebel	Designer
James J. Tidwell	Medical illustrator
Jim Postier	Medical illustrator

Table of Contents

CHAPTER 1

The Neurologic Examination

The neurologic examination is the most important part of the evaluation of a patient who has neurologic symptoms or disease. The information obtained from the history and physical examination is needed to generate a differential diagnosis, to select the appropriate diagnostic tests, and to initiate appropriate therapy.

The neurologic history usually provides all the information needed to understand the disease process. The temporal profile of symptoms is critical (Fig. 1.1). The sudden onset of symptoms suggests a vascular cause of the illness. Patients with symptoms of an infection or inflammatory condition have a subacute (hours to days) course. The temporal profile of neoplastic and degenerative disorders of the nervous system is chronic (months to years). As a general rule, the effects of trauma are maximal at the time of the trauma. A fluctuating temporal profile may indicate demyelinating disease. The disease process in transient disorders (discussed in Chapter 9) cannot be identified from the temporal profile.

The results of the neurologic examination help to localize the problem in the nervous system. If time is limited, an evaluation of the patient's gait, speech, and mental status can provide a relatively complete neurologic examination. The often-reported "neurologic exam grossly intact" or "CN [cranial nerve] II-XII intact" conveys little useful information. However, the report that a patient has a shuffling gait, microphonic speech, and memory difficulty or that a patient has a wide-based staggering gait, slurred (dysarthric) speech, and poor attention provides meaningful neurologic data.

GAIT EXAMINATION

Watch the patient walk. Normal walking depends on several factors that reflect function at every level of the nervous system: motor, sensory, balance, and reflex systems. Gait changes with age and is sensitive to diseases of the nervous system. Gait disorders are common in elderly persons and frequently contribute to the risk of falling.

Normal walking requires equilibrium and locomotion. Equilibrium involves the ability to assume an upright posture and to maintain balance. Locomotion is the ability to initiate and maintain rhythmic stepping. Both components involve sensory input from the vestibular,

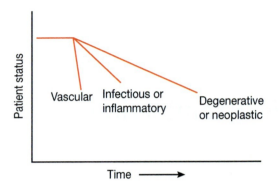

Fig. 1.1. Temporal profile of symptoms.

proprioceptive, tactile, and visual systems and the proper function of motor and reflex systems.

Musculoskeletal and cardiovascular diseases are nonneurologic abnormalities that affect gait. Familiar examples are the slow exercise-intolerant gait of a patient with congestive heart failure and the limp of a patient with degenerative joint disease. The Trendelenburg gait is seen in orthopedic and neurologic diseases (Fig. 1.2). Common causes of this abnormal gait are hip arthropathy and weakness of the gluteus medius muscle from an L5 radiculopathy. Gaits and their typical features and associated diseases are summarized in Table 1.1. The similarities between various gait disorders reflect the limited ways patients adjust to deteriorating performance.

The neurologic examination begins with how the patient is sitting in the waiting room. Secondary gain may be suggested when a patient with work-related low back pain sits comfortably with legs crossed reading a magazine but then walks painfully into the examination room. A patient with proximal muscle weakness needs to push off the chair with the hands to become upright, and a patient with parkinsonism has to make several rocking attempts before being able to stand.

Note how the patient stands. The posture, the position of the extremities, and the position of the head provide important diagnostic

information. Watch how the patient initiates movement. Patients with parkinsonism or certain degenerative disorders have trouble starting (called ignition failure). Does the patient require a gait aid or a companion's arm? Is the stance wide-based, as in cerebellar disorders and peripheral neuropathies? Is the head held perfectly still, as in vestibular disorders? Watch the symmetry of associated movements, such as arm swing. Watching the patient walk to the examination room when the patient does not know he or she is being observed often provides unique information not available when examining the patient's gait when he or she is in a gown in the examination room.

SPEECH

Speech is an integral part of the neurologic examination and can be evaluated when the medical history is being taken. Evaluating the patient's speech provides information about the

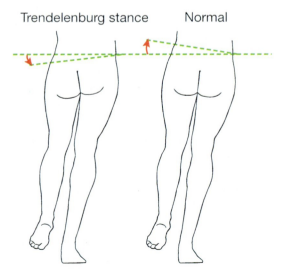

Fig. 1.2. Comparison of Trendelenburg stance with normal stance.

function of most of the lower cranial nerves. The primary lower motor neurons for speech are the trigeminal (CN V), facial (CN VII), vagus (CN X), and hypoglossal (CN XII) cranial nerves. The glossopharyngeal (CN IX) and spinal accessory (CN XI) cranial nerves may also be involved. The phrenic nerve from spinal cord segment C4 innervates the diaphragm, and the spinal intercostal nerves innervate the thoracic intercostal muscles.

Understanding the different types of dysarthria is essential for evaluating speech. Dysarthria, motor speech disorders caused by dysfunction of the peripheral nervous system or brainstem, is the imperfect articulation of speech, and abnormalities are apparent in the speed, strength, range, and timing of speech or in the accuracy of speech movements. The different types of dysarthria are listed in Table 1.2 and include flaccid, spastic, ataxic, hypokinetic, hyperkinetic, and mixed.

MENTAL STATUS EXAMINATION

Most of the mental status examination can be performed while the history is being taken. However, when the patient or the patient's family complains of memory or cognitive difficulty, further evaluation is recommended. Often, formal testing is not performed because of lack of time. Short standardized screening tests such as the Mini-Mental State Examination and the short test of mental status (called the "Kokmen," after its creator) (Fig. 1.3) is a useful screening device for dementia. These tests require time to administer, and often the results are not sufficiently sensitive for recognizing early cognitive dysfunction. Criticisms of these standardized tests include false-positive results in the case of patients with depression and false-negative results for patients of high intelligence. However, the tests are widely used, have normal values

for age and education, and are valuable screening tools. Once baseline function has been determined, the tests can be used for longitudinal monitoring and to suggest whether further testing or referral is needed. Testing is recommended for elderly patients before elective hospitalization because dementia is a major risk factor for delirium in the hospital setting.

Areas of cognitive function that need to be tested include attention, recent and remote memory, language, praxis, visual-spatial relationships, judgment, and calculations. Specific testing is recommended because mildly demented patients with preserved social skills are able to converse superficially and their cognitive deficits can be easily missed. Factors that must be considered in the interpretation of the results include the patient's age, educational level, ethnicity, and primary language (if other than English).

The patient's ability to pay attention is usually the first aspect of mental status testing that is assessed. Inattention can degrade all other mental status functions and is the defining feature of an acute confusional state (delirium). The inability to attend is seen in diffuse brain dysfunction such as toxic encephalopathy or frontal lobe disease. Tests that assess attention include having the patient spell the word "world" backwards or repeat a span of digits. Table 1.3 summarizes tests of specific cognitive functions and provides anatomical and clinical correlations. Mental status testing is discussed in more detail in Chapter 8.

CRANIAL NERVES

Olfactory Nerve (CN I)
Olfactory sense is not routinely tested, but the absence of smell (anosmia) can be a complaint that warrants further investigation. Each nostril is tested with a nonirritating aroma to avoid stimulation of the trigeminal nerve.

Table 1.1. Types of Gait: Characteristics and Associated Diseases

Gait type	Characteristics	Associated diseases
Antalgic	Painful, flexed, slow Patient swings normal leg quickly to avoid weight bearing on affected leg Arm opposite to affected side is held out laterally	Low back pain Degenerative joint disease
Cerebellar ataxia	Wide-based Lateral instability Erratic foot placement	Alcoholism Multiple sclerosis Phenytoin toxicity
Gait apraxia, frontal gait, "lower body parkinsonism"	Wide-based Short stride Trouble with starts and turns Feet glued to the ground	Normal-pressure hydrocephalus Small-vessel disease Multiple strokes
Hemiplegic or hemiparetic	Flexed arm Extended leg with circumduction	Stroke
Myopathic	Waddle Proximal muscle weakness of hip girdle, with excessive pelvic rotation	Polymyositis Muscular dystrophies
Orthopedic	Similar to antalgic and myopathic gaits	Prosthetic joints
Parkinsonian or extrapyramidal	Flexed posture Small steps Shuffling, turning en bloc Trouble initiating movement Festinating	Parkinson disease Drug-induced parkinsonism (phenothiazine)
Psychogenic, astasia-abasia	Odd gyrations Tightrope balancing Inconsistent Near falling Exaggerated effort Atypical postures and weakness	Conversion disorder

Table 1.1   (continued)

Gait type	Characteristics	Associated diseases
Sensory ataxia	Footdrop High steppage gait	Peripheral neuropathy Peroneal palsy L5 radiculopathy Multiple sensory deficits
Spastic, diplegic	Stiff Bouncy Circumduction of legs Scissors-like gait	Cervical myelopathy Vitamin B_{12} deficiency Multiple sclerosis Cerebral palsy
Trendelenburg	Pelvis tilts downward Lateral lurch toward affected side Bilateral waddling	L5 radiculopathy Myopathy Hip arthropathy
Vestibular ataxia	Head held still Cautious gait	Benign positional vertigo

Modified from Adams, AC: Neurology in Primary Care. FA Davis, Philadelphia, 2000, p 5. Used with permission of Mayo Foundation for Medical Education and Research.

Testing agents commonly used are coffee and mint. Frequent causes of anosmia are nasal or paranasal disease and viral infections. Trauma is another frequent cause because of injury to the cribiform plate and the delicate olfactory nerve fibers that pass through it to the ventral surface of the brain (Fig. 1.4). Hyposmia, or decreased olfactory sensation, is associated with several degenerative disorders, including Parkinson disease, Alzheimer disease, and human immunodeficiency virus (HIV)–dementia complex. Frequently, medications and environmental agents decrease olfaction. The perversion of smell (parosmia) and unpleasant odors (cacosmia) occur in psychiatric disease and develop after head trauma. Hyperosmia, or increased olfactory sensation, may occur with migraine headache. Olfactory hallucinations are often an aura in temporal lobe seizures because of involvement of primary olfactory cortex.

Optic Nerve (CN II)

The optic nerve and visual pathway encompass a major portion of the central nervous system; thus, evaluation of the visual system provides considerable information. The pertinent structures are the retina, optic nerve, optic chiasm, optic tract, optic radiations in the temporal and parietal lobes, and primary visual cortex in the occipital lobe. Visual testing should include assessing central and peripheral vision and the pupillary light reflex (Fig. 1.5) and performing an ophthalmoscopic examination. Test visual acuity with correction (glasses on), and test visual fields without correction (glasses off) so the frames do not obstruct vision.

The pupillary light reflex consists of an input (CN II, afferent limb), output (CN III, efferent limb), and intermediate station (interneuron in the midbrain). If a pupil abnormality is found on examination, the next step is to determine

Table 1.2. Types of Dysarthria: Characteristics, Localization of Lesion, Associated Diseases

Type (deficit)	Characteristics	Localization of lesion	Associated diseases
Flaccid (weakness)	Hypernasal, breathy, audible Inspiration (stridor)	Lower motor neuron	Amyotrophic lateral sclerosis Lower motor neuron disease
Spastic or pseudobulbar palsy (spasticity)	Slow rate, strained Reduced variability of pitch and loudness	Bilateral upper motor neuron	Multiple strokes
Ataxic (incoordination)	Irregular, scanning	Cerebellum	Cerebellar degenerative disease
Hypokinetic (rigidity and reduced range of movement)	Rapid rate	Basal ganglia	Parkinson disease
Hyperkinetic (involuntary movement)	Variable rate and loudness Distorted vowels	Basal ganglia	Huntington disease
Mixed	Spastic-flaccid Spastic-ataxic		Amyotrophic lateral sclerosis Multiple sclerosis

From Adams, AC: Neurology in Primary Care. FA Davis, Philadelphia, 2000, p 6. Used with permission of Mayo Foundation for Medical Education and Research.

which arm of the reflex is affected. Anisocoria (unequal pupils) usually is a normal variation, and the asymmetry is slight and both pupils react to light and accommodation. Common pupillary abnormalities and associated clinical conditions are summarized in Figure 1.6. A small pupil (miosis) associated with ptosis (droopy eyelid) and anhidrosis (absence of sweating) is called *Horner syndrome* and results from sympathetic dysfunction on the ipsilateral side. The sympathetic system can be affected at several sites along its extended course (Fig. 1.7).

A central autonomic tract that controls the sympathetic system descends from the hypothalamus through the lateral part of the brainstem.

Infarction of the lateral brainstem, as in Wallenberg syndrome, often interrupts this tract, producing Horner syndrome. Axons in this descending tract synapse in the intermediolateral cell column of the upper thoracic cord, from which preganglionic sympathetic fibers leave the spinal cord and ascend in the sympathetic chain. Tumors at the apex of the lung (Pancoast tumor), thyroid tumors, or any cervical abnormality can cause Horner syndrome by interfering with these sympathetic fibers. The preganglionic sympathetic fibers end in the superior cervical ganglion, from which postganglionic sympathetic fibers leave and join the carotid artery and travel with it to CN III. Involvement of these

1. Orientation

Name, address, current location (bldg), city, state, date (day), month, year

2. Attention/
   Immediate recall

a. Digit span (present 1/second: record longest correct span)

   2-9-6-8-3, 5-7-1-9-4-6, 2-1-5-9-3-6-2

b. Four unrelated words

   Learn: "apple, Mr. Johnson, charity, tunnel"

   (# of trials needed to learn all four: ____)

3. Calculation

5×13, $65 - 7$, $58 \div 2$, $29 + 11$

4. Abstraction

Similarities

   orange/banana, dog/horse, table/bookcase

5. Construction

Draw clock face showing 11:20

Copy

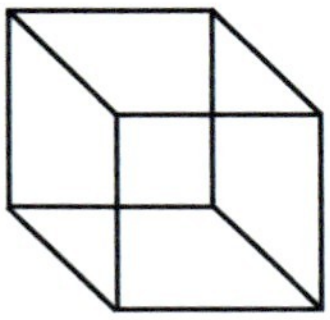

6. Information

President: first President

define an island; # weeks/year

7. Recall

the four words

   "apple, Mr. Johnson, charity, tunnel"

TOTAL SCORE

Subtract 1, 2, or 3 if there was more than 1 trial required to learn the four words.

Fig. 1.3. Short test of mental status, or the "Kokmen." (From Kokmen, E, Naessens, JM, and Offord, KP: A short test of mental status: Description and preliminary results. Mayo Clin Proc 62:281-288, 1987. Used with permission of Mayo Foundation.)

postganglionic fibers in vascular headaches can cause Horner syndrome.

Optic atrophy is characterized by decreased visual acuity, abnormal color vision (dyschromatopsia), afferent pupillary defect, nerve fiber-type visual field defect (eg, altitudinal visual field defect), and swelling or atrophy of the optic nerve (Fig. 1.8). Optic neuritis is the most common cause of optic neuropathy in young adults, and the patients present with acute loss of vision. Anterior ischemic optic neuropathy is the most common cause of optic neuropathy in middle-aged and older adults. An altitudinal visual field defect (eg, the loss of vision in the lower half of the visual field in one eye) often occurs in anterior optic neuropathy, with swelling of the optic disc from nonembolic occlusion of a posterior ciliary artery. Further evaluation is recommended for patients with any visual field defect that suggests optic neuropathy.

Lack of time is often given as a reason for not performing visual field testing; however, confrontation testing can be done relatively quickly and can provide valuable information.

Table 1.3. Tests of Cognitive Function, With Anatomical and Clinical Correlations

Cognitive function	Mental status test	Cortical area involved	Associated disease or feature
Attention	Repeat digit span Spell "world" backwards	Frontal lobe or diffuse	Acute confusional syndrome Metabolic encephalopathy
Memory	Recall	Medial temporal lobe Association cortex	Alzheimer disease
Language	Name objects, repeat phrase, follow commands	Left (dominant) hemisphere	Aphasia
Praxis	Show how to use a hammer	Left (dominant) frontal or parietal lobe	Apraxia
Calculation	Arithmetic	Left parietal lobe	Acalculia
Visual-spatial	Draw a cube or clock	Right parietal lobe	Neglect
Executive function, judgment	Abstractions, proverbs	Frontal lobes	Behavioral changes

Modified from Adams, AC: Neurology in Primary Care. FA Davis, Philadelphia, 2000, p 7. Used with permission of Mayo Foundation for Medical Education and Research.

Patients do not complain of visual field loss unless the onset is abrupt, so visual field testing often can detect clinically silent lesions. It is best to test each eye separately and to ask the patient to look straight at the examiner's eye. Bring the target object (eg, finger or pen) in from the periphery of each quadrant of the eye. In Figure 1.9, the visual field defects are recorded as seen by the patient. The convention is to display visual field defects as seen by the examiner, so make note of whether you are looking at the right or left eye. Monocular loss of vision indicates a lesion of the ipsilateral optic nerve. A bilateral temporal field deficit indicates a lesion at the optic chiasm, for example, compression by a pituitary tumor. Homonymous hemianopia (loss of vision on the same side in each eye) indicates a lesion of the optic tract or optic radiation on the side of the brain opposite that of the patient's deficit (ie, a right visual field loss indicates a left brain lesion). Visual field loss involving the upper quadrant of each eye ("pie in the sky") indicates a contralateral temporal lobe lesion, and a "pie in the floor" deficit indicates a contralateral parietal lobe lesion (Fig. 1.9).

Oculomotor Nerve (CN III)

The oculomotor nerve supplies the levator palpebrae superioris, medial rectus, superior rectus, inferior rectus, and inferior oblique muscles of the eye. It is also the efferent (parasympathetic) limb of the pupillary light reflex. A patient with an eye movement problem may

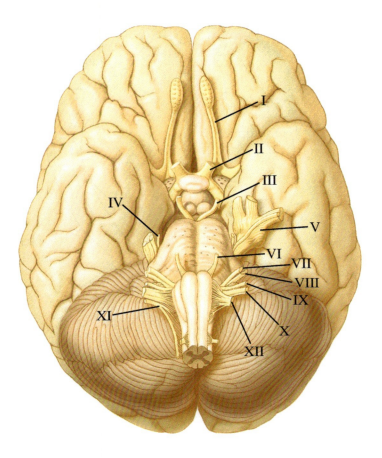

Fig. 1.4. Cranial nerve (I-XII) attachments on the ventral surface of the brain.

complain of double vision (diplopia), blurry vision, and even dizziness, described as dysequilibrium. A third nerve (CN III) palsy is often due to a vascular problem from diabetes mellitus, hypertension, or atherosclerosis. A patient with paralysis of CN III has ptosis, and the eye is positioned down and out (Fig. 1.10). If both pupils are equal and reactive to light (pupil sparing), it is less likely that the paralysis is caused by a compressive lesion.

Test CNs III, IV, and VI by having the patient follow your finger or a light to the right, left, up, down, and diagonally in both directions.

Figure 1.10 indicates which muscle is tested and gives examples of how dysfunction of the extraocular muscles would appear and how it would be recorded. Both eyes are tested together, but if weakness is noted or the patient complains of double vision, then each eye should be tested separately.

Trochlear Nerve (CN IV)

The trochlear nerve supplies the superior oblique muscle, which moves the eye down toward the nose. An isolated CN IV palsy is often due to trauma. Patients generally complain of

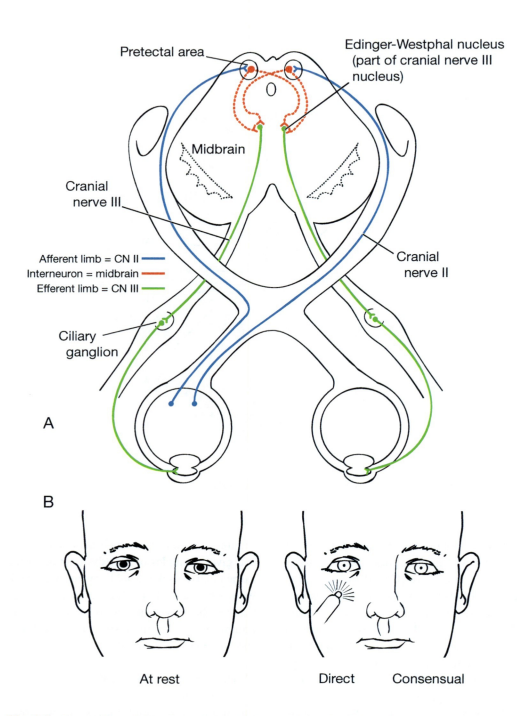

Pretectal area

Edinger-Westphal nucleus
(part of cranial nerve III
nucleus)

Midbrain

Cranial
nerve III

Afferent limb = CN II
Interneuron = midbrain
Efferent limb = CN III

Cranial
nerve II

Ciliary
ganglion

A

B

At rest   Direct   Consensual

Fig. 1.5. The pupillary light reflex pathway (*A*) showing how stimulation of one eye causes pupilloconstriction in both eyes (*B*). (From Adams, AC: Neurology in Primary Care. FA Davis, Philadelphia, 2000, p 8. Used with permission of Mayo Foundation for Medical Education and Research.)

Condition			Pupil abnormality
Anisocoria			Asymmetric Reactive to light and accommodation
Horner syndrome			Reactive to light and accommodation Ptosis, miosis (anhidrosis)
Age			Small, reactive
Argyll Robertson pupil			Small, unreactive to light Responds to accommodation
Opiates			Small, unreactive
Anxiety			Large, reactive
Mydriatic drops or Adie pupil			Large, unreactive

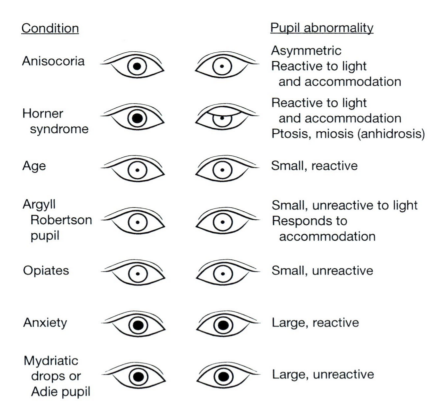

Fig. 1.6. Common pupillary abnormalities. (From Adams, AC: Neurology in Primary Care. FA Davis, Philadelphia, 2000, p 8. Used with permission of Mayo Foundation for Medical Education and Research.)

vertical diplopia and have a tendency to keep their head tilted away from the affected side to reduce double vision.

Trigeminal Nerve (CN V)

The trigeminal nerve, the thickest cranial nerve, is the primary sensory nerve of the face and head. The motor component innervates the muscles of mastication (masseter, temporal, and pterygoid muscles). Test these muscles by having the patient clench the jaw while you palpate the masseter and the temporal muscles on each side and watch the jaw open. Deviation of the jaw indicates muscle weakness; the deviation is toward the side of the involved nerve.

The sensory distribution of the three branches of the trigeminal nerve is shown in Figure 1.11. This anatomical information is helpful in understanding a patient's complaint of facial pain or numbness. A quick screen of facial sensation is to touch each side of the forehead, cheek, and chin and ask if the sensation is "about the same" on both sides. The ophthalmic branch of CN V supplies the upper face, including the cornea, as far as the vertex of the head. This branch is the afferent limb of the corneal reflex (stimulation of the cornea on one side induces tearing and blinking of both eyes). The corneal reflex is useful when evaluating a comatose patient because it can be used to determine whether CN

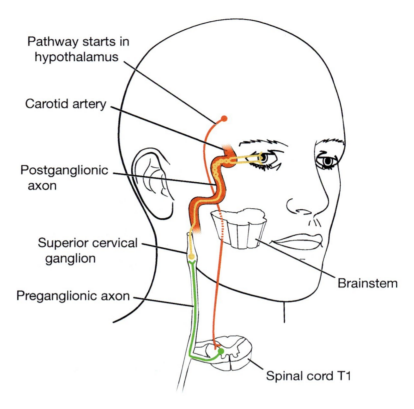

Fig. 1.7. Pathway for sympathetic control of the pupil. (Modified from Patten, J: Neurological Differential Diagnosis. Springer-Verlag, New York, 1977, p 7. Used with permission.)

V and CN VII (the efferent limb of the reflex) and, thus, the pons are intact. In an awake patient, testing the corneal reflex provides objective information about the patient's complaint of facial numbness. With the patient looking to one side (to avoid blinking because of visual threat), lightly touch the edge of the cornea with the corner of a piece of tissue that has been twisted to a point.

The most common clinical syndrome associated with the trigeminal nerve is trigeminal neuralgia, discussed in Chapter 3.

Abducens Nerve (CN VI)

The abducens nerve innervates the lateral rectus muscle, which moves the eye laterally.

Patients with a sixth (CN VI) nerve palsy complain of horizontal double vision that is most prominent when they look to the side of the deficit. To compensate, patients turn their head toward the side of the lesion. A sixth nerve palsy is more frequent than either a third (CN III) or fourth (CN IV) nerve palsy. Neoplasm is a frequent cause of sixth nerve palsy.

Facial Nerve (CN VII)

The facial nerve innervates the muscles of facial expression and contains parasympathetic axons that innervate salivary (submaxillary and sublingual) and lacrimal glands. The nerve also includes sensory axons that innervate taste buds

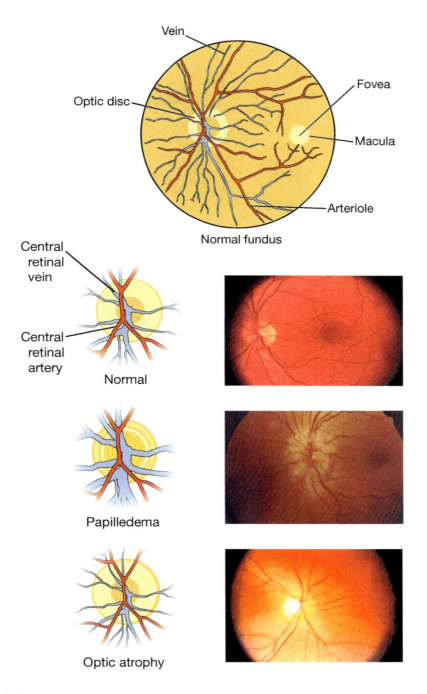

Fig. 1.8. Ophthalmoscopic examination. (*Top*, Modified from Liu, GT: Disorders of the eyes and eyelids. In: Samuels, MA, and Feske, S [eds]: Office Practice of Neurology. Churchill Livingstone, New York, 1996, pp 40-74. Used with permission. *Bottom*, Modified from Patten, J: Neurological Differential Diagnosis. Springer-Verlag, New York, 1977, p 27. Used with permission.)

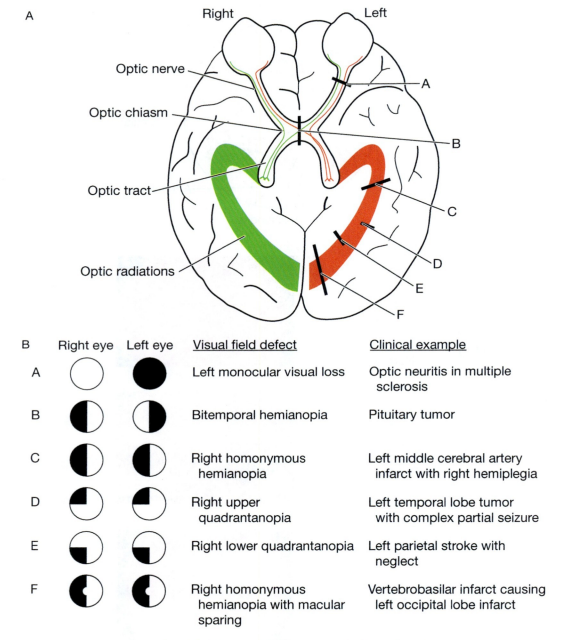

Visual fields are shown as seen by the patient

Fig. 1.9. *A*, Horizontal view of the visual pathway. *B*, Visual field defects resulting from lesions, A-F, of different parts of the visual pathway. Note that visual fields are shown as seen by the patient. (From Adams, AC: Neurology in Primary Care. FA Davis, Philadelphia, 2000, p 10. Used with permission of Mayo Foundation for Medical Education and Research.)

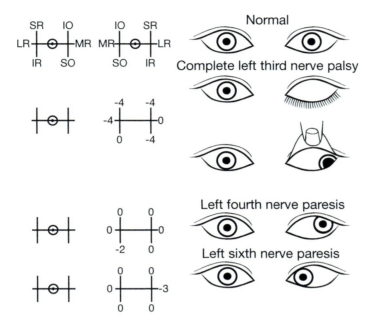

Fig. 1.10. Extraocular muscle dysfunction. Extraocular muscles: IO, inferior oblique; IR, inferior rectus; LR, lateral rectus; MR, medial rectus; SO, superior oblique; SR, superior rectus. (From Adams, AC: Neurology in Primary Care. FA Davis, Philadelphia, 2000, p 11. Used with permission of Mayo Foundation for Medical Education and Research.)

on the anterior two-thirds of the tongue. Test the nerve by asking patients to "wrinkle your forehead," "close your eyes," and "show me your teeth." Note the symmetry of these movements.

In a patient with a seventh (CN VII) nerve palsy, involvement of the forehead and eye indicates a peripheral nerve lesion (distal to the internal auditory meatus) (Fig. 1.12). The phrase "tear, ear, taste, and face" may be helpful in remembering the end points of the branches of the nerve to the lacrimal glands, stapedius muscle, taste buds on the anterior two-thirds of the tongue, and facial muscles. The usual cause of peripheral facial palsy, often called *Bell palsy*, is idiopathic. Approximately 85% of people with this condition recover over a 2- to 3-week period. Most patients require reassurance that they have not had a stroke.

The dry cornea needs to be protected from abrasion. Frequently, patching the eye is not effective because the eye is often open under the patch. Artificial tears help lubricate the eye during the day, and ocular ointments can be used at night in conjunction with patching or taping.

The initial evaluation of facial paralysis often puts clinicians in a difficult position. The most likely diagnosis is idiopathic facial palsy, which resolves spontaneously without unnecessary and expensive testing. However, the risk is that prompt intervention for less common causes, such as tumor, infection, or systemic illness, will be delayed. It is reasonable to allow 2 to 3 weeks for spontaneous recovery.

Corticosteroids are often administered to speed the recovery of patients with a seventh nerve palsy and to avoid complete paralysis. If

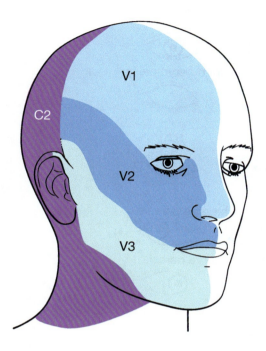

Fig. 1.11. Distribution of the three branches of the trigeminal nerve. V1, ophthalmic branch; V2, maxillary branch; V3, mandibular branch. (Modified from Patten, J: Neurological Differential Diagnosis. Springer-Verlag, New York, 1977, p 41. Used with permission.)

corticosteroid therapy is prescribed, it should be started early. The recommended dose is 1 mg/kg daily for 7 days, and then tapered to zero over the next 10 days. Treatment with acyclovir (or famciclovir) is supported by studies that have suggested idiopathic facial palsy is caused by infection with herpes simplex virus or varicella-zoster virus. For Ramsay Hunt syndrome (varicella-zoster infection with facial paralysis and herpetic eruption in the ear), studies have shown a better outcome after treatment with prednisone and acyclovir at 800 mg 5 times daily for 7 days.

The American Academy of Neurology practice parameter (Grogan PM and Gronseth GS, 2001) indicates that early treatment with

oral corticosteroids is *probably effective* for improving facial functional outcomes, and the combination of prednisone and acyclovir is *possibly effective* for the same outcome.

Vestibulocochlear Nerve (CN VIII)

The vestibulocochlear nerve transmits information from the vestibular apparatus (for balance) and cochlea (for hearing) to the brain. The vestibular portion of the nerve is not routinely tested in the office. Caloric testing is useful for assessing vestibular function. Vestibular deficits found on a neurologic examination include problems with gait and balance and nystagmus. Vestibular function is considered in Chapter 5.

Auditory acuity can be assessed during the interview by noting the patient's response to softly spoken words. Some examiners hold a

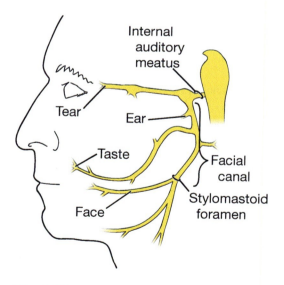

Fig. 1.12. Peripheral distribution of the facial nerve (CN VII). The end points of the branches of CN VII can be summarized by "tear, ear, taste, and face." (From Adams, AC: Neurology in Primary Care. FA Davis, Philadelphia, 2000, p 13. Used with permission of Mayo Foundation for Medical Education and Research.)

ticking watch and measure the distance from which the patient is able to hear it. If a more detailed evaluation is needed, audiology referral is recommended.

A tuning fork can be used to distinguish between hearing loss due to middle ear disease (conductive loss) and that due to sensorineural injury (perceptive loss). In the Rinne test, a vibrating tuning fork is placed on the patient's mastoid process until the patient reports not being able to hear vibrations, after which the tuning fork is held near the ear. When the tuning fork is held by the ear, the vibrations are still audible to normal subjects and to patients with sensorineural hearing loss because air conduction is better than bone conduction. This is not the case in conduction loss (ie, bone conduction is better than air conduction). The Rinne test is used in conjunction with the Weber test, in which the tuning fork is held on the vertex of the head. If the patient has normal hearing or a conductive deficit, the tuning fork vibrations should be heard equally in both ears. However, if the patient has sensorineural hearing loss, the sound appears to be diminished in the affected ear.

Trouble with hearing and noise in the ear (tinnitus) are the most frequent complaints that indicate involvement of the cochlear portion of CN VIII. Common causes of hearing loss are age (presbycusis) and exposure to noise. Anything that affects hearing can cause tinnitus. Ototoxic drugs that clinicians should be aware of include aminoglycoside antibiotics, antineoplastic drugs, antiinflammatory agents, diuretics, and antimalarial drugs.

Glossopharyngeal Nerve (CN IX)

The gag reflex is used to test the glossopharyngeal nerve (and the vagus nerve) clinically. A tongue depressor applied to the posterior pharynx causes the pharyngeal muscles to contract, with or without gagging. This test is unpleasant for patients, and it seldom provides information that cannot be obtained by assessing the patient's speech and watching the patient swallow spontaneously.

Glossopharyngeal neuralgia is an uncommon disorder characterized by paroxysms of lancinating pain in the structures CN IX innervates: the ear, base of the tongue, lower jaw, and tonsillar fossa. Occasionally, syncope is part of glossopharyngeal neuralgia because CN IX innervates the carotid sinus, important in maintaining systemic blood pressure.

Vagus Nerve (CN X)

The gag reflex is also used to test the vagus nerve. The motor component of CN X supplies the muscles of the pharynx and larynx. Although the vagus nerve is the most important of the parasympathetic nerves, it is difficult to assess clinically. It is involved in many reflexes, including coughing, vomiting, and swallowing. Dysphagia and dysarthria are the most common clinical features of vagal dysfunction, because of weakness of the muscles of the larynx and pharynx.

Spinal Accessory Nerve (CN IX)

The spinal accessory nerve innervates the trapezius and sternocleidomastoid muscles. Test this nerve by having the patient turn his or her head, and then assess the strength of each sternocleidomastoid muscle against resistance. To test the trapezius, that is, to assess muscle strength and symmetry, ask the patient to shrug the shoulders. The nerve can be injured by intracranial or cervical trauma. The clinical presentation may include shoulder pain, winging of the scapula, and weak elevation of the shoulder.

Hypoglossal Nerve (CN XII)

The hypoglossal nerve innervates the muscles of the tongue. Test this nerve by asking the patient to stick out the tongue and move it from side to side. Look for weakness, atrophy, fasciculations, and abnormal movements. Unilateral weakness causes the tongue to deviate to the side of the lesion. Hypoglossal dysfunction produces dysarthria. It is important to inspect the tongue for fasciculations if motor neuron disease is suspected. A note of caution: familiarize yourself with how a normal tongue looks before ascribing fasciculations to what may be normal quivering of the tongue. The tongue can also be valuable in "above the neck" assessment of rapid alternating movements when testing coordination.

MOTOR EXAMINATION

Watching the patient stand and walk is a major portion of the motor examination. If an ambulatory patient is able to walk on his or her toes and heels, to hop, and to squat, lower extremity strength is well within normal limits and individual muscle testing may not be needed. Evaluation of the motor system involves assessing the symmetry of muscle strength, bulk, and tone. Abnormal muscle movement such as fasciculations should be noted. All major muscle groups can be tested with the patient seated. For easy comparison of the right and left sides, test both sides simultaneously. Simultaneous testing (done quickly and with encouragement) may also reduce give-way weakness in a patient with a tendency to exaggerate symptoms.

Test the proximal and distal muscles of all four extremities. The deltoid (arms abducted against resistance), biceps, and triceps muscles are good proximal upper extremity muscles to assess. Finger abduction is a good measure of distal upper extremity strength. If proximal muscle weakness is suspected, test neck flexion. Normally, the examiner should not be able to overcome the powerful neck muscles. Test for drift by asking the patient to hold both arms straight out in front, with the palms up. This is useful for detecting subtle weakness of the upper

extremity, which is expressed as pronation and lowering of the weakened arm.

Patients often complain of "weakness," a term they use to imply illness. How weakness limits their ability to perform normal daily activities will reveal more about the complaint of weakness. For example, proximal muscle weakness is suggested when the patient reports difficulty walking up stairs or keeping the arms raised when combing the hair. Fatigable weakness or weakness that is more prominent at the end of the day may suggest myasthenia gravis. If the patient has a history of fatigable weakness, repetitive muscle strength should be tested.

The anatomical features of the motor system important in understanding the physical findings of a motor examination are shown in Figure 1.13. The major tract of the motor system is the corticospinal, or pyramidal, tract, which originates in the precentral gyrus (primary motor cortex) of the frontal lobe. The areas of the body are represented systematically along the precentral gyrus (Fig. 1.14). The leg is represented on the medial surface and the face, arm, and hand on the lateral surface. At the junction between the medulla and spinal cord, the corticospinal tract crosses the midline (pyramidal decussation). Because of this decussation, the right cerebral hemisphere controls the muscles on the left side of the body and the left hemisphere controls those on the right side. The origin, course, and termination of the corticospinal tract constitute the *upper motor neuron*. The clinical features of an upper motor neuron disorder include weakness, spasticity, hyperreflexia, and extensor plantar reflex, or Babinski sign ("up-going toe").

The *lower motor neuron* consists of the motor nerve cell (anterior horn cell) in the spinal cord or brainstem and its axon, which courses through a peripheral nerve to end on a muscle. The lower motor neuron is also called the "final

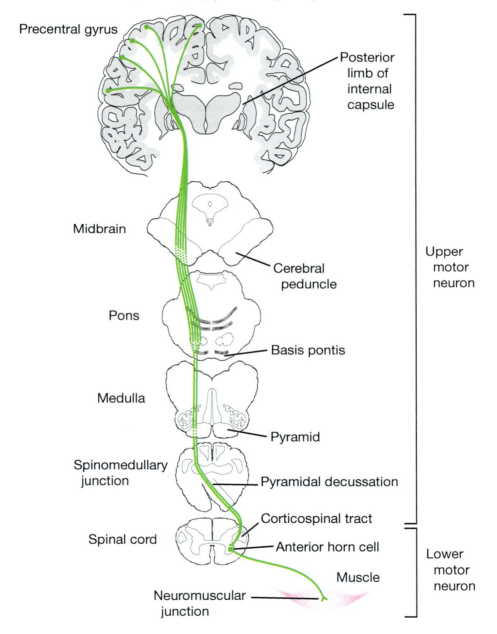

Fig. 1.13. The motor system: upper motor neuron (corticospinal tract) and lower motor neuron (anterior horn cell). (From Adams, AC: Neurology in Primary Care. FA Davis, Philadelphia, 2000, p 15. Used with permission of Mayo Foundation for Medical Education and Research.)

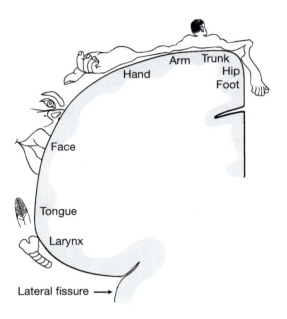

Fig. 1.14. Precentral gyrus (primary motor cortex) motor homunculus.

common pathway." Clinical features of a lower motor neuron lesion include weakness, decreased muscle stretch reflexes (hyporeflexia), loss of muscle bulk or atrophy, and fasciculations. Upper and lower motor neuron disorders are compared in Table 1.4. Other components of the motor system, including the basal ganglia

("extrapyramidal system") and cerebellum, are discussed in Chapter 12.

The pattern of weakness and the associated neurologic findings help localize the lesion in the nervous system. Figure 1.15, from the Mayo neurology examination form, lists the major muscles that are tested in a comprehensive neurologic examination (with the nerve that innervates the muscle in parentheses) and the associated nerve root. Proximal muscle weakness indicates myopathy, whereas distal muscle weakness may indicate peripheral neuropathy, especially if there are associated sensory findings. Weakness of a specific muscle suggests a problem with the nerve that innervates the muscle. For example, a patient with footdrop who has normal strength in the posterior tibial muscle is more likely to have peroneal nerve palsy than a radiculopathy of the L5 root. A patient with footdrop and entirely normal findings on sensory examination may have motor neuron disease. The patterns of weakness that occur with lesions at different levels of the nervous system are summarized in Table 1.5.

SENSORY EXAMINATION

The frequency of sensory complaints such as pain, numbness, and tingling encountered in

Table 1.4. Comparison of Upper Motor Neuron and Lower Motor Neuron Disorders

Clinical feature	Upper motor neuron	Lower motor neuron
Weakness	Yes	Yes
Muscle tone	Increased (spasticity)	Decreased
Muscle stretch reflexes	Increased	Decreased
Muscle bulk	Normal (disuse atrophy)	Atrophy
Fasciculations	No	Yes
Babinski sign	Yes	No

From Adams, AC: Neurology in Primary Care. FA Davis, Philadelphia, 2000, p 16. Used with permission of Mayo Foundation for Medical Education and Research.

Muscle (nerve)	Root*
Neck flexors	C1-6
Neck extensors	C1-T1
Ext. rotators (suprascapular)	C**5,6**
Pectoralis major (pectoral)	C5-T1
Deltoid (axillary)	C**5,6**
Biceps (musculocutaneous)	C5,**6**
Brachioradialis (radial)	C5,6
Supinator (radial)	C5,6
Pronator teres (median)	C6,7
Triceps (radial)	C6,**7**,8
Wrist ext. (radial)	C6,**7**,8
Wrist flex. (median & ulnar)	C6,**7**,8 T1
Digit ext. (radial)	C**7**,8
Digit flex. (median & ulnar)	C7,**8** T1
Thenar (median)	C**8 T1**
Hypothenar (ulnar)	C**8 T1**
Interossei (ulnar)	C**8 T1**
Abdomen	T6-L1
Rectal sphincter	S3,4
Iliopsoas (femoral)	L**2,3**,4
Adductors thigh (obturator)	L2,3,4
Abductors thigh (sup. gluteal)	L4,**5** S1
Gluteus maximus (inf. gluteal)	L5 S**1**,2
Quadriceps (femoral)	L2,**3,4**
Hamstrings (sciatic)	L4,**5** S1
Anterior tibial (peroneal)	L**4,5**
Toe ext. (peroneal)	L4,**5** S1
Extensor hallucis longus	
(peroneal)	L**5** S1
Peronei (peroneal)	L**5** S1
Posterior tibial (tibial)	L**5** S1
Toe flex. (tibial)	L**5** S1
Gastrocnemius-soleus (tibial)	L**5** S**1**,2

Fig. 1.15. The major muscles tested in a comprehensive neurologic examination (part of the Mayo neurology examination form). The corresponding nerve is in parentheses. ext., extensors; flex., flexors; inf., inferior; sup., superior. *Bold indicates the primary root. (Used with permission of Mayo Foundation for Medical Education and Research.)

clinical practice emphasizes the importance of the sensory examination. However, the responses to sensory testing are subjective, and some patients provide misleading or exaggerated responses that complicate the interpretation of the findings. Therefore, it is important to be familiar with the essential anatomy of the sensory system and to correlate the sensory findings with the more objective information obtained from the motor and reflex examinations (Fig. 1.16).

The major types of somatic sensation are exteroceptive sense, including pain and temperature sensations, and proprioceptive sense, including position sense and vibratory sensation. Pain and temperature sensations are conveyed by the spinothalamic system, and vibratory sensation and position sense are conveyed by the dorsal column–medial lemniscus system. Both systems also convey the sensation of touch. A clinically relevant point about the spinothalamic tract (pain and temperature) is that the axons cross the midline near their origin in the spinal cord and ascend laterally in the spinal cord. The dermatomes of the body are represented in a systematic fashion in the tract, with the sacral dermatomes represented laterally (near the surface of the cord) and the cervical segments medially (near the gray matter). The axons that form the dorsal columns do not cross in the spinal cord; instead, they synapse on neurons in caudal medulla, whose axons immediately cross the midline to form the medial lemniscus. Thus, in the spinal cord and medulla, the spinothalamic and dorsal column–medial lemniscal systems are separated, but they come together at the level of mid pons. Because of this arrangement, the sensations of pain and temperature may be lost over part of the body, while vibratory sensation and position sense are spared. This sensory dissociation can occur with lesions only in the spinal cord, medulla, or lower pons. In contrast, all sensory modalities are represented together at the level of the thalamus. This explains why the thalamic syndrome is characterized by

Table 1.5. **Patterns of Weakness by Anatomical Division**

Division (disease)	Clinical example	Examination findings		Other possible associated clinical features
		Motor	**Sensory**	
Muscle (myopathy)	Polymyositis	Proximal weakness	Normal	Diffuse myalgias
Neuromuscular junction	Myasthenia gravis	Fatigable weakness	Normal	Diplopia, ptosis
Peripheral nerve (neuropathy)	Peroneal palsy	Weak peroneal-innervated muscles	Sensory loss in peroneal nerve distribution	Injury at knee
Nerve root (radiculopathy)	L5 radiculopathy	All the above plus weakness of other L5-innervated muscles (posterior tibial, foot inversion)	Sensory loss in dermatomal distribution	Back pain
Anterior horn cell (motor neuron disease)	Amyotrophic lateral sclerosis	Lower motor neuron and upper motor neuron weakness	Normal	Atrophy Fasciculations Increased muscle stretch reflexes
Spinal cord (myelopathy)	Cervical spondylosis	Upper motor neuron weakness	Sensory level	Babinski sign Bladder dysfunction
Brainstem	Brainstem glioma	Upper motor neuron weakness	Variable	Cranial nerve involvement
Cerebral cortex	Cortical infarction	Upper motor neuron weakness	Cortical sensation dysfunction (discriminative sensation, joint position sense, 2-point discrimination, graphesthesia)	Language impairment (if dominant hemisphere) Visuospatial problems

From Adams, AC: Neurology in Primary Care. FA Davis, Philadelphia, 2000, p 17. Used with permission of Mayo Foundation for Medical Education and Research.

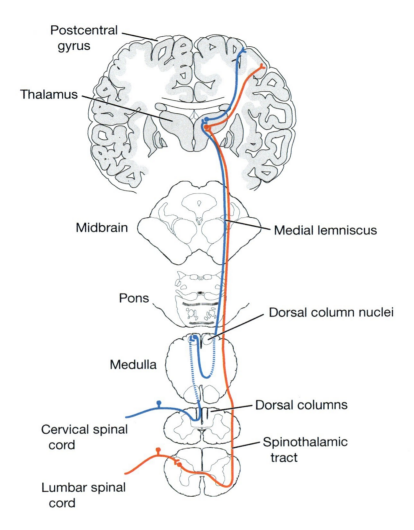

Postcentral gyrus

Thalamus

Midbrain

Medial lemniscus

Pons

Dorsal column nuclei

Medulla

Dorsal columns

Cervical spinal cord

Spinothalamic tract

Lumbar spinal cord

Fig. 1.16. Sensory pathways. *Red*, Spinothalamic system (pain and temperature sensations). *Blue*, Dorsal column–medial lemniscus system (joint position sense and vibratory sensation). Note that the pathways are separate at the level of the spinal cord and medulla but approach one another in the pons.

dense sensory loss of all modalities over an entire half of the body and face.

Lesions of the postcentral gyrus, or primary somesthetic cortex, are associated with the loss of discriminative sensation: joint position sense, two-point discrimination, stereognosis (the appreciation of the form of an object by touch), and graphesthesia (the ability to recognize figures written on the skin). Only a minimal deficit of touch, pain, temperature, and vibratory sensation may be noted with cortical lesions. The sensory pattern typical of lesions at various levels of the nervous system is summarized in Table 1.6 and Figure 1.17.

The minimal sensory examination, in neurologic practice, includes testing pain and/or temperature sensation and joint position sense and/or vibratory sensation in all four extremities. In primary care practice, it may not be necessary to perform a sensory examination unless the patient has a sensory complaint or abnormal gait. While testing a patient's gait and station, determine whether the patient can stand with the feet close together and the eyes open. If the patient is able to do this, then ask him or her to close the eyes (Romberg test). The Romberg test assesses proprioceptive function. A normal person may sway slightly, but marked swaying or falling indicates a proprioceptive deficit (Romberg sign). Patients with a Romberg sign may report difficulty walking to the bathroom in the dark or trouble maintaining their balance in the shower (because reduced visual input accentuates the sensory deficit). In comparison, patients with cerebellar dysfunction sway with the eyes open. Patients with conversion disorder or another factitious illness tend to sway at the hips rather than the ankles and, despite a wide sway arc, maintain their balance. Asking the patient to perform finger-to-nose movements during this examination is a useful distraction.

If there is a sensory complaint, it is useful for the patient to outline the area of deficit so that specific area can be examined more closely. Diagrams of dermatomes and areas supplied by individual peripheral nerves are useful in localizing a specific sensory complaint (Fig. 1.18). To test spinothalamic function, use a disposable straight pin or safety pin. Tell the patient you are going to touch him or her lightly with a pin (it is not necessary to penetrate the skin) and demonstrate what you are going to do before you start. Ask the patient to call the sensation "sharp" when touched with the point of the pin and "dull" when touched with your finger or the head of the pin. Testing at the base of the

nail bed avoids most calluses on the fingers. Assessing whether the patient can distinguish sharp from dull before asking him or her to compare the sensation on the two sides of the body avoids any tendency the patient might have to exaggerate the sensory signs. Asking the question "Is it about the same?" helps the patient avoid over-interpretation of minimal and clinically nonrelevant differences in stimulation. Whether it is necessary to test more than the hands and feet depends on the patient's presenting complaints and if a deficit is found in the hands and feet. If there is a history of spine symptoms, it may be necessary to test several dermatomes or to look for a sensory level. It usually is more convenient to check for sharp versus dull sensation than to test temperature sensation. Temperature sensation can be tested by using a cold reflex hammer or tuning fork; however, it is more difficult for patients to compare temperature sensation on the two sides of the body than to compare sharp and dull sensations.

Proprioception can be assessed with the Romberg test or by testing vibratory sensation or joint position sense. Vibratory sensation is often quicker to test than joint position sense but requires a tuning fork. Use a large tuning fork (128 Hz), especially when testing elderly patients, in whom testing with a small tuning fork may falsely indicate proprioceptive deficit. Hold the tuning fork on the nail bed of a finger and great toe and ask the patient if he or she appreciates the "buzz." Most adults can appreciate vibratory sensation at the toes. If vibration is not appreciated at the toes, move the tuning fork proximally to a bony prominence, for example, the lateral malleolus. Continue to move proximally if no sensation is appreciated. Test both sides. If asymmetry is noted in a patient prone to exaggerate, hold the tuning fork on the side of diminished sensation and ask the patient to report when the buzz is no longer felt; this may minimize the perceived deficit.

Table 1.6. Common Patterns of Sensory Deficit

Anatomy	Clinical example	Sensory loss: pain/temperature or vibratory/joint position	Distribution of sensory abnormality	Associated features
Peripheral nerve (mononeuropathy)	Carpal tunnel syndrome	Both	Precisely in distribution of the median nerve	Weakness of muscles of median nerve Wrist pain
Nerve root (radiculopathy)	L5 radiculopathy	Both	Dermatomal distribution	Weakness of L5-innervated muscles Back pain
Peripheral nerve (peripheral neuropathy or polyneuropathy)	Diabetic neuropathy	Both	Stocking-glove pattern	Painful paresthesias Autonomic neuropathy
Spinal cord				
Commissural syndrome	Syringomyelia	Pain/temperature	Bandlike or capelike pattern	Arnold-Chiari malformation
Brown-Séquard syndrome	Spinal trauma	Both	Contralateral pain/temperature and ipsilateral vibratory/joint position	Ipsilateral motor deficit, Babinski sign
Dorsal cord syndrome	Subacute combined degeneration (vitamin B_{12} deficiency)	Vibratory/joint position	Area distal to level of lesion	Babinski sign
Thalamus	Thalamic infarction	Both	Dense contralateral face and body	Thalamic pain syndrome
Cerebral cortex	Middle cerebral artery infarction	Discriminative sensation, joint position sense, 2-point discrimination, graphesthesia	Contralateral face and upper limb*	Hemiparesis Aphasia if dominant hemisphere

*Also, contralateral lower limb if internal capsule is involved.

From Adams, AC: Neurology in Primary Care. FA Davis, Philadelphia, 2000, p 18. Used with permission of Mayo Foundation for Medical Education and Research.

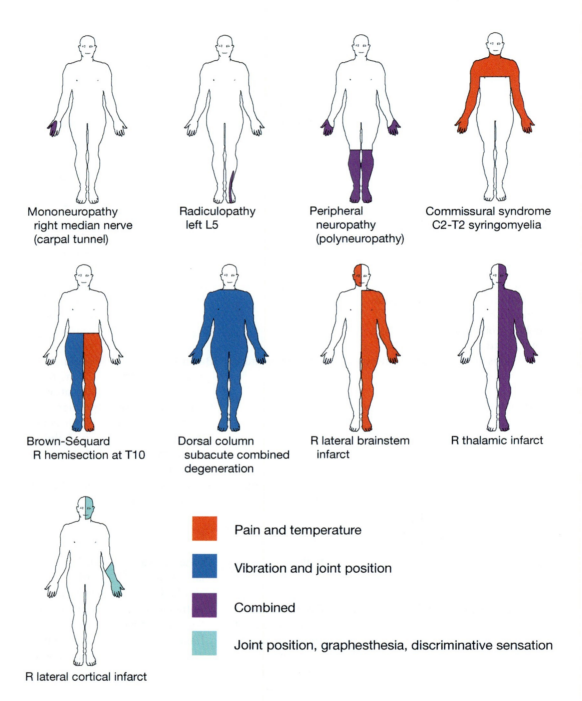

Mononeuropathy
right median nerve
(carpal tunnel)

Radiculopathy
left L5

Peripheral
neuropathy
(polyneuropathy)

Commissural syndrome
C2-T2 syringomyelia

Brown-Séquard
R hemisection at T10

Dorsal column
subacute combined
degeneration

R lateral brainstem
infarct

R thalamic infarct

R lateral cortical infarct

Pain and temperature

Vibration and joint position

Combined

Joint position, graphesthesia, discriminative sensation

Fig. 1.17. Patterns of sensory deficit. (From Adams, AC: Neurology in Primary Care. FA Davis, Philadelphia, 2000, p 20. Used with permission of Mayo Foundation for Medical Education and Research.)

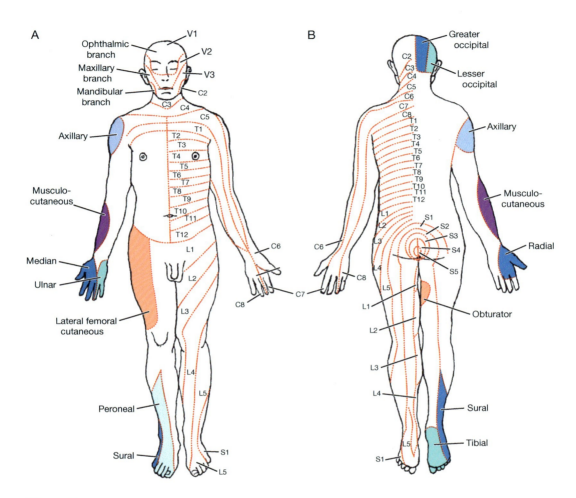

A
V1
Ophthalmic
branch
V2
Maxillary
branch
V3
Mandibular
branch
C2
Axillary
C3   C4
C5
T1
T2
T3
T4
T5
T6
T7
T8
T9
T10
T11
T12
L1
L2
L3
Musculo-
cutaneous
Median
Ulnar
C6
C8
C7
Lateral femoral
cutaneous
L4
L5
Peroneal
Sural
S1
L5

B
Greater
occipital
C2
C3
C4
C5
C6
C7
C8
T1
T2
T3
T4
T5
T6
T7
T8
T9
T10
T11
T12
L1
L2
L3
S1
S2
S3
S4
S5
Lesser
occipital
Axillary
Musculo-
cutaneous
Radial
C6
C8
L1
L2
L3
L4
L5
S1
Obturator
Sural
Tibial
L5

Fig. 1.18. Dermatomes (C2-S5) and area of distribution of peripheral nerves. *A,* Anterior view; *B,* posterior view. (From Adams, AC: Neurology in Primary Care. FA Davis, Philadelphia, 2000, p 21. Used with permission of Mayo Foundation for Medical Education and Research.)

Testing joint position sense is useful for assessing cortical sensory loss. First, demonstrate the test to the patient. Hold one of the patient's distal phalanges laterally, and move the joint up or down a few millimeters. Next, ask the patient to report, without looking, the direction relative to the last position. A coordination test, for example, finger-to-nose test, which the patient is asked to perform with eyes closed, also assesses motion and position sense.

REFLEX EXAMINATION

The examination of reflexes provides the most objective information obtained with neurologic testing. Although reflexes can be reinforced or decreased, they are involuntary motor responses to sensory stimuli and do not depend on voluntary control. Importantly, reflex tests can be performed in a patient who is confused or in coma. Reflex abnormalities may be the first indication of neurologic disease. The major reflexes are muscle stretch reflexes, superficial reflexes, and pathologic reflexes, specifically the plantar (or Babinski) reflex.

Muscle Stretch Reflexes

Routinely tested muscle stretch reflexes are the biceps, brachioradialis, triceps, quadriceps, and gastrocnemius-soleus reflexes, named for the muscle tested. The afferent limb of the reflex arc is a sensory (dorsal) root. The interneuron is in the spinal cord, and the efferent limb is the motor (ventral) root and nerve to the muscle (Fig. 1.19). A process that affects any component of the reflex arc will alter the reflex. For example, the ankle or gastrocnemius-soleus reflex may be absent in a patient with diabetic peripheral neuropathy or with a herniated disk affecting the S1 nerve root. The muscle stretch reflex arc can be affected also by upper motor neuron lesions that reduce inhibitory influences and produce hyperreflexia and by cerebellar or brainstem lesions that reduce facilitation and produce hyporeflexia. Drugs and metabolic factors can also affect reflexes; for example, hyperreflexia occurs with hyperthyroidism and central nervous system stimulants, and hyporeflexia occurs with hypothyroidism.

Several techniques can be used to elicit muscle stretch reflexes. All major muscle stretch reflexes can be tested with the patient seated and the arms resting in the lap. This position allows rapid comparison of the right and left sides and limits patient movement. Testing from side to side can be repeated if there is a question about the symmetry of the reflex. Because it is essential for the patient to be relaxed, talk to the patient during this portion of the examination to divert his or her attention. If the patient remains tense, ask him or her to look up or bite down or to interlock the fingers and pull the hands apart (Jendrassik method) as you tap the tendon with the reflex hammer. The ankle jerk can be elicited easily by having the patient kneel on a chair while you put minimal pressure with one hand on the ball of the patient's foot and then tap the tendon with the reflex hammer.

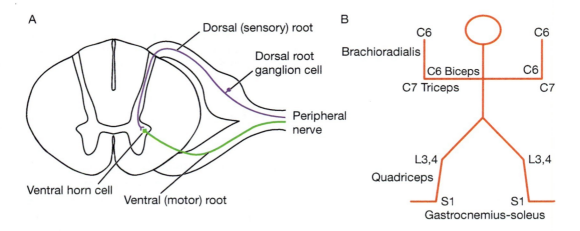

Fig. 1.19. *A*, Anatomy of a muscle stretch reflex arc. *B*, Common muscle stretch reflexes and the associated nerve roots tested.

How the findings are interpreted depends on the results of other parts of the neurologic examination. For example, both the biceps and brachioradialis reflexes test the C5-C6 nerve root, but the biceps is innervated by the musculocutaneous nerve and the brachioradialis muscle by the radial nerve. Thus, if one reflex is abnormal but not the other, the lesion is likely to involve the peripheral nerve and not the C5-C6 nerve root. Information from the reflex examination in conjunction with the results of the motor and sensory examinations is used to localize a problem to the nerve root, plexus, peripheral nerve, and so forth (Table 1.7, Fig. 1.18). Symmetrical hyperreflexia in combination with flexor plantar reflexes may be a normal finding in an anxious patient. However, in an elderly patient, hyperreflexia may indicate cervical spondylosis. Diffuse hyporeflexia can be a normal finding if there is no other abnormality. Ankle jerks that are reduced or absent are common in peripheral neuropathy.

Other muscle stretch reflexes, such as the jaw, internal hamstring, and Hoffman (finger flexor) reflexes, can be tested to aid in the interpretation of the neurologic findings. The internal hamstring reflex tests the L5 nerve root. If the reflex is asymmetric, suspect an L5

Table 1.7. Muscle Stretch Reflexes

Reflex	Root	Nerve	Muscle supplied by nerve only	Other muscles supplied by same root but different nerve
Biceps	C6	Musculocutaneous	Biceps	Pronator teres (median nerve)
Brachioradialis	C5-C6	Radial	Brachioradialis, triceps	External rotator-infraspinatus muscle (supra-scapular nerve)
Triceps	C7	Radial	Triceps, wrist extensors	Pronator teres (median nerve) Wrist flexors (median and ulnar nerves)
Quadriceps	L3-L4	Femoral	Quadriceps, iliopsoas	Adductors of thigh (obturator nerve)
Gastrocnemius-soleus	S1	Tibial	Gastrocnemius-soleus, posterior tibial	Gluteus maximus (inferior gluteal nerve)

From Adams, AC: Neurology in Primary Care. FA Davis, Philadelphia, 2000, p 22. Used with permission of Mayo Foundation for Medical Education and Research.

radiculopathy. However, the value of this reflex is questionable because of the difficulty with eliciting it. The jaw and finger flexor reflexes typically reflect hyperreflexia.

Superficial Reflexes

Superficial reflexes are elicited by stimulating the skin or mucous membranes. These reflexes include the corneal, pharyngeal (gag), abdominal, cremasteric, anal, and bulbocavernosus reflexes. The corneal and gag reflexes are discussed above with the cranial nerves. Although the other reflexes are not routinely tested, they can provide valuable information.

Both the afferent and efferent limbs of the abdominal reflexes are contained in the intercostal nerves at T6-T9 for the epigastric region and T11-L1 for the hypogastric region. The absence of abdominal reflexes can be the result of a segmental or upper motor neuron lesion. Abdominal reflexes are tested with the patient supine and the arms at the sides. Stroke or gently scratch with a blunt object the four quadrants around the umbilicus. Normally, the umbilicus moves toward the stimulus. The reflex may not be present if the patient is obese or multiparous, has had previous abdominal operations, or is tense. Unilateral loss of these reflexes indicates a unilateral upper motor neuron lesion and may be an important clinical clue to early multiple sclerosis. The unilateral absence of abdominal reflexes is sometimes considered a reason to perform magnetic resonance imaging of patients with idiopathic scoliosis to rule out syringomyelia.

The cremasteric reflex tests the L1-L2 nerve root. Stimulation of the inner aspect of the thigh, as in abdominal reflex testing, causes elevation of the testicle. As with the abdominal reflex, loss of the cremasteric reflex may indicate an upper motor neuron lesion or lesion of the L1-L2 segment (reflex arc).

The anal reflex tests segments S2-S4. It is useful for evaluating patients with suspected injury of the sacral spinal cord (conus medullaris or cauda equina). Gently scratch the skin around the patient's anus to produce contraction of the anal ring, which can be detected or palpated with a gloved fingertip. The absence of the reflex indicates a lesion at spinal cord segments S2-4.

Pathologic Reflexes: the Plantar Reflex

The plantar reflex has to be tested carefully to avoid misinterpretation of the results. The lateral aspect of the sole is stroked from the heel toward the toes and across the plantar surface in the direction of the great toe. The normal response is flexion of the toes. An extensor response, or Babinski sign, indicates an upper motor neuron lesion. If there is question about the response, stroke the foot with the leg extended (having the patient extend the leg while seated can be used as a modified straight leg test for eliciting back or root pain). To reduce the problem of withdrawal, divert the patient's attention by discussing unrelated matters and gently pull back on the foot while you apply the stimulus. If excessive withdrawal is encountered, stroke the lateral aspect of the sole (Chaddock maneuver) or run two knuckles down both sides of the tibia (Oppenheim maneuver). The latter is very uncomfortable for the patient and should not be performed unless the results of the other tests are equivocal.

COORDINATION EXAMINATION

Cerebellar function is assessed by testing coordination and rapid alternating movements. The results can serve as a crosscheck for other parts of the neurologic examination. In an ambulatory patient, coordination can be evaluated by heel-to-toe tandem gait and tapping each foot.

The finger-to-nose test is a convenient test of coordination. Ask the patient to extend both arms out in front of the body (observe for static tremor) and then to touch the nose with an index finger, first with the right hand and then with the left, and repeat the action. Abnormalities in the rate, range, direction, and force of movement indicate incoordination. The movement should be symmetric. Next, ask the patient to continue the activity with the eyes closed (this also tests position sense). Apraxia (the inability to execute a skilled or learned motor act not related to weakness) may become apparent in a patient with dementia. A comparable test for the lower extremities is to have the patient place the heel on the opposite knee and run the heel down the shin as smoothly as possible.

Rapid alternating movements of the tongue (wiggling the tongue from side to side), hands (repeatedly turning the hand palm up, palm down), fingers (rapidly tapping the index finger against the thumb), and feet (tapping the foot) also test coordination. Evaluate the rate and range of movement. Movement of the two sides should be symmetric; this is not dependent on hand dominance. The sound that the movement makes (eg, shoe tap on the floor or hand pat on the knee) should be rapid and regular and is often helpful in detecting an abnormality. Occasionally, a "syncopated rhythm" is heard when the abnormality was missed by visual inspection. When movement is slowed by weakness, the rate of movement should be regular. Unilateral abnormalities are consistent with ipsilateral cerebellar lesions. Patients with Parkinson disease may show a decreased range of movement but an increased rate of movement.

PEDIATRIC EXAMINATION

The pediatric neurologic examination needs to be adapted to the age, temperament, and comfort of the child. Generally, observing the child is essential: watch how the child moves and plays while you take the medical history. Playing with the child and making a game of the examination can provide the necessary information and make the encounter a pleasant experience for the child. Finger puppets and other toys are extremely helpful in getting the child's attention and cooperation. The sequence of the examination has to be flexible. Begin the examination with a fun activity like running down the hallway, and reserve the less pleasant parts for the end, after rapport has been achieved. Consult developmental tables for normal motor, language, adaptive, and social behaviors appropriate for age (Table 1.8).

GERIATRIC EXAMINATION

Many abnormalities found on the neurologic examination of elderly patients are attributed to age. The problem is that many of these abnormalities should be attributed to diseases that are common among the elderly. To avoid overlooking findings that indicate neurologic disease, do not expect to find any abnormality on a neurologic examination of the elderly. Do not be cavalier in attributing abnormal results to "ageing." The clinical relevance of physical findings is important to consider. Primitive reflexes such as the snout or suck reflex and gait difficulties are common in the elderly. However, functional implications such as falling are much more important to the patient than the presence or absence of a primitive reflex.

Examining performance-oriented measures of posture and balance is important in the elderly. These include assessing the patient's ability to stand up from a chair, to bend over, to reach, and to respond to a nudge. The pull test is used to test postural instability in parkinsonism. Explain to patients that you will pull them from

Table 1.8. Landmarks for Normal Development of Motor, Language, and Social Skills at 2 to 48 Months

2 Months	24 months
Lifts head up several seconds while prone	Runs
Startle reaction to loud noise	Speaks in 2- to 3-word sentences
Smiles responsively	Kicks ball
Begins to vocalize single sounds	Uses pronouns ("you," "me," "I")
6 Months	36 Months
Lifts head while supine	Rides a tricycle
Sits with support	Copies a circle
Babbles	Repeats 3 numbers or a sentence of 6
Rolls from prone to supine	syllables
12 Months	Plays simple games
Walks with assistance	48 Months
Uses 2-4 words with meaning	Hops on one foot, throws ball overhand
Uses pincer grasp	Identifies the longer of two lines, draws
Understands a few simple commands	a man with 2 to 4 parts
18 Months	Tells a story
Throws ball	Plays with children, with social
Feeds self	interaction
Uses many intelligible words	
Climbs stairs with assistance	

From Adams, AC: Neurology in Primary Care. FA Davis, Philadelphia, 2000, p 24. Used with permission of Mayo Foundation for Medical Education and Research.

behind and they are to maintain their balance. Reassure them that you are ready to catch them if they lose their balance. If the patient is large, there should be a wall behind the examiner. The normal response is to maintain balance in one or two steps. Many of the common findings of an examination of the elderly and diseases associated with these findings are listed in Table 1.9.

Table 1.9. Geriatric Neurologic Examination

Examination	Age-associated changes	Common diseases
Mental status	Reduced visual perception Reduced constructional ability	Dementia, depression
Cranial nerves	Decreased olfaction Decreased pupillary size and reactivity, presbyopia Decreased smooth pursuit movements Limited upward gaze and convergence Presbycusis	Glaucoma, macular degeneration, cataracts Environmental noise damage Positional vertigo from cupulolithiasis
Motor	No age-related weakness	Parkinsonism Stroke Arthritis Reduced cardiovascular fitness
Sensory	Reduced vibratory sensation in lower extremities	Peripheral neuropathy Medication effect Diabetes mellitus
Reflexes	Reduced ankle reflex	Peripheral neuropathy Medication effect Diabetes mellitus
Gait and posture	Reduced balance	Parkinsonism Arthritis Neuropathies Cervical spondylosis

From Adams, AC: Neurology in Primary Care. FA Davis, Philadelphia, 2000, p 25. Used with permission of Mayo Foundation for Medical Education and Research.

SUGGESTED READING

Applegate, WB, Blass, JP, and Williams, TF: Instruments for the functional assessment of older patients. N Engl J Med 322:1207-1214, 1990.

Brazis, PW, Masdeu, JC, and Biller, J: Localization in Clinical Neurology, ed 2. Little, Brown, Boston, 1990.

DeJong, RN: The Neurologic Examination: Incorporating the Fundamentals of Neuroanatomy and Neurophysiology, ed 4. Harper & Row, Hagerstown, Md., 1979.

Diamond, S, and Dalessio, DJ (eds): The Practicing Physician's Approach to Headache, ed 5. Williams & Wilkins, Baltimore, 1992.

Evans, RW: Diagnostic testing for the evaluation of headaches. Neurol Clin 14:1-26, 1996.

Folstein, MF, Folstein, SE, and McHugh, PR: "Mini-mental state." A practical method for grading the cognitive state of patients for the clinician. J Psychiatr Res 12:189-198, 1975.

Galetta, SL, Liu, GT, and Volpe, NJ: Diagnostic tests in neuro-ophthalmology. Neurol Clin 14:201-222, 1996.

Grogan, PM, and Gronseth, GS: Practice parameter: Steroids, acyclovir, and surgery for Bell's palsy (an evidence-based review): Report of the Quality Standards Subcommittee of the American Academy of Neurology. Neurology 56:830-836, 2001.

Kaye, JA, et al: Neurologic evaluation of the optimally healthy oldest old. Arch Neurol 51:1205-1211, 1994.

Knopman, DS, et al: Geriatric neurology: Part A. Continuum: Lifelong Learning in Neurology 2:7-154, 1996.

Mungas, D: In-office mental status testing: A practical guide. Geriatrics 46:54-58, 63, 66, 1991.

Nutt, JG, Marsden, CD, and Thompson, PD. Human walking and higher-level gait disorders, particularly in the elderly. Neurology 43:268-279, 1993.

Odenheimer, G, et al: Comparison of neurologic changes in "successfully aging" persons vs the total aging population. Arch Neurol 51:573-580, 1994.

Samuels, MA, and Feske, S (eds): Office Practice of Neurology, ed 2. Churchill Livingstone, Philadelphia, 2003.

Silberstein, SD, and Lipton, RB: Headache epidemiology: Emphasis on migraine. Neurol Clin 14:421-434, 1996.

Sudarsky, L: Geriatrics: Gait disorders in the elderly. N Engl J Med 322:1441-1446, 1990.

Tangalos, EG, et al: The Mini-Mental State Examination in general medical practice: Clinical utility and acceptance. Mayo Clin Proc 71:829-837, 1996.

Vaughan, VC, III, McCay, RJ, Jr, and Behrman, RE (eds): Nelson Textbook of Pediatrics, ed 11. Saunders, Philadelphia, 1979.

CHAPTER 2

Diagnostic Tests

The diagnostic tests used most often to evaluate patients who have disease of the central nervous system include cerebrospinal fluid (CSF) analysis, electroencephalography (EEG), electromyography (EMG), evoked potentials, computed tomography (CT), and magnetic resonance imaging (MRI). These tests should be used to supplement or to extend the clinical examination. Remember that diagnostic tests have technical limitations and the quality of the results depends on the examiner or laboratory performing the test. The results should always be interpreted in the context of the patient's clinical presentation.

CEREBROSPINAL FLUID ANALYSIS AND LUMBAR PUNCTURE

Usually, CSF is obtained by lumbar puncture. Before performing this straightforward but invasive procedure, know its indications and contraindications. Laboratory evaluation of CSF is indicated for the diagnosis and treatment of intracerebral hemorrhage and infectious, neoplastic, and demyelinating diseases of the central nervous system. With increasing knowledge about degenerative disorders, prions, and other neurologic problems, CSF analysis may become more useful.

Lumbar puncture should not be performed in a patient with a known or suspected intracranial or spinal mass because of the potential for herniation and neurologic compromise with a shift in intracranial pressure. In these patients, CT or MRI is recommended before lumbar puncture is performed. However, neuroimaging should not delay the diagnosis or treatment of suspected meningitis. The risk of missing the diagnosis of meningitis is much greater than the risk of herniation. In this life-threatening illness, empiric treatment with antibiotics may need to be started to avoid delay in therapy (see Chapter 13). Clinical indications that lumbar puncture can be performed safely are nonfocal findings on neurologic examination and the absence of papilledema.

Lumbar puncture is contraindicated in patients who take anticoagulant medication or have a bleeding disorder. Lumbar puncture can cause intraspinal bleeding, which can compress the cauda equina. If CSF analysis is necessary, the patient can be pretreated with fresh frozen plasma, platelets, cryoprecipitate, or the specific factor to correct the hematologic abnormality.

Lumbar puncture should not be performed if there is infection at the puncture site. This is to avoid introducing the infection into the subarachnoid space. In case of infection, a lateral C1-C2 puncture can be performed by a neurosurgeon to obtain the CSF sample. Despite these contraindications, lumbar puncture is a safe and easy procedure.

Explain the procedure to the patient and provide emotional support throughout the procedure to reduce the patient's apprehension. The key to a successful lumbar puncture is proper positioning of the patient. The patient should be in the lateral decubitus position, with the back at the edge of the table or bed to provide back support. The patient's shoulders should be aligned and the spine parallel to the edge of the bed. The patient should assume the fetal position, bringing the knees to the chin. The L3-L4 vertebral interspace is in the middle at the level of the superior iliac crest (Fig. 2.1). In adults, the caudal end of the spinal cord is at vertebral level L1-L2, so vertebral level L3-L4 or the one above or below can be punctured safely. In infants and children, the caudal end of the spinal cord is lower relative to the vertebral column, and it is best to use the L4-L5 or L5-S1 vertebral interspace.

Perform the puncture with strict aseptic technique. Cleanse the skin with an iodine solution three times, starting at the puncture site and washing outward in concentric circles. Often, alcohol is used to remove the iodine to avoid introducing iodine into the subarachnoid space. Apply the sterile drape, and prepare all the equipment before inserting the needle. To anesthetize the skin, use a small intradermal needle to inject lidocaine into a small wheal over the puncture site. Warn the patient that this step can cause a stinging sensation. Deeper structures can be anesthetized, but this may be more uncomfortable for the patient than the spinal needle.

For adults, use a 20-gauge lumbar puncture needle with stylet because 1) it is rigid enough to penetrate the ligamentum flavum, 2) it provides for an accurate pressure reading, and 3) it is large enough to collect CSF rapidly. The stylet needs to be in place on insertion to avoid the rare complication of implanting an epidermoid tumor in the subarachnoid space. The needle with stylet should be directed with the bevel parallel to the long axis of the spine to spread or to split the dural fibers that run longitudinally. This minimizes leakage of the CSF into the subdural space. Steadily direct the needle toward the umbilicus until there is a "give," or a reduction in resistance, as the needle pierces the dura mater.

Remove the stylet, and check for CSF return. If no fluid is obtained, rotate the needle. If no fluid appears, replace the stylet and advance the needle in small, 1- to 2- mm increments, checking for CSF with each advance. Inserting the needle too far injures the venous plexus anterior to the spinal canal; this is the most common cause of a "traumatic tap." If bone is encountered, the needle should be withdrawn to the level of the skin (to avoid the same path of the first puncture) and redirected. Repeated puncture of the skin should be avoided because of the increased risk of infection and subcutaneous bleeding. If the patient complains of pain down the leg, the needle needs to be directed more medially. If the patient cannot tolerate lying on the side or cannot be positioned properly, the procedure can be done with the patient sitting, leaning forward over a table. This position does not permit an accurate pressure reading, but the patient can be repositioned in the lateral decubitus position for this measurement. If the puncture is not successful, a different interspace can be used or the procedure can be performed under fluoroscopic guidance.

After CSF has been obtained, attach the manometer to the hub of the needle and record

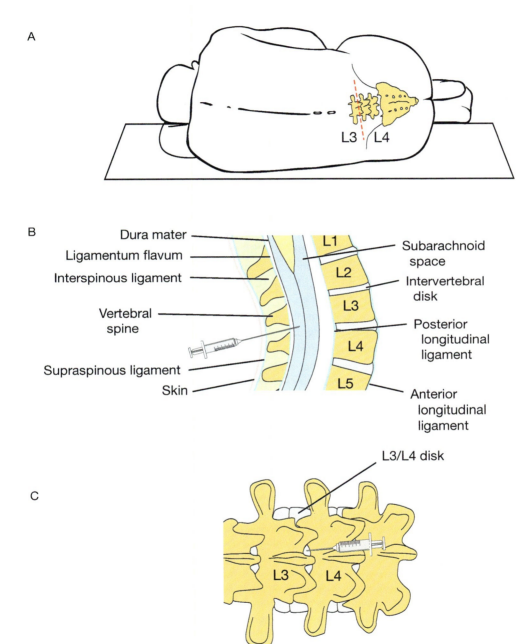

Fig. 2.1. Lumbar puncture. *A*, Position of patient and location of L3-L4 interspace (red dashed line). *B*, Longitudinal section through the vertebral column showing the path of the lumbar needle. *C*, Lumbar needle in the L3-L4 interspace. (Modified from Patten, J: Neurological Differential Diagnosis. Springer-Verlag, New York, 1977, pp 262, 264. Used with permission.)

the opening pressure. The patient should be encouraged to relax and to breathe normally to avoid a falsely high pressure reading. The meniscus should show minimal fluctuation related to pulse and respiration. Collect the CSF in four separate vials (labeled "1" through "4"), and remove the needle without the stylet to avoid trapping any nerve roots. Traditionally, the patient was instructed to remain flat or prone for some time to reduce the risk of post–lumbar puncture headache. However, studies have shown that remaining flat is not an important factor. In a large outpatient study, thin young women had the highest risk for post–lumbar puncture headache. The duration of the recumbence and the amount of CSF obtained did not influence the risk of headache.

Post–lumbar puncture headache is the most frequent complication of lumbar puncture, with a reported frequency of 10% to 38%. The use of an atraumatic spinal needle and a small needle size reduces the risk of post–lumbar puncture headache. The headache usually responds to a short period of bed rest. A persistent headache for more than 2 days can be treated with an epidural injection of autologous blood at the site of the puncture. Other complications of lumbar puncture are rare and include diplopia, infection, backache, and radicular symptoms.

A "traumatic tap," that is, bleeding into the subarachnoid space from injury to small blood vessels, can compromise the interpretation of CSF results. A CSF sample with traumatic blood clears as the fluid is collected, and fewer erythrocytes are found in vial 4 than in vial 1. The opening pressure in a traumatic tap is normal, compared with the pressure in cases of subarachnoid hemorrhage or meningitis. The supernatant of centrifuged CSF should be clear if the tap was traumatic and xanthochromic (yellow) if blood has been present for several hours and has undergone hemolysis. Blood from a traumatic tap will increase the number of erythrocytes and leukocytes and the amount of protein in the CSF. The formula used to estimate the increase is the following: 700 erythrocytes can account for an increase of 1 leukocyte and 1 mg of protein.

Analysis of CSF is essential for diagnosing many disorders of the central nervous system (Table 2.1). Also, the removal of CSF can be therapeutic, as in pseudotumor cerebri and normal-pressure hydrocephalus. In a patient with normal-pressure hydrocephalus, an improvement in gait after removal of CSF indicates that a shunt may be beneficial. The clinical value of CSF analysis is discussed further in relation to neurologic infections and neuro-oncology (Chapters 13 and 14).

ELECTROENCEPHALOGRAPHY

An important feature of EEG is that it is a physiologic test that provides information about function instead of structure. An example that emphasizes this point is the case of a child with a head injury and altered behavior and normal findings on neuroimaging. Normal neuroimaging results cannot explain the child's abnormal behavior. However, EEG identifies the problem, namely, nonconvulsive status epilepticus amenable to anticonvulsant therapy. EEG is noninvasive and relatively inexpensive. It is an extension of the clinical examination, and the information obtained with EEG should be interpreted in the context of the patient's clinical presentation. Normal EEG findings do not exclude neurologic disease, and abnormal EEG findings may be of no clinical consequence.

The quality of the test results depends on the skill of the EEG technician and the electroencephalographer. Accreditation of the EEG laboratory and certification of the technician and electroencephalographer indicate that the recording meets acceptable standards. Eighteen

Table 2.1. Features of the Cerebrospinal Fluid in Various Diseases

Condition	Clinical findings	Appearance	Opening pressure	Protein	Glucose	Cell count
Normal		Clear, colorless	50-200 mm H₂O	15-45 mg/ 100 mL	45-80 mg/mL (2/3 that of serum)	RBCs, 0 WBCs, 0-5 μL (lymphocytes or monocytes)
Subarachnoid hemorrhage	"Worst headache of life," stiff neck, negative CT	Blood tinged, xanthochromic	Increased	Increased	Normal	Same as blood
Bacterial meningitis	Headache, mental status change	Opalescent, purulent	Increased	Increased	Decreased	Increased number of WBCs (PMNs)
Viral meningitis	Headache, mental status change	Normal or opalescent	Increased or normal	Increased	Decreased	Increased number of WBCs (lymphocytes)
Carcinomatous meningitis	Headache, cranial nerve signs, seizures	Cloudy	Increased or normal	Increased	Decreased	Increased number of WBCs, malignant cells
Multiple sclerosis	Multiple signs and symptoms	Normal	Normal	Normal, increased IgG	Normal	Normal or increased number of lymphocytes
Pseudotumor cerebri	Headache, papilledema, normal CT	Normal	Increased	Normal	Normal	Normal
Guillain-Barré syndrome	Ascending paralysis	Normal	Normal	Increased	Normal	Normal

CT, computed tomography; PMNs, polymorphonuclear neutrophils; RBCs, erythrocytes; WBCs, leukocytes. From Adams, AC: Neurology in Primary Care. FA Davis, Philadelphia, 2000, p 31. Used with permission of Mayo Foundation for Medical Education and Research.

to 21 recording channels are recommended. An electrocardiogram line should be used because it provides useful information about cardiac rhythm. This feature is particularly helpful when evaluating a patient who has spells or other transient disorders. Activation procedures, including hyperventilation, intermittent photic stimulation, and sleep, should be part of the EEG study to increase the frequency of epileptogenic activity. Hyperventilation is an activation procedure that is particularly useful in patients with absence seizures. Hyperventilation should be used with care in patients who have cardiopulmonary disease.

EEG is indispensable in the evaluation of patients who have seizures. It can be critical in diagnosing seizures, determining the probability of recurrent seizures, and selecting the best treatment for seizures. The sensitivity of a single EEG recording for identifying specific epileptiform activity is reportedly about 50%. This increases to about 90% with three EEG recordings. Prolonged EEG recording with video monitoring increases diagnostic sensitivity. Ambulatory EEG monitoring can be useful, but excessive artifact can complicate these studies.

EEG can be clinically useful for many transient disorders or "spells." In disorders of altered consciousness, EEG can determine whether the process is diffuse, focal, or multifocal. Serial EEG recordings can help determine prognosis in coma and encephalopathy. EEG may be useful in distinguishing between dementia and pseudodementia, diagnosing sleep disorders, and determining brain death. When requesting an EEG, the clinical question should be stated clearly and the electroencephalographer should attempt to answer the question within the limitations of the test.

The normal awake EEG is characterized by an alpha (8-13 Hz) rhythm recorded over the posterior head region; this rhythm attenuates with eye opening (Fig. 2.2 *A*). EEG sleep activity is illustrated in Figure 2.2 *B* and *C*. Abnormalities seen on EEG include slowing, asymmetry, suppression or loss of EEG activity, and epileptiform activity (spikes, sharp waves, and spike-and-wave). Common EEG findings and their anatomical and clinical correlates are summarized in Table 2.2. EEG abnormalities and abnormal patterns are shown in Figures 2.3 and 2.4.

EVOKED POTENTIALS

An evoked potential is an electrical response of the nervous system to an external stimulus. Evoked potentials measure conduction in nerve pathways from the periphery through the central nervous system. In clinical practice, this includes the visual, auditory (or brainstem), and somatosensory pathways. Evoked potentials are noninvasive tests that provide valuable physiologic information about the nervous system. For example, they are sensitive to demyelination and have been used to detect clinically silent lesions in patients with multiple sclerosis.

Visual evoked potentials extend the physical examination of the visual system and are useful in diagnosing optic nerve disease and determining the likelihood of the recovery of vision. If an ophthalmologic problem has been excluded, abnormal visual evoked potentials reportedly are 100% sensitive in detecting optic neuritis even after the recovery of vision, and can be useful in assessing visual function in infants and uncooperative subjects. The visual evoked potential in response to a pattern reversal stimulus in a patient with left eye optic neuritis is shown in Figure 2.5.

Auditory, or brainstem, evoked potentials are sensitive to anatomical disturbances of brainstem pathways. These potentials are not affected by the level of consciousness, drugs, or metabolic disturbances. Auditory evoked

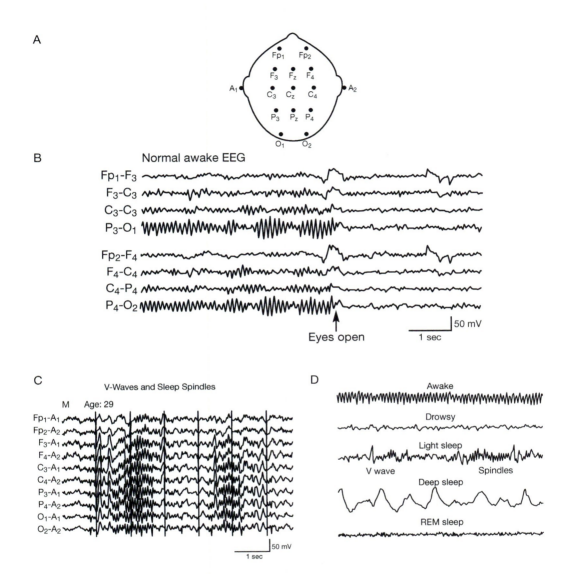

Fig. 2.2. *A*, Placement of EEG electrodes. A, Ear lobe; C, central; F, frontal; O, occipital; P, parietal. Lower case letters: p, polar; z, midsagittal. Even numbers, right hemisphere; odd numbers, left hemisphere. *B*, Normal awake EEG pattern. Note alpha rhythm recorded over the posterior head region (P$_3$-O$_1$ and P$_4$-O$_2$) in an awake patient with eyes closed. The rhythm attenuates when the eyes are opened. *C*, Normal sleep EEG pattern with V waves (these waves are maximal over the vertex region and resemble the letter "V") and spindles (10–14-Hz sinusoidal activity). *D*, Comparison of EEG patterns of wakefulness and different levels of sleep. The awake EEG is recorded from the occipital areas, with eyes closed. The rapid eye movement (REM) sleep pattern resembles the awake EEG pattern with eyes open. (*A* and *B* from Westmoreland, BF: Clinical EEG Manual. Available from: http://mayoweb.mayo.edu/man-neuroeeg/index.html. Used with permission of Mayo Foundation for Medical Education and Research. *C* from Benarroch, EE, et al: Medical Neurosciences: An Approach to Anatomy, Pathology, and Physiology by Systems and Levels. ed 4. Lippincott Williams & Wilkins, Philadelphia, 1999, p 304. Used with permission of Mayo Foundation.)

Table 2.2.   Localization and Clinical Correlates of Common EEG Findings

EEG finding	Localization	Clinical correlate
Generalized spike-and-wave activity	Diffuse cortex	Absence seizure
		Generalized tonic-clonic seizure
Focal spike-and-wave activity, sharp waves	Focal cortex	Partial epilepsy
Diffuse slowing	Diffuse cortex	Encephalopathy
Focal slowing	Focal cortex	Focal structural lesion
Periodic lateralized epileptiform discharges (PLEDs)	Localized or hemispheric dysfunction	Acute or subacute process (eg, herpes encephalitis)
Triphasic waves	Diffuse cortex	Encephalopathy (eg, hepatic)
Generalized periodic and slow wave complex	Diffuse cortex	Creutzfeldt-Jakob disease
Burst suppression	Diffuse cortex	Post-cardiopulmonary arrest

EEG, electroencephalographic.
From Adams, AC: Neurology in Primary Care. FA Davis, Philadelphia, 2000, p 32. Used with permission of Mayo Foundation for Medical Education and Research.

potentials can be used to assess brainstem pathways in infants and in unresponsive or uncooperative patients. They also are helpful in evaluating complaints of vertigo, hearing loss, and tinnitus. Auditory evoked potentials can identify hearing impairment in infants and are used to screen for acoustic neuromas. They also are valuable in intraoperative monitoring during posterior fossa surgery. An abnormal brainstem auditory response on the left side in a patient who had an acoustic neuroma is shown in Figure 2.6.

Somatosensory evoked potentials are useful in assessing peripheral nerves, the spinal cord, and cerebral cortex. They can be used to confirm the presence of an organic disease process in a patient who has sensory complaints. They also are valuable in intraoperative monitoring to protect neural structures.

NERVE CONDUCTION STUDIES AND ELECTROMYOGRAPHY

It cannot be overemphasized that electrophysiologic studies are extensions of the clinical examination and that the quality of the studies is operator dependent. EMG can be indispensable in the evaluation and treatment of patients who have muscle, neuromuscular junction, peripheral nerve, or motor neuron disease. It provides functional information and often supplements structural information from such tests as CT and MRI. EMG may provide the most critical information in the case of a patient with low back pain and radicular symptoms in whom MRI shows multiple-level degenerative changes. Many abnormalities seen on MRI are not clinically significant. The results of an EMG will indicate which level is symptomatic. Also,

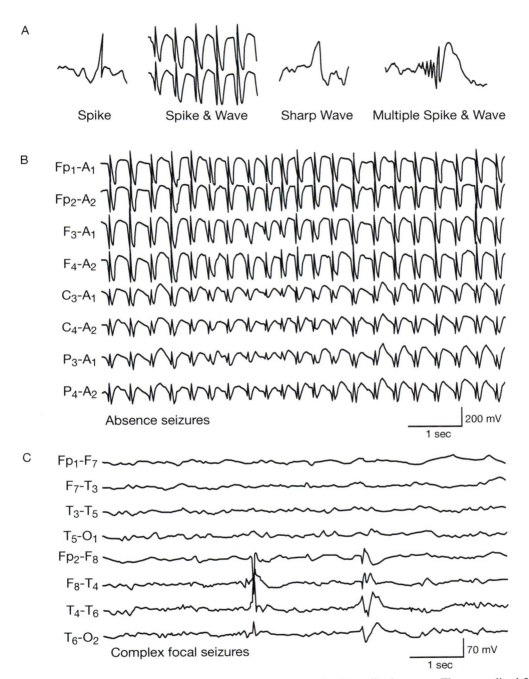

A

Spike   Spike & Wave   Sharp Wave   Multiple Spike & Wave

B

Fp_1-A_1

Fp_2-A_2

F_3-A_1

F_4-A_2

C_3-A_1

C_4-A_2

P_3-A_1

P_4-A_2

Absence seizures

200 mV

1 sec

C

Fp_1-F_7

F_7-T_3

T_3-T_5

T_5-O_1

Fp_2-F_8

F_8-T_4

T_4-T_6

T_6-O_2

Complex focal seizures

70 mV

1 sec

Fig. 2.3. EEG abnormalities. *A,* Epileptiform discharges. *B,* Generalized pattern. The generalized 3 per second spike and wave is the EEG pattern typical of absence seizures. *C,* Focal pattern. Right temporal spike is an EEG pattern seen in complex focal seizures originating on the right. (From Westmoreland, BF: Clinical EEG Manual. Available from: http://mayoweb.mayo.edu/man-neuroeeg/index.html. Used with permission of Mayo Foundation for Medical Education and Research.)

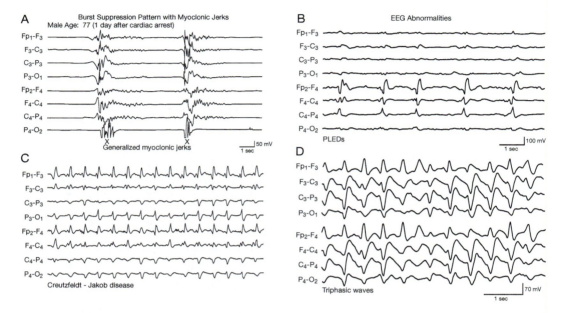

Fig. 2.4. Abnormal electroencephalographic (EEG) patterns. *A*, Burst suppression pattern consists of periodic bursts of abnormal activity separated by periods of electrocerebral silence. This pattern indicates severe brain injury, eg, after cardiopulmonary arrest. *B*, PLEDs (periodic lateralized epileptiform discharges) represent an acute epileptic focus in a focal or lateralized pattern. This pattern often develops after herpes simplex encephalitis or vascular lesions. *C*, Periodic sharp waves are typical of Creutzfeldt-Jakob disease. *D*, Triphasic waves is an EEG pattern associated with hepatic encephalopathy. (*A*, *C*, and *D* from Westmoreland, BF: Clinical EEG Manual. Available from: http://mayoweb.mayo.edu/man-neuroeeg/index.html. Used with permission of Mayo Foundation for Medical Education and Research. *B* from Westmoreland, BF: Epileptiform electroencephalographic patterns. Mayo Clin Proc 71:505-511, 1996. Used with permission of Mayo Foundation for Medical Education and Research.)

EMG is essential for confirming the diagnosis of motor neuron disease.

When ordering EMG, it is important to understand the kind of information that can be obtained and the limitations of the test. EMG results will be more meaningful if the clinical question is clear and the electromyographer knows the clinical question to be answered. The timing of the study is critical. Abnormalities of peripheral nerves may not be demonstrated with EMG until 2 to 6 weeks after an acute injury. It is helpful if the patient is prepared for the test and understands what it involves.

Nerve Conduction Studies

Nerve conduction can be measured in sensory and motor nerves. Nerve conduction studies can test only medium- to large-diameter myelinated fibers. These include motor fibers and the sensory fibers that convey vibratory sensation and proprioception. Small unmyelinated fibers that conduct pain and temperature sensations cannot be evaluated with EMG. Patients with small-fiber neuropathies often have normal EMG findings.

The motor nerves that are commonly tested are the median, ulnar, peroneal, and posterior tibial nerves. A recording electrode is placed on

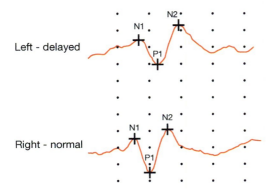

Left - delayed

Right - normal

Fig. 2.5. Visual evoked potential with pattern reversal stimulus. The visual evoked response is prolonged on the left at 116 ms (left eye optic neuritis), compared with 96 ms on the right (right eye normal). (Modified from Mancall, EL [general editor]: Continuum: Lifelong Learning in Neurology. Part A: Clinical Neurophysiology 4:58, October 1998. Used with permission.)

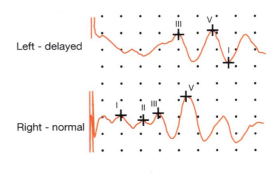

Left - delayed

Right - normal

Fig. 2.6. Brainstem auditory evoked potential. Note the delay of peaks III and V on the left compared with those on the right. This abnormality on the left indicates a brainstem lesion. (Modified from Mancall, EL [general editor]: Continuum: Lifelong Learning in Neurology. Part A: Clinical Neurophysiology 4:57, October 1998. Used with permission.)

the muscle, and the nerve is stimulated with a mild electric shock at distal and proximal sites (Fig. 2.7). Important values include the distal latency, conduction velocity, and conduction amplitude. The time measured from stimulating the nerve at the distal site to contraction of the muscle is the distal latency. The time measured from stimulating the nerve at the proximal site to contraction of the muscle is the proximal latency. For the median nerve, a prolonged distal latency supports the diagnosis of carpal tunnel syndrome. Conduction time is the speed of the nerve impulse. It is calculated by dividing the length of the nerve segment by the difference between the distal and proximal latencies.

Conduction velocity is related to the diameter (myelination) of the nerve. A slow nerve conduction velocity indicates a demyelinating peripheral neuropathy. The amplitude of the motor unit potential is related to the number of axons. A decrease in amplitude indicates an axonal polyneuropathy (Table 2.3).

Muscle Studies

The electrical activity of muscles is recorded by inserting a small needle electrode into the muscle. Information is obtained during the insertion of the needle, with the muscle at rest, and with voluntary contraction. The clinical indication for EMG determines which muscles are tested. To facilitate the study, provide the electromyographer with the necessary clinical information. The electromyographer needs to know if the patient is taking an anticoagulant or has a bleeding diathesis.

The brief discharge that occurs when the needle is inserted into the muscle is called insertional activity. Insertional activity is increased in neurogenic disorders, such as peripheral neuropathies, that cause abnormal excitability of muscle. At rest, a normal muscle has no spontaneous activity (excluding end plate activity). Abnormal spontaneous activity is seen in neurogenic lesions associated with denervation and inflammatory myopathies. Motor unit action potentials are

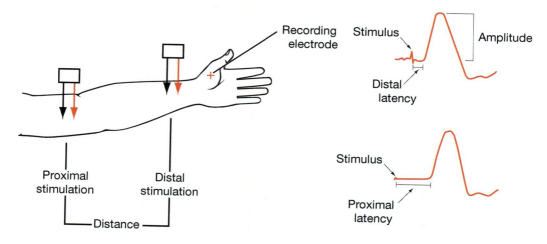

Fig. 2.7. Setup for recording median nerve conduction velocity. Motor nerve conduction velocity, reported in meters per second, $= \dfrac{\text{Distance}}{\text{Proximal latency} - \text{Distal latency}}$. (From Adams, AC: Neurology in Primary Care. FA Davis, Philadelphia, 2000, p 33. Used with permission of Mayo Foundation for Medical Education and Research.)

recorded when the muscle is contracted voluntarily. These potentials are analyzed for amplitude, duration, phases, and recruitment. With continued muscle contraction, the motor units summate and the response is referred to as the interference pattern. EMG features of clinical disorders are summarized in Figure 2.8.

Table 2.3.   Components of Nerve Conduction Studies

Component (unit of measure)	Is a function of	Is abnormal in
Distal latency (milliseconds)	Conduction rate	Compression neuropathies (carpal tunnel syndrome)

Amplitude
  Motor (millivolts)
  Sensory (microvolts)
	Number of axons	Axonal neuropathies (diabetic neuropathy)

Conduction velocity (meters/second)	Axon diameter, myelination	Demyelinating neuropathies (hereditary sensory motor neuropathy, chronic inflammatory demyelinating polyradiculoneuropathy)

From Adams, AC: Neurology in Primary Care. FA Davis, Philadelphia, 2000, p 34. Used with permission of Mayo Foundation for Medical Education and Research.

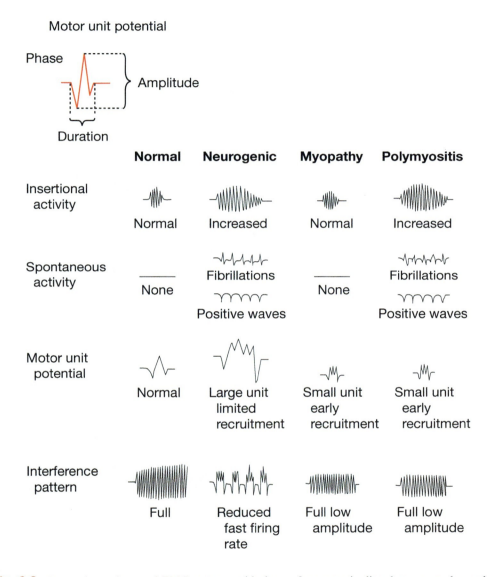

Fig. 2.8. Comparison of normal EMG patterns with those of neurogenic disorders, myopathy, and polymyositis. (Modified from Kimura, J: Electrodiagnosis in Diseases of Nerve and Muscle: Principles and Practice, ed 2. FA Davis, Philadelphia, 1989, p 252. Used with permission.)

MAGNETIC RESONANCE IMAGING

MRI is the imaging test preferred for evaluating the posterior fossa, neoplastic disease, meningeal disease, subacute hemorrhage, seizures, and demyelinating disease. Images can be obtained in several planes, including the coronal, axial, and sagittal planes (Fig. 2.9). Adverse reactions to the contrast agent gadolinium are rare. MRI is more expensive than CT and is insensitive to calcification. The clinical situations for which MRI or CT is the preferred imaging study are summarized in Table 2.4. An absolute contraindication to MRI is the presence of magnetic intracranial aneurysm clips or cardiac pacemakers. Women in the first trimester of pregnancy and metal workers with metal fragments in the eye are usually excluded from the test.

The principles of magnetic resonance are complex, but the images result from the varying intensities of radio wave signals emanating from the tissue in which hydrogen nuclei have been excited by a radiofrequency pulse. The signal intensity (white or dark) on the magnetic resonance image is determined by the way protons revert to the resting state after a radio-frequency pulse (relaxation time, T1 and T2), the concentration of protons in the tissue (proton density), and flow. Contrast on magnetic resonance can be manipulated by changing pulse sequence parameters. The two that are most important are TE (echo time) and TR (repetition time). A discussion of the technique is beyond the scope of this text, but it is important to know from a clinical perspective that different techniques can be used to enhance imaging of the nervous system.

Usually, both T1-weighted images and T2-weighted images are used in imaging the brain and spine. T1-weighted images are useful for analyzing anatomical detail. T2-weighted images are very sensitive to the presence of increased water. Most brain lesions have long T2 and long T1 so they will be of high signal, or white, on T2-weighted images and low signal, or dark, on T1-weighted images (Table 2.5).

Other sequences used in imaging the central nervous system include proton density, fluid-attenuated inversion recovery (FLAIR), and diffusion-weighted imaging (Fig. 2.10). FLAIR sequences minimize signals from CSF and increase the sensitivity for detecting small tumors, vascular malformations, and mesial

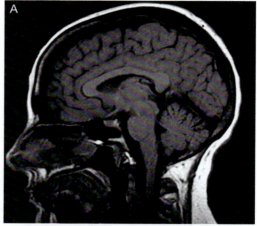

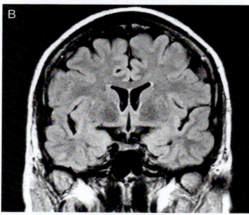

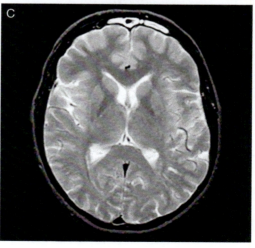

Fig. 2.9. MRI of the brain in the sagittal (*A*), coronal (*B*), and axial (*C*) planes.

Table 2.4. Indication for Selecting Computed Tomography (CT) or Magnetic Resonance Imaging (MRI)

Indication	Preferred test
Acute trauma	CT
Acute stroke (intracranial hemorrhage)	CT
Cost	CT
Bone, calcification	CT
Demyelinating disease	MRI
Mental status changes after trauma	MRI
Seizures	MRI
Tumor	MRI
Metastatic disease	MRI
Meningeal disease	MRI
Dementia	MRI
Uncooperative/medically unstable patient	CT

From Adams, AC: Neurology in Primary Care. FA Davis, Philadelphia, 2000, p 37. Used with permission of Mayo Foundation for Medical Education and Research.

temporal sclerosis. Diffusion-weighted imaging detects random movements of water protons and is sensitive to early cerebral ischemia (Fig. 2.10).

MRI is also advantageous for imaging flowing blood. Magnetic resonance angiography, a noninvasive method for evaluating cerebral vasculature, can detect aneurysms as small as 3 to 4 mm (Fig. 2.11). MRI is a rapidly evolving specialty, and many clinical advances can be anticipated.

ANGIOGRAPHY

Magnetic resonance angiography is becoming the preferred method for evaluating cerebrovascular disease. However, conventional angiography is still a valuable diagnostic test in the assessment of aneurysms, vascular malformations, and vasculitis. Advances have included safer digital imaging, smaller catheters, and improved radiographic contrast agents. The risk of serious morbidity has decreased, and the rate of stroke resulting from the procedure should be less than 0.5% when it is performed by a skilled practitioner. Therapeutic uses have expanded to include use in thrombolytic therapy. The most common adverse effect of angiography is groin hematoma.

Table 2.5. Pathologic Appearance on Different MRI Sequences

Feature	T1-weighted image	T2-weighted image	PD/FLAIR imaging
Acute ischemia	Gray	Dark	Dark
Cyst	Dark	White	Dark
Fat	White	Dark	White
Solid mass	Dark	White	White
Subacute blood	White	White	White

FLAIR, fluid-attenuated inversion recovery; MRI, magnetic resonance imaging; PD, proton density.

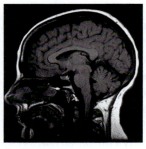

T1WI
  spin lattice
  relaxation time
CSF: dark
Sequence good
  for anatomical
  detail

A Sagittal

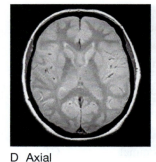

PD
  (proton density)
Sequence mini-
  mizes the effects
  of relaxation time

D Axial

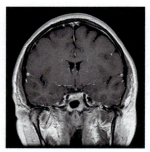

T1WI with
  gadolinium
Gadolinium
  provides greater
  contrast between
  normal and
  abnormal tissue

B Coronal

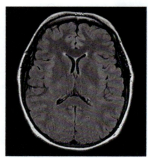

FLAIR
  (fluid-attenuated
  inversion recov-
  ery)
T2WI with CSF
  signal suppressed

E Axial

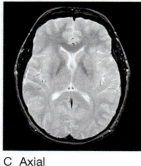

T2WI
Spin-spin
  relaxation time
CSF: white
Sequence
  sensitive to
  increased water
  content

C Axial

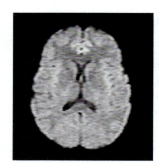

DWI
  (diffusion-
  weighted imaging)
Sequence sensitive
  to early cerebral
  ischemia

F Axial

Fig. 2.10. *A-F,* Normal brain appearance with different MRI sequences. CSF, cerebrospinal fluid; T1WI, T1-weighted image; T2WI, T2-weighted image.

MYELOGRAPHY

Myelography is a radiographic test that allows the spine to be visualized after a radiopaque substance has been injected into the spinal subarachnoid space. The test is helpful in diagnosing disease of the spine, such as herniated disk and spinal stenosis. Myelography is invasive and has the same contraindications as lumbar puncture. MRI of the spine has the

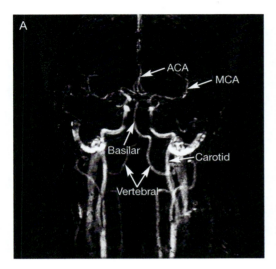 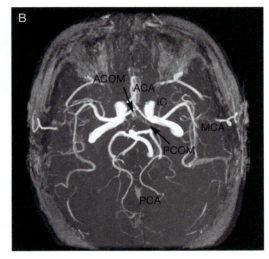

Fig. 2.11. Magnetic resonance angiography of the cerebral circulation. *A*, Anterior-posterior view; *B*, inferior view. ACA, anterior cerebral artery; ACOM, anterior communicating artery; IC, internal carotid artery; MCA, middle cerebral artery; PCA, posterior cerebral artery; PCOM, posterior communicating artery.

major advantage of being noninvasive; also, it may be more sensitive for detecting metastatic disease of the spine and spinal cord compression syndromes. With improvement in contrast agents, myelography has become safer, with fewer adverse reactions. Myelography may provide additional information when the results of MRI or CT are ambiguous.

SUGGESTED READING

Armon, C, Evans, RW, and Therapeutics and Technology Assessment Subcommittee of the American Academy of Neurology. Addendum to assessment: Prevention of post-lumbar puncture headaches: Report of the Therapeutics and Technology Assessment Subcommittee of the American Academy of Neurology. Neurology 65:510-512, 2005.

Daube, JR (ed): Clinical Neurophysiology, ed 2. Oxford University Press, Oxford, 2002.

Evans, RW (guest ed): Diagnostic testing in neurology. Neurol Clin 14:1-254, 1996.

Fishman, RA: Cerebrospinal Fluid in Diseases of the Nervous System, ed 2. Saunders, Philadelphia, 1992.

Gilmore, R (guest ed): Evoked potentials. Neurol Clin 6:649-933, 1988.

Kimura, J: Electrodiagnosis in Diseases of Nerve and Muscle: Principles and Practice, ed 3. Oxford University Press, Oxford, 2001.

Kuntz, KM, et al: Post-lumbar puncture headaches: Experience in 501 consecutive procedures. Neurology 42:1884-1887, 1992.

Members of the Mayo Clinic Department of Neurology: Mayo Clinic Examinations in Neurology, ed 7. Mosby, St. Louis, 1998.

Perkins, CJ, et al: Fluid-attenuated inversion recovery and diffusion- and perfusion-weighted MRI abnormalities in 117 consecutive patients with stroke symptoms. Stroke 32:2774-2781, 2001.

Samuels, MA, and Feske, SK (eds): Office Practice of Neurology, ed 2. Churchill Livingstone, Philadelphia, 2003.

So, EL: Role of neuroimaging in the management of seizure disorders. Mayo Clin Proc 77:1251-1264, 2002.

Wallach, JB: Interpretation of Diagnostic Tests, ed 8. Wolters Kluwer Health/ Lippincott Williams & Wilkins, Philadelphia, 2007.

Westmoreland, BF: Epileptiform electroencephalographic patterns. Mayo Clin Proc 71;501-511, 1996.

CHAPTER 3

Headache

Headache is a universal problem, with a lifetime prevalence of 99%, and it is the most common reason for neurologic referral. Headache may be of little clinical significance or it may represent the onset of a life-threatening illness. To the patient, the symptom is always of major concern, and the relationship you establish with the patient at the initial visit will determine the success of treatment.

The importance of this relationship cannot be overstated. It is essential that you convey to the patient that you believe the patient's symptoms are real and you are concerned about the patient's welfare. You must understand who the patient is, how the headache affects the patient's life, and what the patient's expectations, fears, and concerns are. You must educate the patient about headache, treatment options, and reasonable expectations. The patient must also take responsibility for the treatment plan as both of you work toward the mutual and realistic goal of decreasing the frequency and severity of headache.

HEADACHE RED FLAGS

Most headaches are *primary headaches*, that is, ones without an underlying illness. Primary headaches include migraine, cluster, and tension-type headaches. Although headaches caused by an underlying disease process or condition, called *secondary headaches*, are rare, they are the initial focus in the diagnostic evaluation of headache. An experienced clinician will search for the alarming features in the medical history and examination, and this will direct subsequent work-up. These warnings are summarized in Table 3.1.

The temporal profile of the headache symptoms is important. Sudden onset of headache suggests a vascular cause. In this case, the most serious diagnostic considerations include subarachnoid hemorrhage (Fig. 3.1), hemorrhage from an arteriovenous malformation, pituitary apoplexy, and bleeding into a mass lesion. The characteristic complaint of a patient with a subarachnoid hemorrhage is that it "is the worst headache of my life." Emergency neuroimaging is advised, and computed tomography (CT) without a contrast agent is usually the most expedient test. Negative CT findings do not exclude the possibility of hemorrhage, and if the findings are not diagnostic, lumbar puncture should be performed to examine for blood in the cerebrospinal fluid (CSF). According to estimates, up to 25% of subarachnoid hemorrhages may be

Table 3.1. Headache Warnings ("Red Flags")

Headache warning	Possible diagnoses	Evaluation
Sudden onset of headache	Subarachnoid hemorrhage Hemorrhage from a mass lesion or arteriovenous malformation Pituitary apoplexy Mass lesion (especially in the posterior fossa)	Neuroimaging, lumbar puncture*
New-onset headache after age 50 years	Temporal arteritis Mass lesion	Erythrocyte sedimentation rate, neuroimaging
Papilledema	Mass lesion Pseudotumor cerebri	Neuroimaging, lumbar puncture*
Headache with fever, rash, systemic illness, stiff neck	Meningitis Encephalitis Systemic infection Collagen vascular disease Lyme disease	Neuroimaging, lumbar puncture,* blood tests
New-onset headache in patient with cancer or HIV infection	Metastasis Meningitis Brain abscess	Neuroimaging, lumbar puncture*
Accelerating pattern of headaches	Subdural hematoma Medication overuse	Neuroimaging

HIV, human immunodeficiency virus.
*Lumbar puncture should be performed after neuroimaging. If meningitis is suspected and there are no focal findings and/or papilledema, lumbar puncture should be performed immediately.
From Adams, AC: Neurology in Primary Care. FA Davis, Philadelphia, 2000, p 43. Used with permission of Mayo Foundation for Medical Education and Research.

missed by CT. Other causes of sudden explosive headache can include vasospasm from migraine and an unruptured aneurysm. If subarachnoid hemorrhage is excluded by CT and CSF analysis, angiography or magnetic resonance angiography (MRA), or both, may be needed to complete the evaluation.

Another alarming profile is an accelerating pattern of headaches. Most commonly, this pattern occurs in patients who have been overusing an analgesic medication, but the possibility of an enlarging mass lesion such as a tumor or subdural hematoma needs to be considered. CT with a contrast agent or magnetic resonance imaging (MRI) may be warranted. A "new" headache in a patient with cancer or one who is immunocompromised should always be investigated. In the case of these patients, the diagnostic considerations are metastasis, carcinomatous or infectious meningitis, and brain abscess, and neuroimaging and CSF analysis should be performed.

A patient with headache who also has fever, stiff neck, rash, or other signs of systemic illness

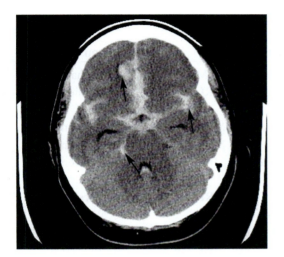

Fig. 3.1. Subarachnoid hemorrhage. CT scan in axial plane showing blood (*arrows*) distributed diffusely in the subarachnoid space.

should be evaluated thoroughly for an infectious disease. Meningitis, encephalitis, Lyme disease, and systemic infections are associated with headache. Collagen vascular disease should also be considered if systemic illness is suspected. The diagnostic evaluation should include neuroimaging, CSF analysis, and blood tests. Focal neurologic symptoms and signs that are not part of a typical migraine aura may indicate a mass lesion and suggest the need to evaluate the patient for a tumor, arteriovenous malformation, stroke, or collagen vascular disease. Papilledema may indicate a mass lesion or pseudotumor cerebri. If imaging study results are negative, lumbar puncture is needed. Pseudotumor cerebri is diagnosed on the basis of negative neuroimaging findings and increased CSF pressure.

DIAGNOSTIC TESTING

Diagnostic testing in headache can be complicated not only by the medical indications but by the demands of cost containment, medical-legal issues, and patient expectations. Diagnostic testing is indicated to confirm the diagnosis, to exclude serious diagnoses, to establish the presence of comorbid disease that may complicate treatment, and to evaluate the patient's status before treatment is initiated. Tests to reassure the patient may be an integral part of the treatment plan. However, diagnostic tests should never replace the clinical evaluation and education of the patient.

Neuroimaging

The diagnostic tests most often used in the evaluation of headache are CT and MRI (Table 3.2). CT is useful in an emergency setting to evaluate for the presence of hemorrhage. With the use of a contrast agent, CT can detect most mass lesions that can cause headache. MRI is more sensitive than CT for detecting tumors and infarcts, and it is also more sensitive for detecting nonspecific abnormalities. Clinically insignificant white matter changes and atrophy have been reported to occur more frequently in patients with migraine than in age-matched controls. The patient's clinical presentation should dictate how much emphasis needs to be put on the imaging studies.

On the basis of a review of the evidence and expert opinion, the American Academy of Neurology issued a summary statement about the use of neuroimaging for patients with headache who have normal findings on neurologic examination. For adult patients with recurrent headache that has been defined as migraine with no recent change in pattern, no history of seizures, and no other focal neurologic signs or symptoms, the routine use of neuroimaging is not warranted. This recommendation was also made for children and adolescents with recurrent headache. For patients with an atypical headache pattern, a history of seizures, or focal neurologic signs or symptoms, CT or MRI

Table 3.2. Indications for Neuroimaging in Headache

Indication	Neuroimaging*	Clinical consideration
First or worse headache	**CT** (without contrast) or MRI	Hemorrhage
Change in clinical features (frequency or severity)	CT (with contrast) or MRI	Mass lesion
Abnormal examination	CT (with contrast) or MRI	Mass lesion
Progressive headache	CT (with contrast) or MRI	Mass lesion
Neurologic symptoms atypical for migraine	CT (with contrast) or MRI	Mass lesion
Persistent neurologic deficits	CT (with contrast) or MRI	Mass lesion
Focal EEG findings	CT (with contrast) or **MRI**	Focal lesion
Seizures	CT (with contrast) or **MRI**	Focal lesion
Orbital bruit	CT (with contrast) or **MRI/MRA**	Arteriovenous malformation
Same-sided pain with focal deficit	CT (with contrast) or MRI	Mass lesion
Anxious or doubting patient	CT (with contrast) or MRI	Reassurance, aid in therapy

CT, computed tomography; EEG, electroencephalography; MRA, magnetic resonance angiography; MRI, magnetic resonance imaging.
*Boldface type indicates preferred method.
From Adams, AC: Neurology in Primary Care. FA Davis, Philadelphia, 2000, p 44. Used with permission of Mayo Foundation for Medical Education and Research.

may be indicated. Headache from an expanding aneurysm, arteriovenous malformation, or vasculitis requires angiography. Noninvasive MRA is useful but can miss aneurysms smaller than 3 mm in diameter. MRA is a reasonable test for patients who have a sudden headache but negative findings on CT and CSF analysis.

Electroencephalography

Electroencephalography (EEG) generally is not useful in the evaluation of headache. However, many associations have been described between migraines and seizures, including postictal headache and migraine aura-inducing seizures. A patient can have both migraine and epilepsy. The indications for EEG

in evaluating headache include alterations in or loss of consciousness, transient neurologic symptoms, suspected encephalopathy, and selection of medications. An anticonvulsant (eg, valproic acid) may be more effective for a patient with migraine and seizures than a medication that potentially could induce seizures (eg, a tricyclic antidepressant).

Lumbar Puncture

After neuroimaging, lumbar puncture is indicated if the patient has the worst headache of his or her life or a severe, recurrent headache with rapid onset. Lumbar puncture can be useful in evaluating a progressive headache and chronic headache that is intractable or atypical.

The diagnosis of CSF hypotension can be made with lumbar puncture in a patient with a postural headache. Patients with postural headache complain that the headache increases when they stand and decreases when they lie down. Lumbar puncture can be used to confirm pseudotumor cerebri in a patient with papilledema and negative neuroimaging studies. Headache from Lyme disease, chronic fungal meningitides, or carcinomatous meningitis requires CSF analysis for diagnostic confirmation.

Other Tests

Other laboratory tests may be needed to evaluate headache. Diagnostic tests are needed to make a diagnosis, to establish a baseline status before initiating treatment, and to monitor for compliance and adverse effects of medications. Some of the diagnostic tests used in the evaluation of headache and the indications for them are summarized in Table 3.3.

CLASSIFICATION

The clinical management of headache is enhanced by a systematic approach to classification and diagnosis. The second edition of the International Classification of Headache Disorders (2004) divides headache into primary headaches, secondary headaches, cranial neuralgias, central and primary facial pain, and other headaches. Primary headaches include migraine, tension-type headache, cluster headache and other trigeminal autonomic cephalalgias, and other primary headaches. Secondary headaches are subdivided according to the underlying disorder. Table 3.4 summarizes the first level of the International Classification of Headache Disorders.

Patients who present with headache often have several types of headache. A meaningful question to ask is, "How many types of

headache do you have?" Frequently, a patient who has head pain is alarmed about the possibility of a brain tumor and is relieved to learn that the brain is not sensitive to pain and that most head pain is the result of a physiologic process, such as vasospasm or muscle contraction, and not a structural problem, such as a tumor. For these patients, the analogy of a "charley horse" is helpful. In this situation, the severe pain results from muscle contraction (a physiologic process) and not a structural problem. Unnecessary neuroimaging may be avoided if the patient understands this point.

Vascular structures are pain-sensitive and include all the intracranial and extracranial arteries and veins and dural venous sinuses. Pain-sensitive nonvascular structures of the head, face, and neck include the arachnoid membrane adjacent to the cerebral arteries and veins; the dura mater adjacent to the meningeal arteries and dural venous sinuses; the mucous membranes of the mouth, nasal cavity, and paranasal sinuses; the teeth; the extracranial muscles and skin; the temporomandibular and zygapophyseal joints; the intraspinous ligaments; and the intervertebral disks. All these pain-sensitive structures can be categorized as musculoskeletal, vascular, or meningeal, and this can simplify the discussion of classification with patients.

PRINCIPLES OF THERAPY

The relationship established with the patient at the initial visit is important for successful management of headache. Patients become frustrated with medical care providers if they perceive that the provider does not listen to them or seems disinterested. The patient's fears and expectations must be considered, and the best way to do this is to educate the patient about the diagnosis and treatment plan. If you establish a

Table 3.3. Diagnostic Testing in Headache

Test	Test is indicated for:			Cause of headache
Complete blood count with differential cell count	Diagnosis	Baseline values	Compliance/toxicity	Anemia, sepsis
Erythrocyte sedi- mentation rate	Diagnosis			Temporal arteritis
Chemistry profile	Diagnosis	Baseline values	Compliance/toxicity	Chronic renal failure, hypo- glycemia, hypercalcemia, hypernatremia
Electrocardiography		Baseline data	Compliance/toxicity*	
Blood gas analysis	Diagnosis			Hypercapnia, hypoxia
Thyroid function	Diagnosis		Compliance/toxicity	Thyrotoxicosis
Serology	Diagnosis			Lyme disease, HIV infection, syphilis
ANA, lupus anticoagulant, anticardiolipin antibodies	Diagnosis			Collagen vascular disease
Drug screen/level	Diagnosis		Compliance/toxicity	Drug abuse

ANA, antinuclear antibody; HIV, human immunodeficiency virus.
*Assess before prescribing β-blockers or vasoconstrictors.
From Adams, AC: Neurology in Primary Care. FA Davis, Philadelphia, 2000, p 46. Used with permis-
   sion of Mayo Foundation for Medical Education and Research.

good relationship at the beginning, the patient is more likely to follow-up with you. Continuity of care is essential for effective management of headache.

Psychologic issues may be prominent in patients with headache. It may be more effec- tive to approach these issues at follow-up visits, after rapport has been established. Depression and anxiety frequently coexist with headache and need to be discussed because of the implications for treatment. A discussion of the potential side effects of a medication may be helpful in approaching the topic of depression. For exam- ple, a migraineur with depression may prefer a tricyclic antidepressant medication to a β-block- er when given a choice of prophylactic agents.

Table 3.4. First Level of the International Classification of Headache Disorders

I. The primary headaches

    1. Migraine

    2. Tension-type headache

    3. Cluster headache and other trigeminal autonomic cephalalgias

    4. Other primary headaches

II. The secondary headaches

    5. Headache attributed to head and/or neck trauma

    6. Headache attributed to cranial or cervical vascular disorder

    7. Headache attributed to nonvascular intracranial disorder

    8. Headache attributed to a substance or its withdrawal

    9. Headache attributed to infection

    10. Headache attributed to disorder of homeostasis

    11. Headache or facial pain attributed to disorder of cranium, neck, eyes, ears, nose, sinuses, teeth, mouth, or other facial or cranial structures

    12. Headache attributed to psychiatric disorder

III. Cranial neuralgias, central and primary facial pain, and other headaches

    13. Cranial neuralgias and central causes of facial pain

    14. Other headache, cranial neuralgia, central or primary facial pain

From Headache Classification Subcommittee of the International Headache Society: The International Classification of Headache Disorders, ed 2. Cephalalgia 24 Suppl 1:9-160, 2004. Used with permission.

Before a therapeutic regimen is established, it is important to know all the medications the patient is taking, including over-the-counter drugs, and the dosages, the duration of use, and the specific side effects the patient has had. Knowing what over-the-counter drugs the patient is taking is critical because patients select them on the basis of advertising information and not because of medical or pharmaceutical advice. For example, patients may mistakenly take "sinus" medicine for migraine. Overuse of over-the-counter analgesic drugs leads to rebound headache and makes prophylactic treatment less effective.

If a patient is not able to provide information about the dose of the drug and how long it has been taken, it generally indicates that the patient was not educated appropriately about the drug. Treatment with the same medication could be attempted again, with education and adequate dosing and duration of treatment. Frequently, the lack of patient compliance, insufficient dose, inadequate duration of treatment, and side effects are the culprits when therapy fails. Patients and clinicians both need to know that few patients react the same way to a treatment and that medication regimens need to be individualized. The patient's coexisting conditions such as hypertension, heart disease, and pregnancy need to be determined when reviewing treatment options.

The goals of treatment must be defined clearly. It is unrealistic to expect that the headache will be eliminated completely or that the medication will not have side effects. A reasonable goal is to decrease the frequency and severity of the headache so there is minimal disruption of the patient's work and quality of life. The patient must be an active participant in the treatment program and may need to make substantial lifestyle changes to accomplish the goal. The patient needs to stop smoking and needs to exercise regularly, avoid certain foods and alcohol, consume caffeine in moderation, and maintain regular schedules of eating and sleeping. Encourage patients to keep a headache log to monitor their response to medication and to reveal potential modifiable headache triggers. If biofeedback, relaxation techniques, and cognitive therapies are part of the therapeutic regimen, they need to be practiced and performed regularly. When patients are actively engaged in

their health care, they are more compliant, have more realistic expectations, and have better results. Some of the major pitfalls of effective headache treatment are listed in Table 3.5.

Medication regimens, as mentioned above, need to be individualized. Initially, give all medications at a low dose to reduce the chance of adverse effects. Increase the dosage to the highest dose that is tolerable and effective without causing ill effects. The patient should have an active role in the selection of medications. The cost of a medication is an important factor, but the cost of loss of work time and visits to the emergency department also should be considered. An emergency department is not the place to treat recurrent headache.

The frequency of a headache is the major factor in determining whether to prescribe an abortive or a prophylactic medication. For

Table 3.5. Major Pitfalls of Headache Treatment

Clinician
  Rapport not established with patient
  No patient education provided
  Recurrent headache treated with narcotics, leading to rebound headache
  Abortive medications prescribed for frequent headache, leading to rebound and chronic
    daily headache: butalbital-analgesic-caffeine combination products
  Initial dose of medication too high
  Dose of medication not changed on basis of patient's response
  Medication discontinued before an adequate trial is achieved
Patient
  Overuse of over-the-counter analgesics
  Overuse of caffeine
  Smoking
  Avoidance of exercise
  Inadequate sleep
  Improper diet
  Unrealistic expectations

From Adams, AC: Neurology in Primary Care. FA Davis, Philadelphia, 2000, p 48. Used with permission of Mayo Foundation for Medical Education and Research.

infrequent headache, many abortive medications are effective. The patient needs to know that overuse of analgesics can cause rebound headache. Overuse (more than 2 days/week) of aspirin, acetaminophen, ergotamines, butalbital products, caffeine, or opioids can cause frequent headaches. Rebound headache is less likely with long-acting nonsteroidal antiinflammatory drugs and dihydroergotamine. Prophylactic medication is recommended when the frequency of the headache is two or more times per month or when the headache causes extended disability (more than 3 days). When prescribing prophylactic medication for women of child-bearing age, be aware of the possibility of pregnancy and the potential of the medication for teratogenic effects. Many of the common abortive and prophylactic medications used in headache are listed in Tables 3.6 and 3.7.

SUBSTANCE-INDUCED HEADACHES

It is important to recognize that many medications and other substances can cause headache. Substance-induced headache is not to be confused with analgesic overuse headache. Medication is often unrecognized as a cause of headache, but it is estimated to cause 8% of headaches. The International Headache Society classifies these headaches as headaches associated with substances, including use or withdrawal as well as acute or chronic exposure.

Table 3.6. Abortive Medications for Vascular and Tension-Type Headaches

Drug	Initial dose	Rebound headache*
Acetaminophen	1,000 mg PO	+++
Acetaminophen-isometheptene mucate-dichloralphenazone combination) (Midrin)	65 mg PO	+++
Aspirin	1,000 mg PO	+++
Butalbital combination (Fiorinal)	2 tablets PO	+++
Butorphanol nasal spray (Stadol)	1 mg IN	+++
Codeine	30 mg PO	+++
Dihydroergotamine (DHE 45 or Migranal)	1 mg IM, SC, or IV, or 2 mg IN	+
Ergotamine (Ergomar)	1 mg PO or 2 mg PR	+++
Ibuprofen (Motrin)	800 mg PO	+++
Indomethacin (Indocin)	50 mg PO	+
Meperidine (Demerol)	100 mg PO or IM	+++
Naproxen (Naprosyn)	500 mg PO	+
Sumatriptan (Imitrex)	6 mg SC, 50 mg PO, or 10 mg IN	++

IM, intramuscular; IN, intranasal; IV, intravenous; PO, oral; PR, rectal; SC, subcutaneous.
*+++, high rebound potential; ++, medium rebound potential; +, low rebound potential.
From Adams, AC: Neurology in Primary Care. FA Davis, Philadelphia, 2000, p 49. Used with permission of Mayo Foundation for Medical Education and Research.

Table 3.7. Prophylactic Medications for Headache

Drug	Dose*, daily	Type of headache	Contraindications	Adverse effects
β-Blockers		Vascular	Asthma, heart block, insulin-dependent diabetes	Fatigue, impotence, reduced exercise tolerance, depression
Atenolol (Tenormin)	50-100 mg			
Metoprolol (Lopressor)	50-200 mg			
Nadolol (Corgard)	80-240 mg			
Propranolol (Inderal)	80-240 mg			
Tricyclic anti-depressants		Migraine, tension-type, mixed	Glaucoma, prostatism, acute recovery phase from myocardial infarction	Drowsiness, dry mouth, constipation, weight gain
Amitriptyline (Elavil)	10-100 mg			
Nortriptyline (Pamelor)	10-100 mg			
Calcium channel blockers		Cluster and other vascular headaches	Heart disease, depression	Constipation, weight gain, edema, depression
Verapamil (Calan)	180-320 mg			
Anticonvulsants		Migraine		
Divalproex (Depakote)	250-1,000 mg		Liver disease, disorders of urea cycle	Weight gain, tremor, alopecia
Gabapentin (Neurontin)	900-2,400 mg		Renal insufficiency	Fatigue, edema
Topiramate (Topamax)	100-400 mg		Behavioral disorders	Weight loss, cognitive disturbance, renal stones
NSAIDs		Migraine, tension-type	Allergic reactions to aspirin and other NSAIDs	Gastrointestinal irritation
Naproxen sodium (Naprosyn)	200-1,000 mg			
Antiserotonin		Vascular		
Methysergide (Sansert)	4-8 mg		Renal disease, liver disease, cardiovascular disease	Fibrotic complications, rebound on withdrawal

Table 3.7   (continued)

Drug	Dose*, daily	Type of headache	Contraindications	Adverse effects
MAO inhibitor		Migraine,	Concomitant use of	Vasopressor reac-
Phenelzine	45 mg	tension-type,	many drugs,	tions with some
(Nardil)		mixed	liver disease	foods and drugs

MAO, monoamine oxidase; NSAID, nonsteroidal antiinflammatory drug.
*Doses need to be individualized, and all potential adverse effects and contraindications should be
  reviewed. Start at the lowest dose and advance according to the patient's response.

An important exclusion in the classification is the worsening of a preexisting type of headache from a medication or substance. The mechanism of substance-induced headache often is not known. A partial list of the many substances that can cause or contribute to headache is given in Table 3.8. It is important to obtain from patients a list of all the substances they take and any potential relation to their headache. If possible, eliminate any medication or substance that could cause or contribute to the headache.

MIGRAINE HEADACHE

Migraine is an episodic headache with neurologic, gastrointestinal, and autonomic changes. Genetic factors are important in migraine, but the specific inheritance pattern has not been defined. The International Headache Society classifies migraine into five major categories, of which the two most important are migraine without aura and migraine with aura.

Migraine Without Aura

The diagnostic criteria for migraine without aura require at least five attacks, each lasting 4 to 72 hours, associated with two of four pain features (unilateral location, pulsating quality, moderate or severe pain intensity, aggravated by or causing avoidance of routine physical activity) and either one of two associated symptoms (nausea/vomiting or photophobia/phonophobia). The criterion for chronic migraine is the headache attack occurs on 15 or more days per month.

Migraine With Aura

Migraine with aura is the same type of headache as migraine without aura but is preceded or accompanied by focal neurologic symptoms. Auras include visual, sensory, motor, and language symptoms. Visual auras are the most common and can include positive symptoms such as flickering spots and lines or a negative phenomenon such as scotomata. Sensory symptoms may be negative (numbness) or positive (tingling). The migraine with aura classification includes the typical aura with migraine headache, typical aura with nonmigraine headache, and typical aura without headache. Other subtypes of migraine with aura include familial hemiplegic migraine, sporadic hemiplegic migraine, and basilar migraine.

A typical aura that occurs in the absence of any headache has been called migraine equivalents and acephalic migraines. All types of auras can occur, but visual symptoms are the most common. If patients present with these symptoms but have no previous history

Table 3.8. Substances That Can Cause or Contribute to Headache

Alcohol
Anesthetic agents
    Nitrous oxide
    Ketamine
Anticonvulsants
    Divalproex
    Gabapentin
Antibiotics and antimalarials
    Amphotericin
    Chloroquine
    Ethionamide
    Griseofulvin
    Linezolid
    Mefloquine
    Metronidazole
    Agents causing idiopathic intracranial
      hypertension
        Ampicillin
        Minocycline
        Nalidixic acid
        Nitrofurantoin
        Ofloxacin
        Tetracycline
        Trimethoprim-sulfamethoxazole
    Agents causing drug-induced aseptic
      meningitis
        Amoxicillin
        Cephalosporins
        Ciprofloxacin
        Cotrimoxazole
        Isoniazid
        Penicillin
        Pyrazinamide
        Sulfasalazine
Antihistamines and histamines
Antiparkinsonian agents
    Bromocriptine
    Dopamine
    Pramipexole
Asthmatic agents
    Aminophylline
    Beclomethasone
    Terbutaline
    Theophylline

    Zafirlukast
Caffeine
Cardiovascular agents
    Amiodarone
    Atenolol
    Captopril
    Dipyridamole
    Isosorbide
    Methyldopa
    Metoprolol
    Nifedipine
    Nitroglycerin
    Pentoxifylline
    Propranolol
Foods and additives
    Aspartame
    Citrus fruits
    Chocolate
    Dairy products
    Monosodium glutamate (MSG)
    Sodium chloride
    Sodium nitrate
    Tyramine-containing foods
Gastrointestinal agents
    Cimetidine
    Omeprazole
    Ranitidine
Hormones
    Estrogens
    Danazol
    Corticosteroids
Illicit drugs
    Amphetamines
    Cocaine
    Heroin
    Marijuana
Neuropsychiatric agents
    Benzodiazepines
    Lithium
    Selective serotonin reuptake inhibitors
Nonsteroidal antiinflammatory drugs
    Diclofenac
    Ibuprofen
    Indomethacin
    Ketoprofen
    Naproxen
    Piroxicam

of migraine, the diagnosis can be difficult. Transient ischemic attacks are the most important differential diagnosis and should be excluded before these symptoms are attributed to migraine.

Familial Hemiplegic Migraine

Familial hemiplegic migraine is the first migraine symptom to be linked to a specific set of genetic polymorphisms. Patients have migraine with aura with motor weakness and at least one first- or second-degree relative who has migraine with aura with motor weakness. For patients who have this type of headache but no family history of the disorder, the classification is sporadic hemiplegic migraine.

Basilar Migraine

Basilar migraine is a migraine type that suggests involvement of the posterior fossa. Patients with familial hemiplegic migraine have basilar-type symptoms, so basilar migraine should be diagnosed only when weakness is not present. Basilar migraine occurs more frequently in children and young adolescents than in adults. Clinical characteristics include brainstem symptoms of ataxia, diplopia, vertigo, tinnitus, dysarthria, bilateral sensory disturbances, and depressed level of awareness. Also, visual field defects can occur in basilar migraine.

Migraine Phases

The five phases of migraine are the following: 1) premonitory, 2) aura, 3) headache, 4) headache resolution, and 5) postdromal. The premonitory phase affects 40% to 60% of patients who have migraine and includes behavioral, emotional, autonomic, and constitutional disturbances that occur 1 or 2 days before the headache. These disturbances may include sleep disruption, food cravings, fatigue, yawning, depression, and euphoria. Common migraine triggers are possible components of the premonitory phase.

The aura usually precedes the headache but can accompany it. The aura symptoms are reversible and develop over 5 minutes or more but last no more than 60 minutes. The headache of migraine is usually unilateral but can be bilateral in up to 40% of patients. Many symptoms can accompany the headache, such as nausea, vomiting, and visual disturbances. Autonomic symptoms include hypertension, hypotension, nasal stuffiness, peripheral vasoconstriction, tachycardia, and bradycardia. Other symptoms include fatigue, emotional changes, mental dullness, sensory abnormalities, and fluid retention. The length of time for the headache phase can vary from 4 to 72 hours. The postdromal phase often includes symptoms of fatigue and mental confusion that last for 1 or 2 days.

The pathogenesis of migraine is not completely known. Evidence indicates that neuronal events mediate the migraine aura and headache phase. Cortical hyperexcitability, activation of the trigeminovascular system and its central projections, and abnormal modulation of brain nociceptive systems are involved. More is being learned about the pathogenesis of migraine, and this knowledge should lead to the development of more effective treatments for this common disorder.

Associations of Migraine

A strong association between migraine and estrogen is suggested by the increased incidence of migraine with menarche, menstruation, use of oral contraceptive agents, pregnancy, and menopause. Menstrual migraine is defined as migraine attacks that occur regularly on or between days −2 to +4 of the menstrual cycle. The proposed mechanism of these headaches is related to decreased levels of estrogen. If patients with menstrual migraine do not have a response to the usual migraine therapies, hormonal treatment may be effective (Table 3.9).

The frequency of migraine generally changes during pregnancy, but 25% of pregnant women who have migraine experience no change. Headaches may increase in frequency during the first trimester and decrease in the last two trimesters, perhaps in relation to the sustained high level of estrogen. Despite this decrease in headache frequency, the management of migraine during pregnancy is complicated. Potential adverse effects of drug therapy on the fetus need to be balanced with the frequency of the headache and the complications. Although medications should be limited during pregnancy, they need to be considered if the headache poses a risk to the fetus. Nonpharmacologic treatment should be attempted first, for example, massage, ice packs, intravenous hydration, and inhalation of oxygen. Analgesic medications should be administered on a limited basis if the patient does not have a response to other measures. Prophylactic medication should be prescribed only as a last resort. The various migraine medications and associated risks during pregnancy are listed in Table 3.10. It is important to remember that several serious causes of headache can occur during pregnancy, including stroke, cerebral venous thrombosis, eclampsia, and subarachnoid hemorrhage.

The use of oral contraceptive agents can influence migraine, but no consistent pattern has been detected. Women who take oral contraceptive agents have reported an increase, a decrease, or no change in the frequency of migraine attacks. This emphasizes the importance of individualized treatment.

The prevalence of migraine decreases with advancing age, but some women experience an increase in migraine frequency during menopause. Hormone replacement therapy can also increase the frequency of migraine attacks. Strategies to treat estrogen-replacement headache include decreasing the estrogen dose. A change in the type of estrogen is recommended, that

Table 3.9. Suggested Treatment of Menstrual Migraine

Nonsteroidal antiinflammatory drugs for 5-7 days around vulnerable period
Estrogen therapy
　Percutaneous estradiol 1.5 mg daily starting on day −3 of menses for 6 days
　Transdermal estradiol 1 × 100-μg patch on day −3, day −1, and day +2 of menses
Synthetic androgens
　Danazol 200-600 mg daily started before onset of headache and continued through menses
Antiestrogens
　Tamoxifen 5-15 mg daily for days 7 through 14 of 28-day cycle
Dopamine agonists
　Bromocriptine 2.5 mg 3 times daily

From Adams, AC: Neurology in Primary Care. FA Davis, Philadelphia, 2000, p 51. Used with permission of Mayo Foundation for Medical Education and Research.

is, changing from a conjugated estrogen to estradiol, synthetic estrogen, or a pure estrone. Continuous dosing may be preferable to interrupted dosing. Compared with an oral preparation, a parenteral preparation may reduce the headache. Also, adding an androgen to the medication regimen may prevent estrogen-replacement headache.

The relation of migraine and stroke is complicated and can be confusing to clinicians. Migraine and stroke can coexist. Furthermore, migraine can induce stroke, and stroke can occur with clinical features of migraine (symptomatic migraine and migraine mimic [Chapter 11]). A large-scale epidemiologic study showed an association between migraine and stroke and concluded that migraine should be considered

Table 3.10. Migraine Medication and Pregnancy Risk

Risk	Abortive medications	Prophylactic medications
Class A—controlled studies in humans show no risk	None	None
Class B—no controlled human studies, but no evidence of risk to humans	Acetaminophen (Tylenol) Ibuprofen (Motrin) Meperidine (Demerol) Metoclopramide (Reglan) Naproxen sodium (Naprosyn)	Naproxen sodium (Naprosyn)
Class C—risk to humans has not been ruled out	Aspirin Acetaminophen-isometheptene mucate-dichloralphenazone (Midrin) Codeine Ketorolac (Toradol) Neuroleptics Triptans	Gabapentin (Neurontin) MAO inhibitors Metoprolol (Lopressor) Nadolol (Corgard) Propranolol (Inderal) Topiramate (Topamax)
Class D—animal or human studies have shown risk to humans	Corticosteroids Intravenous valproate (Depacon)	Atenolol (Tenormin) NSAIDs near term Tricyclic antidepressants Valproate (Depakote)
Class X—absolutely contra-indicated in pregnancy	Dihydroergotamine (Migranal) Ergotamine (Ergomar)	Methysergide (Sansert)

MAO, monoamine oxidase; NSAID, nonsteroidal antiinflammatory drug.
Modified from Edmeads, J: Migraine. In Noseworthy, JH (ed): Neurological Therapeutics: Principles and Practice. Vol 1. Martin Dunitz, London, 2003, pp 73-88. Used with permission of Mayo Foundation for Medical Education and Research.

a risk factor for stroke. The risk of stroke in a young woman is low, even if she is taking an oral contraceptive. However, if the patient has a prolonged aura, it is best to avoid oral contraceptives or vasoconstrictive agents that make the risk of stroke unacceptably high. This emphasizes the importance of avoiding other risk factors for stroke, especially smoking.

Treatment of Migraine

The pharmacologic management of migraine includes acute and prophylactic therapies. Many abortive medicines are available for treating migraine. Treatment of acute migraine should be done rapidly and should restore the patient's ability to function, minimize the need for backup or rescue analgesia, optimize self-care, have minimal or no adverse events, and be cost-effective.

Emphasize to the patient that the frequent use of abortive medications can cause rebound headache (Table 3.6). Abortive medications that are more likely to cause rebound headache include aspirin, acetaminophen, butalbital products, ergotamines, ibuprofen, and narcotics. These agents should not be taken more often than twice a week. The long-term use of any medication should be scrutinized for the possibility of habituation and renal and liver disease. The elimination of medications used long term may obviate prophylactic therapy.

Failure to administer an effective treatment rapidly may increase the pain and disability of the headache. Triptans and dihydroergotamine (DHE) should be prescribed for moderate or severe migraine and for mild-to-moderate headaches that respond poorly to nonsteroidal antiinflammatory drugs (NSAIDs) or aspirin-acetaminophen-caffeine combinations. Consider antiemetics and medications with nonoral routes of administration for patients with nausea and vomiting.

Acetaminophen is not recommended as a sole agent for the treatment of acute migraine. However, this treatment is reasonable to try in a patient with migraine who is pregnant. NSAIDs can be useful in treating symptoms of mild-to-moderate migraine. Overuse (more than 2 weeks) of NSAIDs can lead to rebound headache, which is less likely with longer-acting medications. Contraindications to NSAIDs are hypersensitivity to the drug or a history of allergy to aspirin or other antiinflammatory agents. NSAIDs should be prescribed carefully for patients with a history of gastrointestinal ulceration, bleeding, or perforation or renal or liver dysfunction. Nausea, abdominal pain, diarrhea, and fluid retention are some common adverse effects of NSAIDs. Ketorolac can be given parenterally in the emergency department for migraine. However, it has a high incidence of adverse effects and should be used sparingly. Naproxen sodium and ibuprofen have a strong safety profile and are available as over-the-counter drugs.

The combination of acetaminophen, isometheptene mucate, and dichloralphenazone (Midrin) is effective for symptomatic relief of mild-to-moderate migraine. It is contraindicated for patients with glaucoma, renal disease, hypertension, heart disease, or liver disease and for patients receiving treatment with a monoamine oxidase inhibitor. The few adverse reactions reported include transient dizziness and skin rash in sensitive patients. Overuse of this product can cause rebound headache.

Since the introduction of sumatriptan in the early 1990s, 5-hydroxytryptamine (5-HT_1) receptor agonists, or triptans, have revolutionized the acute treatment of migraine. Currently available 5-HT_1 receptor agonists include sumatriptan, zolmitriptan, naratriptan, rizatriptan, almotriptan, eletriptan, and frovatriptan (Table 3.11). The effect these agents have on 5-HT_1 receptors on intracranial blood vessels and peripheral sensory nerve endings produces cranial vasoconstriction and decreases the release of inflammatory neuropeptides. The most common adverse effects are paresthesias, a feeling of chest tightness, nausea, dizziness, and somnolence. Because of the possibility of cardiovascular and cerebrovascular disease, these medications should be avoided if the patient has ischemic heart disease or uncontrolled hypertension. Manufacturers recommend that these agents be prescribed with caution for men older than 40 years, postmenopausal women, and persons with other cardiac risk factors such as diabetes mellitus, obesity, cigarette smoking, hypercholesterolemia, or a family history of coronary artery disease. An ergot-containing drug should not be taken within 24 hours before or after a 5-HT_1 receptor agonist is taken because of the potential for increasing the prolonged vasoconstrictive action of the drug. Similarly, monoamine oxidase A inhibitors should not be taken within 2 weeks of taking a 5-HT_1 receptor agonist. Caution should be used for patients who take selective serotonin reuptake inhibitors. This combination of drugs can

Table 3.11. 5-Hydroxytryptamine Receptor Agonists for Treatment of Acute Migraine

Drug	Dose
Sumatriptan (Imitrex)	
Subcutaneous, 6-mg self-dose kit	6 mg at onset, can repeat in 1 hour; maximum 2 injections/day
Oral, 25- and 50-mg tablets	50 mg at onset, can repeat in 2 hours; maximum 300 mg/day
Nasal spray, 5- and 20-mg spray	5 mg in each nostril at onset, may repeat in 2 hours, maximum 40 mg/day
Almotriptan (Axert)	
Oral, 6.25- and 12.5-mg tablets	6.25 or 12.5 mg at onset, can repeat in 2 hours; maximum 2 doses/day
Eletriptan (Relpax)	
Oral, 20- and 40-mg tablets	20 or 40 mg at onset, can repeat in 2 hours; maximum 80 mg/day
Frovatriptan (Frova)	
Oral, 2.5-mg tablets	2.5 mg at onset, can repeat in 2 hours; maximum 7.5 mg/day
Naratriptan (Amerge)	
Oral, 1- and 2.5-mg tablets	1 or 2.5 mg at onset, can repeat in 2 hours; maximum 5 mg/day
Rizatriptan (Maxalt)	
Oral, 5- and 10-mg tablets, disintegrating tablets	5 or 10 mg at onset, can repeat in 2 hours; maximum 30 mg/day
Zolmitriptan (Zomig)	
Oral, 1.25- and 2.5-mg tablets, disintegrating tablets	1.25 or 2.5 mg at onset, can repeat in 2 hours; maximum 10 mg/day
Nasal spray, 5 mg	5 mg one nostril at onset, may repeat in 2 hours; maximum 10 mg/day
Dihydroergotamine (DHE 45)	
Intramuscular, 1 mg = 1 ampule	1 mg at onset, can repeat in 1 hour; maximum 3 mg/day
Intravenous, 1 mg = 1 ampule	0.5 or 1 mg at onset, can repeat in 8 hours; maximum 3 mg/day
Intranasal (Migranal) 0.5-mg spray	0.5 mg each nostril at onset, can repeat in 15 minutes; maximum 3 mg/day
Ergotamine tartrate (Ergomar, Ergostat) 2-mg rectal suppositories	1/4 to 1 suppository at onset, can repeat in 1 hour; maximum 4 mg/day, 10 mg/week

Modified from Adams, AC: Neurology in Primary Care. FA Davis, Philadelphia, 2000, p 54. Used with permission of Mayo Foundation for Medical Education and Research.

cause serotonin syndrome (ie, restlessness, hyperthermia, hyperreflexia, and incoordination). Cimetidine and oral contraceptives may increase the serum concentration of $5\text{-}HT_1$ receptor agonists.

Patients with migraine may complain of allodynia (pain caused by a nonnoxious stimulus). Allodynia is considered a manifestation of central sensitization. Patients may complain that their "hair hurts" and report that brushing or combing the hair can be painful. Patients who experience allodynia with their migraine attacks are more likely to have pain relief if the triptan is administered before the onset of allodynia.

The choice of which triptan to prescribe can depend on different circumstances. Price and availability are a concern. If the patient has nausea or vomiting early in the course of the migraine or difficulty taking oral medications, then subcutaneous injections or nasal sprays should be used. Although naratriptan has been shown to be tolerated better, it has a slower effect than other triptans. For headache recurrence, almotriptan, eletriptan, and naratriptan have been recommended. A patient may have a response to another triptan if the first one is not effective or is poorly tolerated.

Ergotamine tartrate and DHE, $5\text{-}HT_1$ receptor agonists, have been available for more than 50 years to treat acute migraine. Ergotamine tartrate is available in oral, sublingual, inhalation, and rectal suppository dosage forms (with and without caffeine). Because of the poor oral absorption of ergotamine and the frequent association of nausea and vomiting with migraine, the rectal suppository preparation is recommended. These suppositories can be hardened in the refrigerator and sliced across their length into halves and quarters. The dose that does not cause nausea should be taken at the onset of headache. Ergotamine tartrate in appropriate doses is safe and effective in the treatment of migraine in adults. Contraindications to the use of ergotamine tartrate include pregnancy, sepsis, coronary artery disease, cerebral or peripheral vascular disease, liver or renal insufficiency, and uncontrolled hypertension. The major adverse reactions are paresthesias, nausea, and cramps. If the patient has a feeling of chest tightness, treatment with the medication needs to be discontinued and possible heart disease investigated. Ergotamine should be limited to no more than 10 mg/week. Overuse (more than 2 weeks) can lead to rebound headache and ergotism, consisting of vomiting, diarrhea, muscle cramps, peripheral ischemic gangrene, muscle tremors, and headache.

Unlike ergotamine, DHE is a potent venoconstrictor that minimally constricts peripheral arteries. Its advantages over ergotamine include the absence of physical dependance and little or no problem with rebound headache. The contraindications are similar to those for ergotamine. DHE is an effective abortive therapy for migraine and can be administered by several routes, including subcutaneously, intramuscularly, intravenously, and by nasal spray. An antiemetic (25 mg promethazine, 5 mg metoclopramide, or 10 mg prochlorperazine) is frequently given in conjunction with DHE to avoid nausea. Repetitive intravenous injections of the drug are indicated in the management of status migrainosus and transformed migraine.

Status migrainosus is a prolonged migraine attack that lasts longer than 72 hours and is associated with nausea and vomiting. Hospitalization is often required. Repetitive intravenous injections of DHE are indicated for status migrainosus and provide relief in up to 90% of patients in 2 to 3 days (Fig. 3.2). Fluids given intravenously and oxygen therapy are useful adjunctive measures. Corticosteroids are prescribed sometimes, but their effectiveness has not been firmly established.

The contraindications to DHE include pregnancy, history or suspicion of ischemic heart disease, coronary artery disease, chest pain following the test dose of DHE, uncontrolled hypertension, previous use of a triptan within 24 hours, basilar or hemiplegic migraine, and use of a monoamine oxidase inhibitor within 2 weeks. Metoclopramide (Reglan) can cause dystonia, akathisia, and oculogyric crisis. Benztropine mesylate has been used to treat these extrapyramidal effects.

Antiemetics and other medications that improve gastric motility and facilitate drug absorption are helpful during an acute migraine attack. Intravenous injections of prochlorperazine (Compazine) and chlorpromazine (Thorazine) have been given in emergency departments to avoid treatment with narcotic analgesics. Prochlorperazine, 10 mg, is given by slow intravenous infusion over 5 minutes. The most frequent adverse effects are dizziness and drowsiness. Dystonic reactions may occur and are treated with benztropine mesylate (Cogentin), 1 mg given intramuscularly. Pretreatment with 500 mL of isotonic saline is recommended before intravenous injection of 12.5 mg chlorpromazine. The dose can be repeated every 30 minutes, to a total dose of 37.5 mg. Orthostatic blood pressure should be monitored after every dose and 1 hour after treatment has been completed. Hypotension is the primary adverse reaction, and it is best to keep patients supine for at least 4 hours. Dystonic reactions may occur and are treated with benztropine mesylate or diphenhydramine (Benadryl).

Most migraine attacks can be treated without narcotic analgesics. Narcotics should be avoided because more effective agents are available; also, narcotics produce rebound headache and can cause habituation. However, for patients with headaches unresponsive to 5-HT_1 receptor agonists or for whom these agents are contraindicated, narcotics can be prescribed.

Intravenous meperidine (Demerol) is often given in conjunction with an antiemetic medication. Occasionally, butorphanol (Stadol), an opioid agonist-antagonist available in an intranasal dosage form, is prescribed. The abuse potential for this medication is reportedly low because of its dysphoric effect. Treatment with narcotic analgesics requires that you carefully discuss the possible risks with the patient. Guidelines for the treatment of nonmalignant pain with narcotics are discussed in Chapter 10. Steps in the abortive treatment of migraine are listed in Table 3.12.

The decision to treat migraine prophylactically should be based on several factors, including the frequency of the headaches, the severity of the attacks, prolonged time of attack, inadequate symptomatic treatment, and the patient's ability to cope with migraine. If the patient is overusing analgesics, prophylactic treatment may not be needed when the patient stops taking the agents. Also, overusing analgesics makes prophylactic medication less effective. Prophylactic therapy should not be considered for patients who anticipate becoming pregnant.

The choice of prophylactic medication should be individualized on the basis of the adverse effects and contraindications. The various medications and potential side effects should be discussed with the patient. If the patient is an active participant in the selection process, then he or she is more likely to be compliant with the medication. It is very useful for the patient to maintain a headache log or calendar to follow the frequency and severity of the headache in response to medication. If the medication is successful, it is reasonable to withdraw it after 1 year to determine whether it is still necessary. The knowledge that the medication is to be used for a limited time is often reassuring to the patient. Steps in the prophylactic treatment of migraine are listed in Table 3.13.

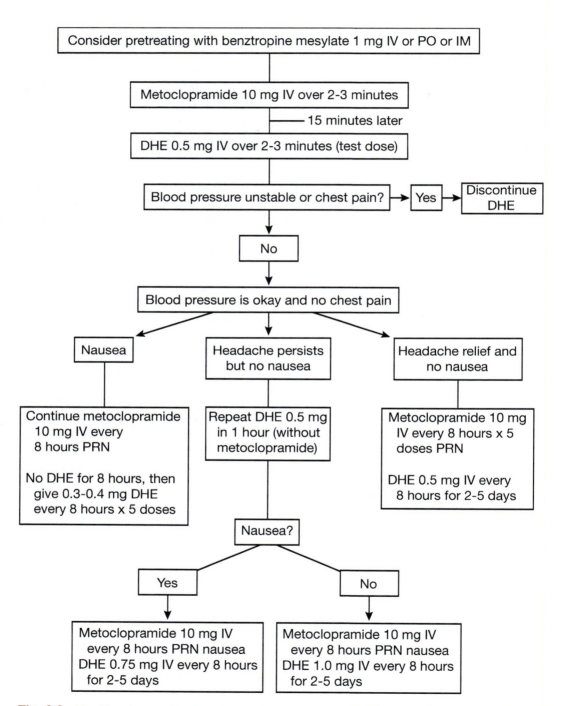

Fig. 3.2. Algorithm for repetitive intravenous dihydroergotamine (DHE) therapy for status migrainosus. IM, intramuscular; IV, intravenous; PO, oral; PRN, as needed. (Data from Raskin, NH: Repetitive intravenous dihydroergotamine as therapy for intractable migraine. Neurology 36:995-997, 1986.)

Table 3.12. Steps in the Abortive Treatment of Migraine*

---

1. **Nonsteroidal antiinflammatory agents**
   Naproxen sodium (Naprosyn)
   Ibuprofen (Motrin)
   Indomethacin (Indocin)
   Ketorolac (Toradol)
          or
   Combination products
   Acetaminophen-isometheptene mucate-dichloralphenazone (Midrin)
2. **5-HT$_1$ agonists**
   Almotriptan (Axert)
   Dihydroergotamine (DHE 45, Migranal)
   Eletriptan (Relpax)
   Frovatriptan (Frova)
   Naratriptan (Amerge)
   Rizatriptan (Maxalt)
   Sumatriptan (Imitrex)
   Zolmitriptan (Zomig)
3. **Neuroleptic agents**
   Chlorpromazine (Thorazine)
   Prochlorperazine (Compazine)
4. **Parenteral narcotics**
   Meperidine (Demerol)

The first choice is "1." If it is ineffective, try second choice ("2") and so on to last choice ("4").
Modified from Adams, AC: Neurology in Primary Care. FA Davis, Philadelphia, 2000, p 55. Used with permission of Mayo Foundation for Medical Education and Research.

Certain β-blockers are effective in the prophylactic treatment of migraine headache. The ones that are effective lack partial agonist activity. These include propranolol, atenolol, metoprolol, nadolol, and timolol. Failure of the headache to respond to one β-blocker does not imply a failure to respond to all β-blockers. For example, if the headache does not respond to propranolol, it is reasonable to try atenolol. Contraindications to β-blockers include cardiogenic shock, sinus bradycardia, heart block greater than first-degree, bronchial asthma, and congestive heart failure. Remember that β-blockers can mask symptoms of hypoglycemia in patients with diabetes mellitus. Potential adverse effects include fatigue, cold extremities, dizziness, and depression. There is no standard dose, and it is reasonable to start low and increase to the highest tolerated dose without side effects. Propranolol should be given twice a day. A long-acting preparation is available and is more convenient for patients. If β-blocker therapy needs to be discontinued, gradually withdraw the drug over 1 week.

Tricyclic antidepressants that inhibit the uptake of serotonin and norepinephrine (eg, amitriptyline and nortriptyline) are effective for prophylactic treatment of migraine. They

Table 3.13. Steps in the Prophylactic Treatment of Migraine*

1. **β-Blockers**
      Propranolol (Inderal)
      Atenolol (Tenormin)
      Metoprolol (Lopressor, Toprol)
      Nadolol (Corgard)
      Timolol (Blocadren)
            or
   Tricyclic antidepressants
      Amitriptyline (Elavil)
      Nortriptyline (Aventyl, Pamelor)
2. **Anticonvulsants**
      Valproate (Depakote)
      Gabapentin (Neurontin)
      Topiramate (Topamax)
            or
   Nonsteroidal antiinflammatory drugs
      Naproxen sodium (Naprosyn)
      Indomethacin (Indocin)
            or
   Calcium channel blockers
      Verapamil (Calan)
3. **Monoamine oxidase A inhibitor**
      Phenelzine (Nardil)
            or
   Ergot derivative
      Methysergide maleate (Sansert)

*The first choice is "1." If it is ineffective, try second choice ("2") and then third choice ("3").
Modified from Adams, AC: Neurology in Primary Care. FA Davis, Philadelphia, 2000, p 56. Used with permission of Mayo Foundation for Medical Education and Research.

are most useful for patients with mixed headaches or those who have features of vascular and tension-type headaches. It is extremely important for the patient to understand that it will take at least 6 weeks of continuous treatment before the therapeutic effect can be judged.

The time spent educating the patient about the potential side effects is worthwhile and greatly improves compliance. The common side effect of drowsiness can be beneficial for patients who also have difficulty sleeping. Dry mouth, constipation, and weight gain are common with these agents. Special attention should be given to patients with urinary retention, seizures, angle-closure glaucoma, or cardiovascular abnormalities because the medication potentially can aggravate these conditions. Amitriptyline can be started at 10 to 25 mg at bedtime and increased as tolerated. For most adults, 100 mg is the maximal amount. Nortriptyline is as efficacious as amitriptyline and has fewer anticholinergic side effects. The dose of nortriptyline is the same as that for amitriptyline.

Several anticonvulsants have been shown to be effective prophylactic agents for the treatment of migraine. The benefit of these medications in epilepsy may make them preferred agents for patients who have migraine and coexisting seizure disorders. In 1996, divalproex sodium was approved for the treatment of migraine and has been used to treat anxiety and mania. The dose recommended for migraine prophylaxis is 250 mg twice a day, up to 1,000 mg daily. An extended release preparation is available. An intravenous preparation has been used in the acute management of migraine. Common adverse effects include tremor, weight gain, and alopecia. More serious problems are hepatitis and pancreatitis, and the guidelines for monitoring should be followed. Anticonvulsant levels do not correlate with clinical efficacy. Women of child-bearing age should be reminded of the potential teratogenic effects of this medication. Patients should be encouraged to take a vitamin with folate concomitantly with the anticonvulsant.

Gabapentin has been used effectively in the treatment of migraine. The recommended dose is 2,400 mg daily in three divided doses.

Common adverse effects include peripheral edema, somnolence, dizziness, and fatigue.

The recommended dose of topiramate for migraine headache prophylaxis is 100 mg daily in two divided doses. The agent usually is titrated by starting at 25 mg once daily and increasing weekly by 25 mg. Precaution should be taken for patients with behavioral or cognitive deficits and for conditions or therapies that predispose to acidosis, such as renal disease or severe respiratory disease. Common adverse effects include nausea, inability to concentrate, and anorexia.

NSAIDs can be given for migraine prophylaxis (eg, naproxen sodium 500 mg twice daily or indomethacin 25 mg three times daily). For menstrual migraine, naproxen sodium 1 week before and the week of the menstrual period can be effective. Several primary headache syndromes such as paroxysmal hemicrania are particularly responsive to indomethacin, and, except for these syndromes, NSAIDs are best prescribed for short-term therapy.

The efficacy of calcium channel blockers in the prophylactic treatment of migraine is disappointing. Nifedipine often causes a dull, persistent headache. Nimodipine, approved for the treatment of vasospasm in subarachnoid hemorrhage, is not a practical long-term agent because it is expensive. Verapamil may be helpful for patients with migraine and coexisting Prinzmetal angina or Raynaud phenomenon. It should be considered for patients who have a prolonged aura or complicated migraine or who have not had a response to other, more efficacious medications. Contraindications include severe left ventricular dysfunction, hypotension, sick sinus syndrome, second- to third-degree atrioventricular block, and atrial flutter or fibrillation. Constipation, hypotension, edema, congestive heart failure, and heart block are potential adverse effects. The starting dose of verapamil is 40 mg three times daily, with

gradual 40-mg increments per week, to a maximum of 480 mg/day. Two to 3 months may be needed to assess its therapeutic effect.

Treatment with multiple medications increases the risk of untoward adverse effects, but combination therapy may be reasonable for migraine. The combination of a β-blocker and a tricyclic antidepressant may be successful when monotherapy fails. β-Blockers, tricyclic antidepressants, anticonvulsants, and calcium channel blockers can all be given in combination. Product information guidelines should be consulted for possible drug interactions.

Treatment of migraine and tension-type headache with botulinum toxin has had favorable results. This treatment may be an option for patients who cannot tolerate or whose headache is refractory to oral medications.

Methysergide, an ergot medicine, is effective in preventing migraine attacks. Its potential serious adverse effect of fibrotic complications limits its value. To avoid this complication, a 1-month drug holiday is recommended after 6 months of continuous therapy. Contraindications include pregnancy, peripheral vascular disease, arteriosclerosis, hypertension, coronary artery disease, pulmonary disease, collagen disease, and valvular heart disease. In addition to fibrotic complications, patients may experience weight gain, peripheral ischemia, hallucinations, or peptic ulcer disease. The initial dose can be 0.5 mg twice daily, with a gradual increase to a maximum of 2 mg four times daily.

Monoamine oxidase inhibitors can be effective treatment for migraine headaches refractory to more standard treatment. Some headache specialists refer to phenelzine sulfate as "pharmacologic last rites." The list of foods and medications that cannot be taken in conjunction with this medication is extensive, and patients should be made aware of these interactions. Phenelzine can potentiate sympathomimetic substances and cause a hypertensive crisis. Contraindications include liver disease, pheochromocytoma, and congestive heart failure. Constipation, orthostatic hypotension, and weight gain are side effects. The initial dose is 15 mg at bedtime, and this is increased to a maximum of 60 mg/day.

The treatment of migraine headache in children has not been universally established. The problem is that many drugs have not been studied in younger age groups. The American Academy of Neurology concluded that for children younger than 6 years, ibuprofen is effective and acetaminophen is probably effective for the acute treatment of migraine. For adolescents older than 12 years, sumatriptan nasal spray is effective for acute treatment of migraine. However, because of insufficient or conflicting data, recommendations could not be made about preventative therapy of migraine in children and adolescents. Children have been treated with other agents described for treating adult migraine, but appropriate precautions about dosage and effect on growth and development should be considered for the pediatric age group.

TENSION-TYPE HEADACHE

The most common type of primary headache is the tension-type headache. Other designations for this headache type include tension, stress, muscle contraction, and psychogenic headache. The revised classification system distinguishes three subtypes on the basis of frequency of headache: infrequent (less than 1 attack per month), frequent (1 to 14 attacks per month), and chronic (headache for more than 15 days per month). Tension-type headaches are usually bilateral in location, have a nonpulsating pressure or tightening quality, are mild to moderate in intensity, and are not aggravated by routine physical activity. Nausea and vomiting are not associated with this type of headache,

but anorexia may occur. In the revised classification, the headache can include either phonophobia or photophobia but not both.

Abnormal neuronal sensitivity and pain facilitation are thought to cause tension-type headaches. Myofascial pain receptors may become hypersensitive and respond to both noxious and nonnoxious stimuli.

The diagnostic criteria suggest that migraine and tension-type headache are separate entities, and many authors contend that the headaches are distinct, with separate causes and comorbid conditions. The distinction has not been clearly defined. Other authors, however, argue that migraine and tension-type headaches are the same, distinguished only by the intensity of the pain. Both these headaches have similar symptoms and many patients have features of both types. The response to medications may be similar. Whatever the difference is between these two types of headache, the clinical emphasis should always be on the patient.

The principles of treating tension-type headache are similar to those discussed above for migraine. Patients with tension-type headache are most likely to self-medicate with over-the-counter analgesics. General health measures should be discussed with the patient. Regular exercise is important and should become part of the patient's everyday routine. Most patients have a response to exercise, stretching, and simple analgesics. The most important factor to emphasize to patients is the risk of chronic daily headache from the overuse (more than 2 weeks) of medication. If a patient does not have a response to these measures, prophylactic treatment should be considered. Tricyclic antidepressants are efficacious for tension-type headache. Patients with depression may have a response to other antidepressant agents, including selective serotonin reuptake inhibitors. The prophylactic agents described above for migraine are all reasonable alternatives for patients with difficult-to-control episodic tension-type headache (Table 3.7).

CHRONIC DAILY HEADACHE

Chronic daily headache includes both primary and secondary varieties. Primary chronic daily headaches include chronic tension-type headache, chronic migraine, new daily-persistent headache, and hemicrania continua. Short-duration headaches that can become daily include cluster headache, paroxysmal hemicranias, hypnic headache, and idiopathic stabbing headache.

New daily-persistent headache is like chronic tension-type headache but becomes daily and unremitting from or very soon (less than 3 days) after onset. For diagnosis, the headache must persist for more than 3 months and medication overuse must be excluded as a cause. Hemicrania continua is an infrequent headache disorder characterized by mild to moderately severe unilateral pain that is continuous and fluctuating, with occasional jabs and jolts of pain. This type of headache responds to indomethacin.

Chronic daily headache can be secondary. Causes include trauma, cervical spine disease, vascular conditions such as subdural hematoma, nonvascular disorders such as infection or neoplasm, temporomandibular joint disease, and sinusitis. These potential causes should be examined for and treated accordingly.

Patients with chronic daily headache are the most challenging headache patients to treat. Overused symptomatic medication needs to be discontinued. Frequently, this results in a withdrawal syndrome, with an increase in headache. However, if the patient can endure this process, the headache will improve and be more responsive to prophylactic agents. Hospitalization may be necessary if detoxification from symptomatic medication is severe. If so, repetitive intravenous injections of DHE can be effective (Fig. 3.2).

The frequency of depression, personality disorder, emotional dependency, or low frustration tolerance may be increased for patients with chronic daily headache. The patient's emotional and psychologic needs must be addressed. Psychiatric or psychologic consultation may be necessary.

CLUSTER HEADACHE

Cluster headache is a distinct primary headache characterized by severe, excruciating, unilateral periorbital pain that can last from 15 to 180 minutes. Associated autonomic symptoms include conjunctival injection, lacrimation, nasal congestion, rhinorrhea, forehead and facial sweating, miosis, ptosis, and eyelid edema. The frequency of the attacks can vary from one every other day to eight per day. The attacks occur in "clusters," which can last for weeks or months, separated by remissions.

Cluster headache is distinct from migraine in many ways. Cluster headache is not associated with an aura, nausea, vomiting, photophobia, or phonophobia. A patient with cluster headache is up and active during an attack, unlike the migraine patient, who prefers to lie down in a quiet, dark room. Cluster headache occurs more frequently in men than in women and attacks can continue into late life. In most patients with cluster headache, the pain remains on the same side of the head. Autonomic symptoms readily differentiate cluster headache from tension-type headache and trigeminal neuralgia. The autonomic symptoms and periodicity of the attacks often lead patients with cluster headache to attribute their symptoms to sinus disease or allergies. Unlike migraine or trigeminal neuralgia, nocturnal attacks of cluster headache are more frequent than daytime attacks.

Cluster headache is categorized as a trigeminal autonomic cephalalgia because of the distribution of pain and the associated autonomic signs. Other trigeminal autonomic cephalalgias are chronic paroxysmal hemicrania, episodic paroxysmal hemicrania, and SUNCT syndrome (short-lasting, unilateral, neuralgiform headache with conjunctival injection and tearing). The individual attacks of these disorders are more frequent and of shorter duration than those of cluster headache.

The pathophysiologic mechanism of cluster headache is not known. The location of the pain suggests involvement of the ipsilateral trigeminal nociceptive pathway. Involvement of the parasympathetic pathway is suggested by the lacrimation and rhinorrhea, and involvement of the sympathetic pathway is suggested by the ptosis and miosis. The role of the hypothalamus is suggested by the periodicity of cluster headache and supported by functional and morphometric neuroimaging studies.

The management of cluster headache should include both symptomatic and prophylactic treatments (Table 3.14). The observation that high altitude and strenuous exercise precipitated cluster attacks led to the use of oxygen inhalation for abortive therapy. Although oxygen is very effective, it can be inconvenient. The oxygen should be administered by face mask at 7 L/minute until the attack is aborted. The time should not exceed 20 minutes, but if the attack is not aborted during this time, the treatment can be repeated after a 5-minute break.

Triptans have been used for abortive therapy, with the subcutaneous and intranasal preparations preferred because of the more rapid onset of action. Triptans with longer half-lives, such as naratriptan and frovatriptan, have been used in the transition between abortive and prophylactic therapy and as add-on agents with preventative therapy.

Prophylactic treatment is essential to decrease the length of the cluster period and to avoid overtreatment with abortive medications. The selection of medication depends on many factors, including the patient's previous experience, contraindications, frequency and timing of attacks, and expected length of the cluster period. Corticosteroids such as prednisone and dexamethasone can rapidly suppress an attack during the time required for the longer-acting maintenance prophylactic agents to take effect. Long-term corticosteroid therapy is not recommended.

Verapamil is often considered the drug of choice for the treatment of cluster headache. Other medications are lithium, indomethacin, ergotamines, methysergide maleate, divalproex sodium, topiramate, and melatonin. For at least 2 weeks after the cluster stops, maintain treatment with the prophylactic medication, followed by gradual taper of the agent. Combination therapy may be needed for chronic cluster, for attacks lasting 1 year without remission, or for a remission shorter than 14 days.

Medically refractory cluster headache has been treated surgically. The results of preliminary studies on deep brain stimulation with the electrode placed in the ventroposterior hypothalamus are encouraging.

OTHER PRIMARY HEADACHES

Headaches Triggered by Common External Stimuli

Several headache syndromes are triggered by common external stimuli and characterized by relatively brief attacks of head pain. They are benign and often respond to treatment with indomethacin. The diagnosis of these disorders is by exclusion of serious secondary causes of headache, and the appropriate evaluation should be performed. The classification of these headaches includes primary stabbing headache,

Table 3.14. Therapies for Cluster Headache

Therapy	Clinical comment
Abortive therapy	
Oxygen inhalation—7 L/minute by face mask	Patient should be seated leaning forward
Sumatriptan (Imitrex)—6 mg SC, may repeat in 1 hour; maximum 12 mg/day	Do not use concomitantly with ergotamines Contraindicated in hypertension; heart, vascular, liver, or renal disease; and pregnancy
Dihydroergotamine (DHE 45, Migranal)—0.5-1 mg SC, IM, IV, IN; maximum 3 mg/day	Administer with an antiemetic Contraindicated in hypertension; heart, vascular, liver, or renal disease; and pregnancy
Ergotamine—1 inhalation, may repeat in 5 minutes; maximum 6/day and 15/week	Contraindicated in hypertension; heart, vascular, liver, or renal disease; and pregnancy
Lidocaine 4% nasal spray—4 sprays ipsilaterally	Adjunctive therapy
Prophylactic therapy	
Verapamil (Calan)—Titrate up to 720 mg/day	Higher doses may be required Side effects: constipation, hypotension, edema, congestive heart failure, heart block
Lithium carbonate (Lithobid, Eskalith)—300-1,200 mg/day	Lithium level below 1.5 mEq/L to avoid toxicity, use divided dosing Avoid in renal or cardiovascular disease or tremor
Indomethacin (Indocin)—75-150 mg/day	Use lowest effective dose Gastrointestinal side effects
Ergotamine tartrate (Ergomar)—1-2 mg every night or 1 mg twice daily	Effective in nocturnal cluster, use more as transition agent, watch for ergotism
Methysergide maleate (Sansert)—2-8 mg/day	Watch for fibrotic complications, peripheral ischemia, hallucinations, peptic ulcer disease
Divalproex sodium (Depakote)—250-2,000 mg/day	Check liver function before treatment Side effects: tremor, weight gain, alopecia
Prednisone—40 mg/day tapered over 3 weeks	Transition agent, observe general precautions with corticosteroids
Topiramate (Topamax)—100-400 mg/day	Somnolence and cognitive disturbance
Melatonin—3-10 mg/day at night	Preparation variability for this over-the-counter agent

IM, intramuscular; IN, intranasal; IV, intravenous; SC, subcutaneous.
Modified from Adams, AC: Neurology in Primary Care. FA Davis, Philadelphia, 2000, p 60. Used with permission of Mayo Foundation for Medical Education and Research.

primary cough headache, primary exertional headache, primary headache associated with sexual activity, hypnic headache, primary thunderclap headache, hemicrania continua, and new daily persistent headache (Table 3.15).

Posttraumatic Headache

The symptom that occurs most frequently after mild head injury is posttraumatic headache. The diagnosis is difficult and often complicated by equivocal clinical findings, limited objective information, and medical-legal issues. Posttraumatic headache is one of the major features of posttraumatic syndrome, which is characterized also by fatigue, dizziness, anxiety, nausea, weakness, insomnia, depression, cognitive disturbance, impaired concentration, and temperature intolerance. These standard symptoms of the syndrome cannot be correlated with the extent of the head injury.

The specific mechanism of posttraumatic headache is not known. Evidence suggests that head trauma causes injury to neurons, disruption of cerebral blood flow, and neurochemical changes in transmission of nociceptive stimuli to the central nervous system. Whiplash injuries, or flexion-extension injuries of the cervical spine, can cause neuronal dysfunction from the acceleration and deceleration of the brain, as opposed to direct impact of the head. Damage to cervical roots, facet joints, and temporomandibular joints contributes to the symptoms of posttraumatic syndrome and posttraumatic headache.

The symptoms of posttraumatic headache may not develop or be recognized immediately after the injury. Head symptoms may be delayed up to 48 hours after injury. The pain patterns of posttraumatic headache include tension-type, migraine, neuralgia-like, cluster, and mixed. The most frequent type is tension-type posttraumatic headache. The pain is dull, bilateral or generalized, and of variable intensity. Next most frequent is the mixed headache type, which has features of tension-type and migraine headaches.

After a head injury, patients are confronted with several issues that increase emotional distress. The injury affects their health, relationships with family and friends, and employment. It is difficult for the clinician to determine whether the psychologic symptoms that develop are related to the injury or to the patient's premorbid personality traits. The interpretation and treatment of posttraumatic headache are complicated further by the role of litigation. Despite these controversial issues, most patients seek a health care professional who will believe their symptoms and explain the cause.

The diagnostic evaluation of a patient with posttraumatic headache is performed to exclude structural and physiologic disturbances of the nervous system. Also, many diagnostic tests are performed for medical-legal reasons. However, these tests do not distinguish between patients who have legitimate complaints and those who feign injury, although the latter are in the minority. The diagnostic considerations that need to be excluded are subdural and epidural hematomas, CSF hypotension from a dural tear, posttraumatic hydrocephalus, cerebral vein thrombosis, cavernous sinus thrombosis, and cerebral hemorrhage (Fig. 3.3).

Posttraumatic headache is considered chronic if it persists longer than 8 weeks. Posttraumatic headache is diagnosed in 90% of patients with mild head injury at 1 month after injury, in 35% at 1 year, and in 20% at 3 years. The diagnosis of posttraumatic headache should not be made unless analgesic rebound headache has been excluded.

The treatment principles for posttraumatic headache are the same as those for any type of headache. Be vigilant about the problem of analgesic overuse. Patients often need support and reassurance, and they need to know that you believe them. Medications for tension-type

Table 3.15. Other Primary Headaches

Headache	Clinical features	Evaluation	Treatment
Primary stabbing headache	Sharp jabs, V1 distribution	MRI, ESR	Indomethacin
Primary cough headache	Transient head pain with cough or other Valsalva maneuver	MRI with attention to posterior fossa	Indomethacin
Primary exertional headache	Triggered by exercise, lasts 5 minutes to 48 hours, pulsating	CT or MRI and CSF to exclude subarachnoid hemorrhage, MRA to exclude aneurysm or dissection	Indomethacin, propranolol
Primary headache associated with sexual activity	Dull bilateral, intense at orgasm	CT or MRI and CSF to exclude subarachnoid hemorrhage, MRA to exclude aneurysm or dissection	Indomethacin, propranolol
Hypnic headache	Short attacks that awaken patient from sleep	MRI to exclude mass lesion	Lithium, indomethacin, caffeine
Primary thunderclap headache	Severe headache of abrupt onset	CT or MRI and CSF to exclude subarachnoid hemorrhage, MRA to exclude aneurysm or dissection	Nimodipine
Hemicrania continua	Trigeminal autonomic cephalalgia	Primary headache evaluation	Indomethacin
New daily persistent headache	Resembles chronic tension-type headache	Primary headache evaluation	See Table 3.7

CSF, cerebrospinal fluid; CT, computed tomography; ESR, erythrocyte sedimentation rate; MRA, magnetic resonance angiography; MRI, magnetic resonance imaging; V1, ophthalmic division of trigeminal nerve.

headache and migraine are effective for posttraumatic headache. Antidepressant medications, including tricyclic agents and selective serotonin reuptake inhibitors, are useful when depression is part of the posttraumatic syndrome. Anticonvulsant medications (eg, carbamazepine and gabapentin) are helpful if there is a neuralgic component to the head pain. Psychologic counseling, biofeedback, relaxation therapy, physical therapy, and cognitive retraining exercises may all be useful in the management of posttraumatic headache.

TEMPORAL ARTERITIS

Temporal arteritis, also called *giant cell arteritis* or *cranial arteritis*, is an important diagnosis to consider whenever a patient older than 50 years complains of headache. The disease causes inflammation of the medium- and large-sized arteries, which can lead to stenosis and occlusion of the arteries. Temporal arteritis can cause severe neurologic problems, but the most significant complications are stroke and blindness.

One-third of the patients who have temporal arteritis have headache as the presenting symptom, and it is the most common symptom. The headache can be throbbing, bitemporal to generalized, and associated with scalp tenderness. Other symptoms of this systemic illness include malaise, fatigue, jaw claudication, fever, cough, neuropathy, dysphagia, vision loss, and limb claudication. Physical findings may include erythema and tenderness to palpation of the temporal arteries, with reduced pulses (Fig. 3.4). The erythrocyte sedimentation rate is usually increased at 85±32 mm/hour (Westergren). Anemia and thrombocytosis may occur. A large study demonstrated that an abnormal temporal artery on physical examination and the presence of anemia were the best predictors for severe ischemic manifestations.

The erythrocyte sedimentation rate can be normal in 3% to 10% of patients; temporal artery biopsy should be performed to confirm the diagnosis. However, the patchy nature of the disease process may result in negative biopsy results. If the diagnosis is suspected, it is recommended that corticosteroid therapy be started immediately to avoid the risk of blindness. Prednisone, 60 mg daily, eliminates the headache and systemic symptoms. The dose can be tapered gradually over several months on the basis of the patient's clinical response and erythrocyte sedimentation rate. Temporal arteritis is self-limited, and corticosteroid therapy can be discontinued after 6 months to 2 years.

There is a strong relation between temporal arteritis and polymyalgia rheumatica. Polymyalgia rheumatica is characterized by diffuse proximal and axial joint pain and proximal myalgias. Whether it is part of the same vasculitic syndrome as temporal arteritis or a related disorder has not been decided. Evidence suggests that temporal arteritis and polymyalgia rheumatica may be more benign than originally thought.

FACIAL PAIN

Several conditions distinct from headache are associated with facial or head pain. Frequent nonneurologic causes of facial pain are sinusitis and temporomandibular joint syndrome. Common neurologic causes of facial pain are trigeminal neuralgia and herpes zoster. Other neurologic facial pain disorders are glossopharyngeal neuralgia, occipital neuralgia, tumors or aneurysms that compress the trigeminal nerve, infiltrative disease (eg, lymphoma), trauma, post-endarterectomy syndrome, and carotid dissection. A striking aspect of pain in the head and face is the pronounced psychologic effect it has on the patient. Strong emotional factors need to be considered when treating a patient who has facial pain.

The diagnostic approach to a patient who has facial pain can be complicated because of referred pain. The location of the pain may be misleading. Cranial and spinal nerve lesions can be referred to any region of the head and neck. For example, right thoracic and abdominal pain can be referred to the right face and ear. Intracranial pain is represented extracranially. The character of the pain can be helpful in making the diagnosis. Paroxysmal pain suggests neuralgic pain. Musculoskeletal pain has a dull quality, and movement or palpation can elicit pain. Physical medicine modalities are helpful in the treatment of somatic or musculoskeletal pain. Medication is often needed for neurogenic pain.

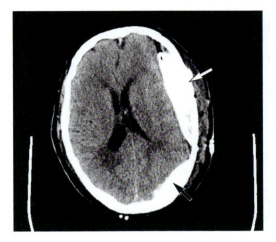

A   Noncontrast CT of head showing large sub-dural hematoma (*arrows*) overlying left cerebral hemisphere.

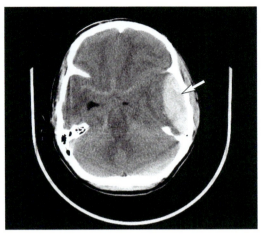

B   Noncontrast CT of head showing left epidural hematoma (*arrow*).

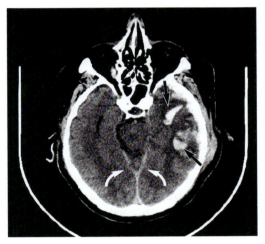

C   Posttraumatic intracerebral hemorrhage (*black arrows*) in left temporal lobe and blood in subarachnoid space (*white arrows*).

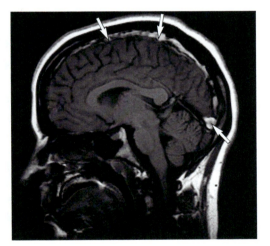

D   Cerebral vein thrombosis. Sagittal MRI showing blood clot in the superior sagittal sinus (*top arrows*) and transverse sinus (*bottom arrow*).

Fig. 3.3. Posttraumatic neuroimaging. CT, computed tomography; MRI, magnetic resonance imaging.

Trigeminal Neuralgia

The most common facial pain syndrome is trigeminal neuralgia. The pain is brief, lancinating, and located in the distribution of one or more branches of the trigeminal nerve (Fig. 3.5). The repetitive jolts of pain can be triggered by tactile stimulation such as brushing the teeth, talking, chewing, kissing, or shaving. Patients often describe a dull ache between the paroxysms of shocklike pain. Pain in the second

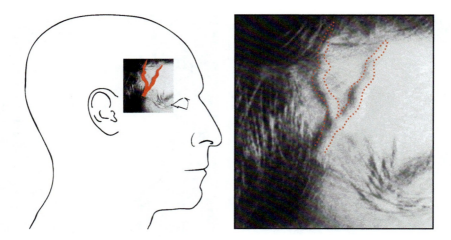

Fig. 3.4. Temporal arteritis. *Left*, Position of the temporal artery. *Right*, Enlarged view of the artery (dotted lines). The artery is thickened and tender.

(maxillary [V2]) or third (mandibular [V3]) division of the trigeminal nerve often causes the patient to visit a dentist.

Most cases of trigeminal neuralgia occur in persons older than 40 years. A secondary cause is suggested if the person is younger than 40 years or an abnormality is found on neurologic examination. Investigation involves MRI to exclude the secondary causes of trigeminal neuralgia, such as multiple sclerosis, a mass lesion in the posterior fossa, or an abnormal arterial loop (anterior inferior cerebellar or superior cerebellar artery).

Many options are available for treating trigeminal neuralgia (Table 3.16). Patients need to be reminded that spontaneous remissions occur, and after 2 months of successful therapy, it is reasonable to begin a slow drug taper over the same length of time. Most of the medications are anticonvulsants that are sodium channel blockers or γ-aminobutyric acid derivatives that inhibit nerve impulses. Carbamazepine has often been the first option for treatment. It is recommended that baseline values of a complete

blood count and chemistry panel be established before treatment commences. The medication should be started at the lowest dose and gradually titrated to the lowest effective dose. Monotherapy usually is effective, but occasionally a combination of medications is needed for adequate results.

For trigeminal neuralgia refractory to medical therapy, several surgical treatments are available. Ablative procedures include percutaneous radiofrequency and glycerol trigeminal rhizotomy. The infrequent complications include corneal anesthesia, anesthesia dolorosa, and dysesthesias. Microvascular decompression is successful but requires craniotomy in which the trigeminal nerve is separated from an adherent or juxtaposed vessel by a synthetic material. Gamma knife radiosurgery, in which gamma rays can perform the equivalent of ablative surgery without craniotomy, is rapidly becoming the favored surgical procedure for trigeminal neuralgia. Neurosurgical consultation is recommended for patients with medically refractory trigeminal neuralgia.

Glossopharyngeal Neuralgia

Glossopharyngeal neuralgia, less common than trigeminal neuralgia, is characterized by paroxysmal pain in and around the ear, jaw, throat, tongue, and larynx. The pain can be triggered by swallowing cold liquids, chewing, talking, or yawning. Another pain trigger is tactile stimulation around the ear. Although the glossopharyngeal nerve innervates the carotid sinus (which contains receptors important for regulating blood pressure), syncope is rare in glossopharyngeal neuralgia. Evaluation and treatment are similar to those for trigeminal neuralgia.

Occipital Neuralgia

Occipital neuralgia is characterized by paroxysms of pain in the distribution of the greater occipital nerve (Fig. 3.6). The back of the head may be tender, but it also may be painful in migraine, tension-type headache, and disease of the upper cervical spine. Occipital neuralgia is much less common than primary headache disorders and myofascial pain syndromes. The pharmacologic treatment of occipital neuralgia is the same as for trigeminal neuralgia. Occipital nerve blocks are often effective in treating occipital neuralgia.

Atypical Facial Pain

Facial pain that is not consistent with the neuralgic syndromes described above and is of unknown cause is designated *atypical facial pain*. The location of the pain can vary from being confined to one area of the face to including both sides of the face and neck. The pain is deep and poorly localized. It has no associated physical, neurologic, laboratory, or radiographic abnormalities. Atypical facial pain can be a manifestation of serious disease, and a thorough diagnostic investigation should be completed. Diagnostic testing should include a complete blood count, chemistry panel, erythrocyte sedimentation rate, chest radiography, and MRI with gadolinium, with attention to the brain, posterior fossa, jaw, and neck. Dental and otolaryngologic evaluation should be obtained. Atypical facial pain is difficult to manage, and pain specialty consultation may be needed.

Herpes Zoster and Postherpetic Neuralgia

Reactivation of latent varicella-zoster virus in cranial nerve ganglia can cause facial pain. When this involves the first division of the trigeminal nerve, it is called *herpes zoster ophthalmicus*. If the facial nerve is involved, there may be facial weakness and vesicular eruption in the external ear canal; this is called *Ramsay Hunt syndrome*. Pain that persists longer than 3 months after the herpetic eruption meets the criterion for *postherpetic neuralgia*.

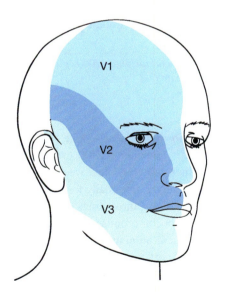

Fig. 3.5. Distribution of the three divisions of the trigeminal nerve (CN V): V1, ophthalmic division; V2, maxillary division; V3, mandibular division. (Modified from Patten, J: Neurological Differential Diagnosis. Springer-Verlag, New York, 1977, p 41. Used with permission.)

Table 3.16. Medications for Neuralgic Pain

Drug and dosage	Adverse effects (clinical comment)
Baclofen (Lioresal)—5-10 mg, three times daily; maximum 20 mg 4 times daily	Sedation, dizziness (withdraw slowly)
Carbamazepine (Tegretol)—100 mg twice daily, increase to maximum 1,200 mg/day	Drowsiness, dizziness, diplopia, ataxia (decreasing response)
Clonazepam (Klonopin)—0.5 mg twice daily, titrate as needed	Central nervous system depression, tolerance can develop (withdraw gradually)
Divalproex sodium (Depakote)—250 mg twice daily, titrate as needed	Tremor, weight gain, alopecia (check liver function before treatment)
Gabapentin (Neurontin)—100-300 mg/day, titrate up to 3,600 mg/day in 3 divided doses	Drowsiness, weight gain (renal metabolism, few drug interactions, high tolerability)
Lamotrigine (Lamictal)—25 mg/day, increase 25 mg every 3rd day to maximum 400 mg/day	Dizziness, ataxia, somnolence, headache, rash
Oxacarbazepine (Trileptal)—300 mg twice daily, increase to maximum 2,400 mg/day	Drowsiness, dizziness, diplopia, ataxia
Phenytoin (Dilantin)—300 mg/day, titrate as needed	Allergic reaction, dose-related ataxia
Pregabalin (Lyrica)—50 mg, three times daily; maximum 600 mg/day	Dizziness, ataxia, weight gain

Modified from Adams, AC: Neurology in Primary Care. FA Davis, Philadelphia, 2000, p 64. Used with permission of Mayo Foundation for Medical Education and Research.

Fever, malaise, and gradual onset of paresthesias of the affected dermatome may precede the acute illness. The rash may erupt 2 to 3 days later and consist of erythematous macules, papules, and vesicles. Serious complications of herpes zoster ophthalmicus include eye damage, cranial nerve palsies, meningoencephalitis, and stroke.

Acute treatment of cephalic herpes zoster may include antiviral agents, analgesics, local anesthetic creams, antidepressants, anticonvulsants, and corticosteroids. Administration of antiviral medication within the first 72 hours after the onset of herpes zoster can decrease the intensity and duration of the acute illness and prevent postherpetic neuralgia. The suggested regimen is famciclovir, 500 to 750 mg orally three times daily for 1 to 2 weeks, or acyclovir, 800 mg orally 5 times daily for 10 days, or valacyclovir, 100 mg three times daily for 1 week. For immunocompromised patients, parenteral antiviral medication may need to be considered. The use of corticosteroids for this condition has not been established. Many clinicians restrict corticosteroid treatment to immunocompetent patients who have severe pain or patients with zoster complicated by meningitis or vasculitis. Tricyclic antidepressants (amitriptyline, nortriptyline, desipramine, and maprotiline), gabapentin, pregabalin, opioids, and lidocaine patch are

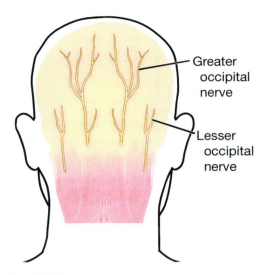

Greater
occipital
nerve

Lesser
occipital
nerve

Fig. 3.6. Distribution of the greater occipital nerve. Occipital neuralgia is characterized by paroxysms of pain in the distribution of this nerve.

effective in reducing the pain of postherpetic neuralgia. The treatment of postherpetic neuralgia is discussed further in Chapter 10.

Temporomandibular Joint Dysfunction

Temporomandibular joint dysfunction can be a source of facial and head pain. The patient may complain of pain of the jaw, face, ear, and surrounding area. The diagnostic criteria for temporomandibular joint disease include two of the following: pain in the jaw precipitated by movement, decreased range of motion, noise during joint movement, and tenderness of the joint capsule.

The temporomandibular joint should be palpated while the patient opens and closes the jaw. Inflammation of the joint will be painful, and any crepitus or noise can be observed. The normal opening range of the jaw is approximately the width of three fingers.

Treatment of temporomandibular joint dysfunction includes bite guards, soft diet, local heat, NSAIDs, and relaxation therapies. Dental and orthodontic consultation may be needed if none of these treatments is effective.

The major headache types are summarized in Figure 3.7.

Headache	Quality and duration	Associated symptoms
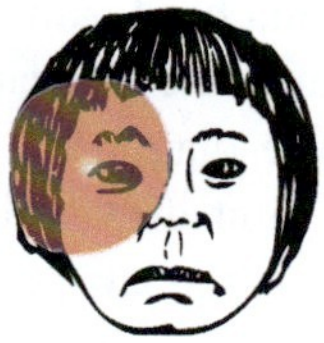 Migraine	Throbbing (unilateral to bilateral); 6-48 hours	Nausea, vomiting, photophobia, phonophobia, worse with physical exertion
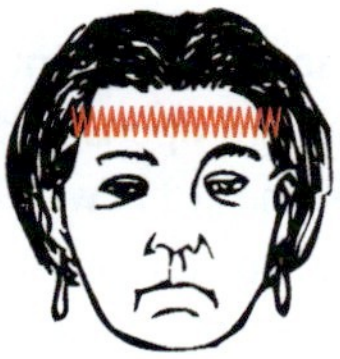 Tension-type	Dull pressure (diffuse to bilateral); hours to days	Depression
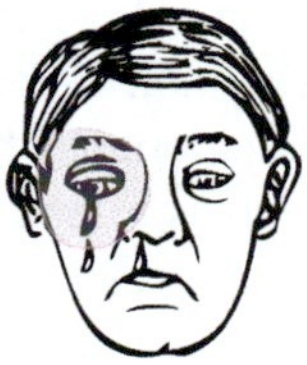 Cluster	Boring, sharp periorbital; 15-120 minutes	Ipsilateral tearing, nasal stuffiness, Horner syndrome
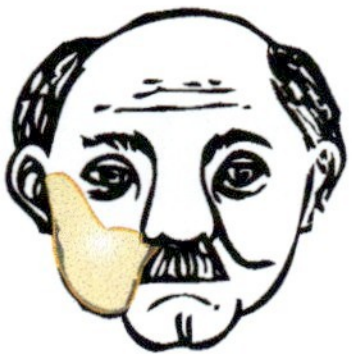 Trigeminal neuralgia	Lancinating, paroxysmal (trigeminal distrtibution) 15-60 seconds	Trigger zones
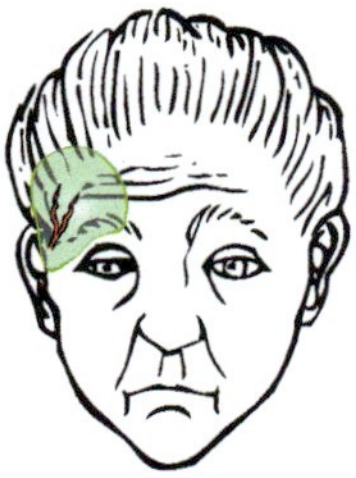 Temporal arteritis	Dull, intense (temporal to diffuse) increasing in frequency to continuous	Systemic symptoms Elevated sedimentation rate

Fig. 3.7. Summary of major headache types. (From Adams, AC: Neurology in Primary Care. FA Davis, Philadelphia, 2000, p 65. Used with permission of Mayo Foundation for Medical Education and Research.)

SUGGESTED READING

Bartolini, M, et al: Efficacy of topiramate and valproate in chronic migraine. Clin Neuropharmacol 28:277-279, 2005.

Brandes, JL: The influence of estrogen on migraine: A systematic review. JAMA 295:1824-1830, 2006.

Burstein, R, Collins, B, and Jakubowski, M: Defeating migraine pain with triptans: a race against the development of cutaneous allodynia. Ann Neurol 55:19-26, 2004.

Capobianco, DJ, Cheshire, WP, and Campbell, JK: An overview of the diagnosis and pharmacologic treatment of migraine. Mayo Clin Proc 71:1055-1066, 1996.

Diener, HC: Advances in the field of headache 2003/2004. Curr Opin Neurol 17:271-273, 2004.

Dubinsky, RM, et al, Quality Standards Subcommittee of the American Academy of Neurology. Practice parameter: Treatment of postherpetic neuralgia: An evidence-based report of the Quality Standards Subcommittee of the American Academy of Neurology. Neurology 63:959-965, 2004.

Evers, S, and Goadsby, PJ: Hypnic headache: Clinical features, pathophysiology, and treatment. Neurology 60:905-909, 2003.

Gonzalez-Gay, MA, et al: Giant cell arteritis: Disease patterns of clinical presentation in a series of 240 patients. Medicine (Baltimore) 84:269-276, 2005.

Headache Classification Subcommittee of the International Headache Society. The International Classification of Headache Disorders, ed 2. Cephalalgia 24 Suppl 1:9-160, 2004.

Hentschel, K, Capobianco, DJ, and Dodick, DW: Facial pain. Neurologist 11:244-249, 2005.

Herzog, AG: Continuous bromocriptine therapy in menstrual migraine. Neurology 48:101-102, 1997.

Howard, L, et al: Are investigations anxiolytic or anxiogenic? A randomised controlled trial of neuroimaging to provide reassurance in chronic daily headache. J Neurol Neurosurg Psychiatry 76:1558-1564, 2005.

Leone, M, et al: Hypothalamic deep brain stimulation for intractable chronic cluster headache: A 3-year follow-up. Neurol Sci 24 Suppl 2:S143-S145, 2003.

Leone, M, Franzini, A, and Bussone, G: Stereotactic stimulation of posterior hypothalamic gray matter in a patient with intractable cluster headache. N Engl J Med 345:1428-1429, 2001.

Lewis, D, et al, American Academy of Neurology Quality Standards Subcommittee; Practice Committee of the Child Neurology Society: Practice parameter: Pharmacological treatment of migraine headache in children and adolescents: Report of the American Academy of Neurology Quality Standards Subcommittee and the Practice Committee of the Child Neurology Society. Neurology 63:2215-2224, 2004.

Lewis, DW, et al, Quality Standards Subcommittee of the American Academy of Neurology; Practice Committee of the Child Neurology Society: Practice parameter: Evaluation of children and adolescents with recurrent headaches: Report of the Quality Standards Subcommittee of the American Academy of Neurology and the Practice Committee of the Child Neurology Society. Neurology 59:490-498, 2002.

Lipton, RB, et al: Classification of primary headaches. Neurology 63:427-435, 2004.

Lipton, RB, Bigal, ME, and Stewart, WF: Clinical trials of acute treatments for migraine including multiple attack of studies of pain, disability, and health-related quality of life. Neurology 65 Suppl 4:S50-S58, 2005.

Lu, SR, et al: Nimodipine for treatment of primary thunderclap headache. Neurology 62:1414-1416, 2004.

MacGregor, EA: Menstruation, sex hormones, and migraine. Neurol Clin 15:125-141, 1997.

Mathew, NT, Kailasam, J, and Seifert, T: Clinical recognition of allodynia in migraine. Neurology 63:848-852, 2004.

McGeeney, BE: Cluster headache pharmacotherapy. Am J Ther 12:351-358, 2005.

Mokri, B: Headaches caused by decreased intracranial pressure: Diagnosis and management. Curr Opin Neurol 16:319-326, 2003.

Nordborg, E, and Nordborg, C: Giant cell arteritis: Strategies in diagnosis and treatment. Curr Opin Rheumatol 16:25-30, 2004.

Noseworthy, JH (ed): Neurological Therapeutics: Principles and Practice. Martin Dunitz, London, 2003.

Porta, M, and Camerlingo, M: Headache and botulinum toxin. J Headache Pain 6:325-327, 2005.

Ramadan, NM: Targeting therapy for migraine: What to treat? Neurology 64 Suppl 2:S4-S8, 2005.

Raskin, NH: Repetitive intravenous dihydroergotamine as therapy for intractable migraine. Neurology 36:995-997, 1986.

Samuels, MA, and Feske, SK (eds): Office Practice of Neurology, ed 2. Churchill Livingstone, Philadelphia, 2003.

Silberstein, SD: Practice parameter: Evidence-based guidelines for migraine headache (an evidence-based review): Report of the Quality Standards Subcommittee of the American Academy of Neurology. Neurology 55:754-762, 2000. Erratum in: Neurology 56:142, 2000.

Silberstein, SD, and Lipton, RB: Headache epidemiology: Emphasis on migraine. Neurol Clin 14:421-434, 1996.

Toth, C: Medications and substances as a cause of headache: A systematic review of the literature. Clin Neuropharmacol 26:122-136, 2003.

Welch, KM: Contemporary concepts of migraine pathogenesis. Neurology 61 Suppl 4:S2-S8, 2003.

Zwart JA, et al: Analgesic use: A predictor of chronic pain and medication overuse headache: The Head-HUNT Study. Neurology 61:160-164, 2003.

CHAPTER 4

Back and Limb Pain

Back (spine) pain is a common problem. Low back pain is estimated to occur in up to 80% of adults and is the greatest cause of lost workdays in the United States. The cause of acute back pain is usually musculoskeletal. The differential diagnosis of back pain is listed in Table 4.1. Most patients with back pain can be cared for by their primary care provider, without the need for specialist consultation or diagnostic tests.

Chronic back pain is caused most often by degenerative disease of the spine. Neurologists are frequently consulted about back pain and asked about involvement of the nerve roots, spinal cord, spinal stenosis, and the need for surgery. Neurologic consultation is often requested for patients who have intractable back pain.

Pain in the upper and lower extremities is often related to problems of the spine. In addition to limb pain from spinal disease, this chapter reviews limb pain due to plexopathy. Common mononeuropathies are discussed in Chapter 6.

SPINAL ANATOMY

The spinal column consists of 7 cervical, 12 thoracic, 5 lumbar, 5 sacral (the sacrum), and 4 coccygeal (the coccyx) vertebrae. The vertebral segments are numbered from rostrally to caudally (Fig. 4.1). The pain-sensitive structures of the spine include the ligaments, facet joint capsules, peripheral fibers of the anulus fibrosus, periosteum of the vertebral bones, spinal nerves, and muscle (Fig. 4.2).

The relation of the spinal nerves to the vertebrae is important in understanding disk protrusion and its effect on the exiting nerve roots. Cervical roots C2 through C7 exit above their respective vertebrae, and the C8 nerve roots exit between vertebrae C7 and T1 (because there are 8 cervical nerve roots but only 7 cervical vertebrae). Cervical nerve root C1 usually has no dorsal root (sensory component). Nerve roots T1 through Coc 1 exit below their respective vertebrae (Fig. 4.3). Thus, lateral protrusion of the intervertebral disk at the C5-C6 level usually affects the C6 nerve roots, and lateral protrusion of the intervertebral disk at the L4-L5 level may affect the L5 and sacral nerve roots (Fig. 4.4).

In adults, the spinal cord terminates as the conus medullaris at the level between vertebrae L1 and L2. The conus medullaris consists of the lower lumbar and sacral segments of the spinal

Table 4.1. Causes of Back (Spine) Pain

Musculoskeletal/mechanical
Muscle strain
Degenerative spondylosis
Degenerative disk disease
Osteoarthritis

Tumor
Primary spinal cord tumor
Metastatic tumor
Plasmacytoma of multiple myeloma
Primary bone tumor
Retroperitoneal tumor

Vascular lesion
Arteriovenous malformation
Spinal dural arteriovenous fistula

Infection
Diskitis
Osteomyelitis
Epidural abscess
Urinary tract infecton

Intra-abdominal or pelvic disease
Abdominal aortic aneurysm
Posterior perforating duodenal ulcer
Endometriosis

Metabolic bone disease
Osteoporosis
Paget disease

Rheumatologic disease
Ankylosing spondylitis
Rheumatoid arthritis

Congenital
Spina bifida
Tethered cord
Intraspinal lipoma

Trauma
Fracture
Dislocation

From Adams, AC: Neurology in Primary Care. FA Davis, Philadelphia, 2000, p 70. Used with permission of Mayo Foundation for Medical Education and Research.

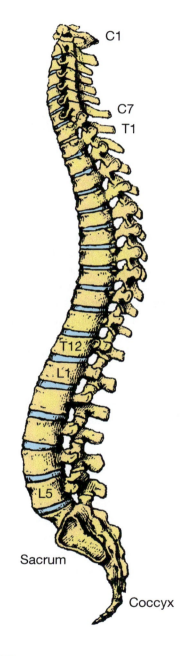

Fig. 4.1. The vertebral column (lateral view). (Modified from The Care of the Back. Mayo Foundation for Medical Education and Research, Rochester, MN, 1999, p 3. Used with permission.)

cord. This anatomical relation is important to remember when performing lumbar puncture and in understanding spinal cord syndromes that involve the conus medullaris and cauda equina. The clinical syndrome of cauda equina must be recognized because it requires emergent surgical treatment (Fig. 4.5).

EVALUATION OF BACK PAIN

The first step in evaluating a patient who has back pain is to determine whether the problem is complicated or uncomplicated. Most back pain is uncomplicated in that it does not require immediate attention or diagnostic testing.

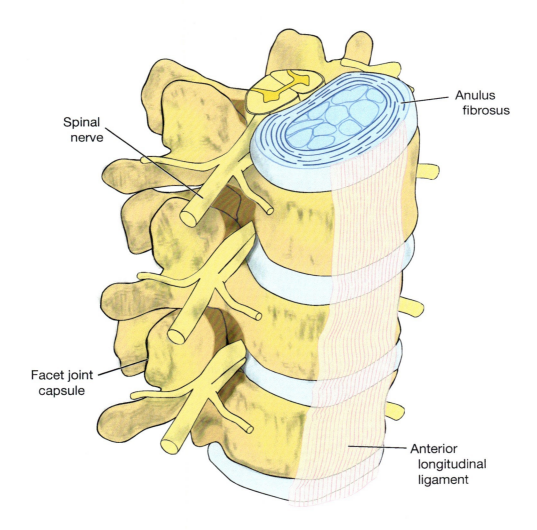

Spinal nerve

Facet joint capsule

Anulus fibrosus

Anterior longitudinal ligament

Fig. 4.2. Pain-sensitive structures of the spine. (Modified from The Care of the Back. Mayo Foundation for Medical Education and Research, Rochester, MN, 1999, p 4. Used with permission.)

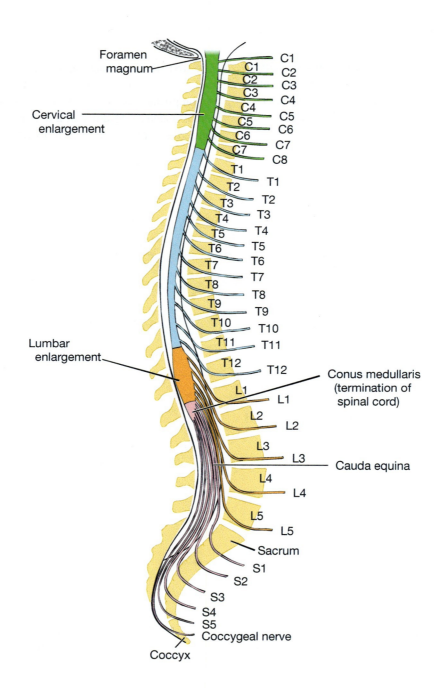

Fig. 4.3. Relation of spinal roots to the corresponding vertebral level. (Modified from Parent, A: Carpenter's Human Neuroanatomy. ed 9. Williams & Wilkins, Baltimore, 1996, p 328. Used with permission.)

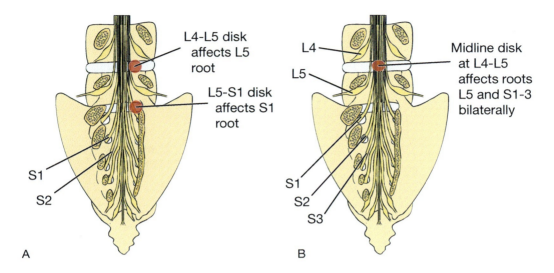

Fig. 4.4. Herniated nucleus of vertebral disk compressing spinal roots. *A,* Lateral herniation of a lumbar or sacral disk compresses the nerve root below the disk (eg, lateral herniation of L4-L5 disk compresses ipsilateral spinal root L5). *B,* In comparison, midline herniation of a lumbar disk compresses several spinal roots bilaterally (eg, midline herniation of disk L4-L5 compresses spinal roots L5 and S1-S3 bilaterally).

Complicated back pain, which includes fractures, cancer, infection, systemic diseases, and back pain associated with neurologic deficit, requires further attention. The diagnosis of uncomplicated or complicated back pain can be determined from a careful history and physical examination. The important points, or red flags, associated with complicated back pain are summarized in Table 4.2.

The history of a patient with back pain should include special references to the quality of the pain, location, radiation, and factors and activities that exacerbate or relieve the pain. Nerve root pain is usually sharp, "shooting," and brief and is increased by coughing or straining. Pain from the nerve or plexus is described as "burning," "pins and needles," "asleep," or "numb." Other important characteristics of back pain are listed in Table 4.3. It is essential to ask questions about weakness and bowel and bladder control. Ask about work

activity, trauma, disability, and litigation. Inconsistencies of activity and overreaction may indicate a problem that is more psychologic than physical.

The temporal profile and the presence or absence of red flags determine whether further diagnostic evaluation is needed. Acute back pain of less than 6 weeks' duration is usually caused by musculoskeletal factors and will resolve without further investigation. Back pain that persists after 6 to 12 weeks warrants further investigation. Subacute back pain raises the possibility of osteomyelitis, neoplasm, or spondylosis. The evaluation at this time may include laboratory testing, spine radiography with oblique views, bone scans, and other spine imaging. If chronic pain lasts longer than 12 weeks, magnetic resonance imaging (MRI) and specialist consultation may be needed.

The sudden onset of symptoms in relation to lifting, bending, or twisting is usually the

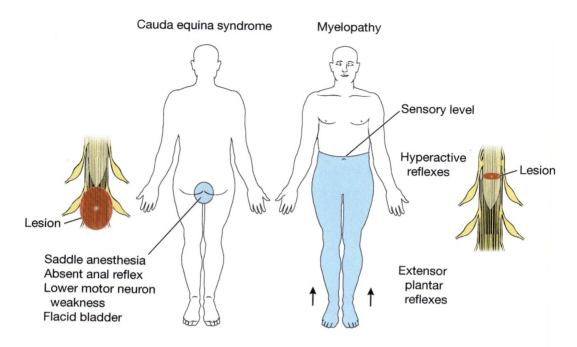

Fig. 4.5. Comparison of deficits associated with cauda equina syndrome and myelopathy. (From Adams, AC: Neurology in Primary Care. FA Davis, Philadelphia, 2000, p 73. Used with permission of Mayo Foundation for Medical Education and Research.)

result of stress on musculoskeletal structures, as in lumbosacral strain or acute disk herniation. Mechanical pain is suggested when the pain is associated with movement. Radicular pain radiates down the extremity and is aggravated by an increase in intra-abdominal pressure (eg, cough or sneeze). An increase in pain with spinal extension may suggest spinal stenosis. If the pain increases with rest, malignancy or infection needs to be considered.

Most back pain is musculoskeletal; however, back pain can be a feature of serious systemic disease. Be aware of the signs and symptoms of serious back pain (Table 4.2). Aggressively evaluate any elderly patient who has constitutional symptoms or any patient with immunosuppression. Back pain associated with a neurologic deficit needs to be evaluated. Evaluate for inflammatory spondyloarthropathy

when the clinical history suggests that the back pain began before the patient was 30 years old, has lasted several months, increases with rest, and decreases with activity.

It is crucial to ask about any change in bowel or bladder control. Incontinence or retention can occur with any lesion that involves the cauda equina or spinal cord bilaterally. If the patient has bowel or bladder problems and back pain, the sacral dermatomes and anal reflex should be examined. To test the anal reflex, gently scratch the skin around the anus and either observe the contraction of the anal ring or palpate with a gloved fingertip. Spinal cord segments S2-S4 in the conus medullaris and sacral nerve roots of the cauda equina supply the anal sphincter. If a lesion involves the conus medullaris or the sacral nerve roots bilaterally, the anal reflex will be absent, the lower

Table 4.2. Causes and Red Flags of Complicated Back Pain

Cause	Red flags
Fracture or dislocation	Trauma: major in young patients, minor in elderly
	Bone disease: osteoporosis, osteomalacia, Paget disease
	Corticosteroid therapy
	Congenital anomalies
Infection	Fever
	Immunosuppressed status
	Intravenous drug user
	Urinary tract infection
	Spinal surgery
	Penetrating wound
Neoplasm	History of cancer
	Pain at rest, causing movement
	Weight loss
	Unexplained blood loss
	Constitutional symptoms
Neurologic deficit	Major strength loss
	Bowel and bladder symptoms
Cauda equina syndrome	Bowel and bladder symptoms
	Saddle anesthesia
Inflammatory spondyloarthropathy	Pain increases with rest, pain decreases with activity, onset before age 30 years, several months' duration

From Adams, AC: Neurology in Primary Care. FA Davis, Philadelphia, 2000, p 74. Used with permission of Mayo Foundation for Medical Education and Research.

extremities will be weak, the lumbosacral area will be anesthetic, and ankle reflexes (S1) will be reduced or absent. In comparison, a more proximal lesion of the spinal cord is associated with a spastic bladder and long tract signs, including hyperreflexia, bilateral extensor plantar reflexes (Babinski sign), and a sensory level (Fig. 4.5). Flaccid and spastic types of neurogenic bladder occur in patients with disorders of the spine. The three types of neurogenic bladder are summarized in Table 4.4.

The physical examination of a patient who has back pain should include a general evaluation, with attention to the neurologic, joint, abdominal, and rectal examinations. Observing the patient sitting, standing, and walking before the formal evaluation is often more revealing than it is during the examination. The gait of a patient with spine pain frequently is described as painful, or *antalgic*. A patient with an antalgic gait walks slowly, taking small steps, while holding the back stiffly in a specific position. A patient with lower extremity pain lists to the asymptomatic side while standing and walking. A patient with L5 weakness may walk with a foot slap because

Table 4.3. Types of Back Pain and Associated Clinical Conditions

Pain type	Cause
Pain at rest	Neoplasm, infection, primary bone disease
Pain increases with movement	Mechanical (eg, musculoskeletal problem)
Pain increases with rest, decreases with activity	Inflammatory spondyloarthropathy
Pain with fever	Vertebral osteomyelitis, subacute bacterial endocarditis
Pain that causes movement (eg, writhing to alleviate pain)	Neoplasm, visceral disease (ulcers, pancreatic disease)
Acute pain in a patient with cancer	Metastasis
Pain with urinary incontinence or retention	Cauda equina syndrome, myelopathy
Pain radiating down an extremity, increases with Valsalva maneuver	Radiculopathy
Pain increases with spine extension (standing, walking) and decreases with flexion (sitting)	Spinal stenosis

From Adams, AC: Neurology in Primary Care. FA Davis, Philadelphia, 2000, p 74. Used with permission of Mayo Foundation for Medical Education and Research.

of weakness of the anterior tibialis muscle. With weakness of the gluteus medius muscle, another L5 muscle, the contralateral pelvis drops on stance phase, producing a Trendelenburg gait (Fig. 4.6). The Trendelenburg gait involves lurching of the trunk to the weakened side in an attempt to keep the pelvis level. Subtle weakness of muscles innervated by L5 can be detected by having patients walk on their heels. If the muscles innervated by S1 are weak, patients have

Table 4.4. Comparison of Flaccid, Spastic, and Uninhibited Neurogenic Bladder

Feature	Flaccid	Spastic	Uninhibited
Incontinence	Yes	Yes	Yes
Location of lesion	Cauda equina, sacral segments of conus medullaris	Spinal cord (distal to pontine micturition center)	Medial frontal cortex
Retention	Yes	Yes	No
Anal reflex	Absent	Present	Present
Clinical condition	Cauda equina lesion, disk protrusion, tumor	Myelopathy, spinal cord trauma	Hydrocephalus, dementia

From Adams, AC: Neurology in Primary Care. FA Davis, Philadelphia, 2000, p 75. Used with permission of Mayo Foundation for Medical Education and Research.

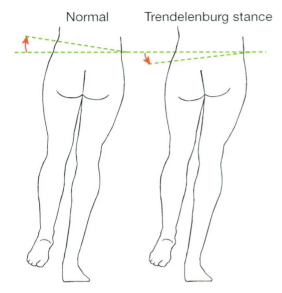

Normal   Trendelenburg stance

Fig. 4.6. Trendelenburg stance. Weakness of the gluteus medius muscle (eg, L5 radiculopathy) results in the pelvis tilting down on the opposite side. In an attempt to keep the pelvis level while walking, the trunk lurches to the weakened side.

difficulty walking on their toes. Hysterical or malingering gait tends to be bizarre, with excessive movements of the trunk and arms.

Inspect and palpate the spine for localized tender points and examine for muscle consistency. Hair tufts, dimples, or scoliosis may suggest congenital spine defects. The patient's posture can be revealing. Patients with spinal stenosis often stand with flexed posture. Those with radiculopathy may list to one side or keep the knee of the symptomatic leg bent; also, they avoid putting weight on the affected heel. Assess spinal mobility. An increase in pain with any movement indicates musculoskeletal injury. A "corkscrew" motion with forward flexion suggests radiculopathy. Difficulty bending to one side (side flexion) and bending the symptomatic knee with forward flexion also suggest radiculopathy.

Ask a patient with neck and arm pain to flex, extend, rotate, and bend the neck laterally. These maneuvers often increase musculoskeletal neck pain. An increase in arm pain or paresthesias suggests radiculopathy.

The stretching of irritated or inflamed nerve roots causes pain. This is the principle of several provocative tests, including the straight leg raising, or sciatic stretch, test. The straight leg raising test is useful for determining whether a patient with low back pain has an L5 or S1 radiculopathy. With the patient supine, ask him or her to keep the symptomatic leg straight and raise it to a 90-degree angle. This maneuver stretches the nerve root, and the test is considered positive if the patient feels pain before the leg reaches 90 degrees. The smaller the angle of elevation needed to elicit pain, the greater the likelihood that a herniated disk is compressing the root. The location of the pain is meaningful. Pain in the leg or buttock is more suggestive of radiculopathy than is pain in the back. When the asymptomatic leg is raised, pain in the opposite leg or buttock is an excellent indication of radiculopathy (the crossed straight leg raising test). A feeling of tightness in the hamstrings is not a positive result. Other methods for stretching the L5-S1 nerve roots is to ask a patient who is seated to dorsiflex the foot or, during the straight leg raising test, ask the patient to dorsiflex the foot of the raised leg when the leg is at an angle that pain would not be felt if the foot were not dorsiflexed. Both of these methods help assess the consistency of patients who exaggerate their symptoms. Similarly, the L2, L3, and L4 nerve roots can be tested by stretching the femoral nerve, for example, by having the patient flex the knee while supine.

While evaluating back and limb pain, also evaluate the hip joint if the patient has low back pain or the shoulder joint if he or she has neck pain. Referred pain from the hip frequently causes low back pain and leg pain. Pain due to flexion, abduction, and external rotation of the lower extremity may indicate a hip lesion. Shoulder disease frequently causes arm and neck pain. If abduction, flexion, extension, or rotation of the shoulder elicits pain, shoulder disease is likely.

The evaluation of muscle strength can be complicated by pain that inhibits function or the conscious or unconscious attempt of the patient to appear weak. The best way to assess strength is to watch the patient move. Toe flexor and extensor weakness usually precedes foot weakness. Watching the patient walk on the toes and heels is useful in assessing the strength of these muscles. If a patient is not able to walk on the toes or heels, determine if he or she can stand on the toes and heels while you offer support. A good way to assess proximal muscle strength is to have the patient squat. By encouraging the patient to "break through the pain," you may be able to determine his or her strength. If root pain prevents testing the quadriceps muscle with the leg extended, the muscle can be tested with the patient prone. Atrophy is rare unless the weakness has been present for more than 3 weeks. If atrophy is severe, consider an extradural spinal tumor. Sudden giving way, jerkiness, or involvement of many muscle groups is characteristic of nonorganic weakness.

On sensory examination, a patient with spine pain may have sensory loss that has a dermatomal distribution. Because the overlap of root distributions is wide, involvement of a single nerve root may cause minimal sensory loss. Assess for a sensory level if there is a question of myelopathy. Nonanatomical sensory loss is a functional sign of back pain but should be correlated with more objective signs.

Muscle stretch reflexes are useful in evaluating patients who have back pain, because these reflexes are not influenced by subjective factors.

The symmetry of muscle stretch reflexes is important. If the ankle reflex is difficult to elicit, test this S1 reflex while the patient kneels.

Psychologic dysfunction can be prominent in patients with back pain. Depression, anxiety, and stress can cause and aggravate pain. Several signs suggest that the pain is nonorganic. Waddell and colleagues described five features that suggest nonorganic pain: palpation tenderness, simulation, distraction, regional distribution, and overreaction. The presence of three of the five is considered significant. Palpation tenderness is excessive if it is widespread or caused by light touch. Simulation involves mimicking but not performing painful tests. An example is elicitation of pain while you rotate the patient's shoulders and hips together or while you push down on the patient's head (axial loading). An example of distraction is when a straight leg raising test yields a positive result when the patient is supine but a negative result when the patient is sitting or being "distracted." Regional distribution involves nonanatomical motor or sensory loss. Disproportionate verbalization, wincing, collapsing, and tremor are examples of overreaction.

DIAGNOSTIC TESTS

Two points deserve emphasis: 1) the history and physical examination are the most important diagnostic tests, and 2) asymptomatic imaging abnormalities of the spine are common. The patient's clinical presentation determines which diagnostic tests are needed and the significance of the findings of imaging studies. Common structural abnormalities are degenerative changes, disk narrowing and bulging, spurs, and spondylolisthesis. The high frequency of back complaints has the potential of causing expensive and unnecessary testing. Finding asymptomatic structural abnormalities may impede recovery from an episode of uncomplicated back pain. For this reason, the clinical question must be specific before any diagnostic studies are performed. Diagnostic tests should not be performed for uncomplicated back pain if it has not persisted for 7 weeks.

Plain radiographs of the spine are useful for examining the vertebral bodies for bony abnormalities, including fracture, neoplasm, congenital deformity, and rheumatic disease (Fig. 4.7). Oblique views are useful in assessing spondylolisthesis and spondylolysis. Spondylolisthesis is forward displacement of a vertebral body onto the body below it. Spondylolysis, often associated with spondylolisthesis, is the condition in which the posterior portion of the vertebral unit (pars interarticularis) is split (Fig. 4.8). It can be due to abnormal development, trauma, or degenerative disease. If the borders of the split are sclerotic, the fracture is likely chronic and unlikely to heal. A bone scan can also determine whether the spondylolysis is active or chronic. Plain radiographs with the patient in flexion and extension can help assess the stability of the spine. Flexion and extension views are helpful in evaluating the stability of the spine in spondylosis and in patients who have had previous back operations. Plain radiography of the spine is the standard test for the initial evaluation of trauma.

Disks, nerve roots, and the spinal cord are evaluated best with computed tomography (CT), MRI, and myelography with CT. CT is useful for imaging bony detail and can be a reasonable test for detecting spinal stenosis and disk herniation. The addition of contrast dye (myelography with CT) provides better visualization of the nerve roots and spinal cord. The disadvantages of myelography are the invasion of the cerebrospinal fluid space and the associated complications.

MRI is superior to CT for evaluating all conditions of the spine (Fig. 4.9). The images can be viewed in several planes, and the variable signal capability provides better images than CT does. MRI is noninvasive, uses nonionizing radiation, and is extremely sensitive for detecting tumors and infection. MRI with gadolinium contrast is valuable in distinguishing between scar tissue and recurrent disk protrusion in patients with previous back surgery. This highly sensitive test often shows abnormalities that need to be correlated with clinical findings. MRI can be expensive and is best used when the anticipated findings will alter management. The diagnostic imaging tests used to image the spine are summarized in Table 4.5.

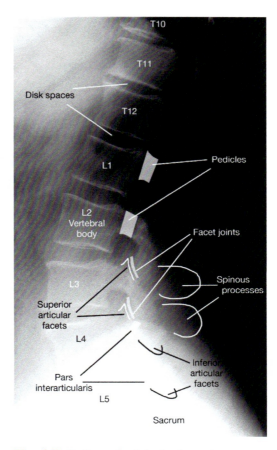

Fig. 4.7. Radiograph of the lumbar spine.

Electromyography (EMG) is a useful extension of the clinical examination and provides physiologic information. It can be helpful when imaging studies show abnormalities at multiple levels. EMG can localize a radiculopathy and determine whether it is active or chronic. This information may be essential if surgical treatment is considered. For a patient with footdrop, EMG can distinguish between a lesion of the L5 root and peroneal nerve palsy. (EMG is discussed in more detail in Chapter 2).

RADICULOPATHY

Radiculopathy is disease of a nerve root. One of the questions neurologists are asked most frequently is whether a patient with back and limb pain has radiculopathy. The diagnostic approach to the patient depends on the answer to this question (Fig. 4.10).

A spinal nerve consists of a motor component (ventral root), whose axons arise from ventral horn cells, and a sensory component (dorsal root), whose axons rise from cell bodies

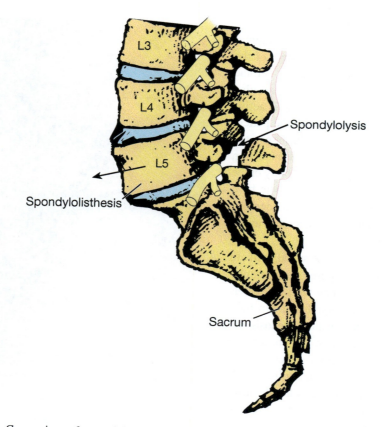

Fig. 4.8. Comparison of spondylolisthesis and spondylolysis. (Modified from Hinton, RC: Backache. In Samuels, MA [ed]: Manual of Neurologic Therapeutics, ed 5. Little, Brown and Company, Boston, 1995, pp 78-88. Used with permission.)

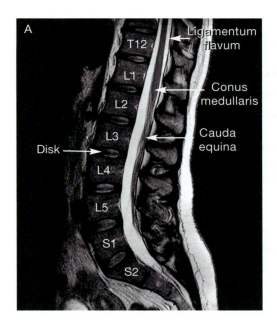
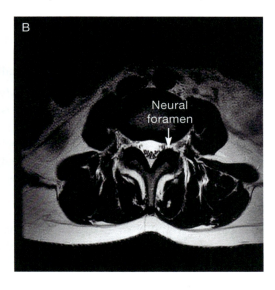

Fig. 4.9. MRI of the lumbar spine. *A*, Midsagittal view. *B*, Axial view through vertebral body.

in the associated dorsal root ganglion. Most diseases of the spinal roots affect both of these components. An exception is herpes zoster, which causes a radiculitis of the sensory root. Another, but rare, exception is pure motor polyradiculoneuropathy.

The common causes of radiculopathy are disk herniation and degenerative changes of the spine. Acute radiculopathy can occur in diabetes mellitus, suggesting a vascular cause. Herpes zoster and other infections can affect the nerve roots. A chronic temporal profile suggests degenerative changes or, rarely, a neoplastic cause.

The clinical features of radiculopathy include pain and paresthesia in a sensory dermatome and weakness of the muscles innervated by the nerve root. The history and physical examination findings suggest radiculopathy. The important root syndromes are summarized in Table 4.6. Features suggestive of cervical radiculopathy and lumbar radiculopathy on clinical examination are listed in Tables 4.7 and 4.8, respectively.

More than 95% of herniated disks of the lower back affect either the L5 or S1 nerve roots and cause the clinical syndrome of sciatica. The term *sciatica* is used to describe pain in the hip and buttock area that radiates down the posterolateral aspect of the leg. This term is not synonymous with *radiculopathy*. Because patients frequently use sciatica incorrectly, it is important to have them describe their symptoms without the use of medical terminology.

Conservative treatment is reasonable for a patient who has a radiculopathy due to a herniated disk but does not have neurologic deficit. Most patients with acute back pain, with or without radiculopathy, have improvement after 6 weeks. Bed rest, if any, should be brief and probably less than 2 days. Physical medicine may include exercise and the use of modalities such as heat, cold, ultrasound, or massage to

Table 4.5. Diagnostic Imaging Tests for Back Pain

Test	Indications	Advantages and disadvantages

Plain radiographs
  Oblique views
  Flexion and extension
	Trauma, spondylosis, spinal stability (postsurgical)	Inexpensive
		Disks and nerve roots are not visualized

Bone scan	Infection, neoplasm, bone disease, spondylosis	Often adjunctive test
CT	Spinal stenosis, disk herniation	Poor contrast without myelography Bone detail is good
Myelography with CT	Disk herniation, spinal stenosis, cord compression, myelopathy	Invasive Postmyelogram headache Entire spinal cord can be evaluated Can obtain CSF sample
MRI with gadolinium	Disk herniation, scar tissue vs. disk, spinal stenosis, cord compression, myelopathy infection/inflammation, neoplasm	Sensitive, multiplanar, contrast of different tissues Expensive Claustrophobia

CSF, cerebrospinal fluid; CT, computed tomography; MRI, magnetic resonance imaging.
From Adams, AC: Neurology in Primary Care. FA Davis, Philadelphia, 2000, p 78. Used with permission of Mayo Foundation for Medical Education and Research.

reduce the pain. Patients, especially those with occupational back pain, may benefit from ergonomic education.

SPINAL STENOSIS

Spinal stenosis is narrowing of the spinal canal (Fig. 4.11). It has several causes, including congenital narrowing of the canal, bulging intervertebral disks, spondylolisthesis, or degenerative osteoarthropathies of the spine, or a combination of these. The narrowed spinal canal compresses the nerve roots and, presumably, their vascular supply.

The diameters of the spinal canal and spinal foramina decrease with standing and walking (extension) and increase with flexion of the spine. Comments the patient may make that support the diagnosis of spinal stenosis are 1) being able to walk farther when using a shopping cart, 2) leaning on the sink when doing dishes or shaving, and 3) having no difficulty with bicycling. Any activity that flexes the spine reduces the symptoms of neurogenic claudication.

When a patient presents with the complaint of pain in the legs with walking, the possibility of vascular ischemia (claudication) versus spinal stenosis (neurogenic claudication or pseudoclaudication) is raised. The differences

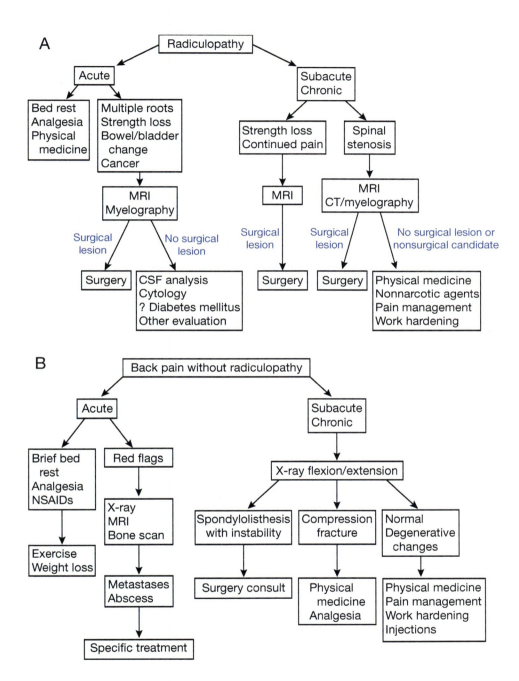

Fig. 4.10. Algorithms for evaluation and treatment of, *A*, radiculopathy and, *B*, back pain without radiculopathy. CSF, cerebrospinal fluid; CT, computed tomography; MRI, magnetic resonance imaging; NSAID, nonsteroidal antiinflammatory drug. (From Adams, AC: Neurology in Primary Care. FA Davis, Philadelphia, 2000, p 79. Used with permission of Mayo Foundation for Medical Education and Research.)

Table 4.6. Summary of Root Syndromes

Segment	Sensory loss and pain	Motor weakness	Reflex loss
C3-C4	Shoulder	Diaphragm	
C5	Lateral shoulder	Deltoid	
C6	Radial side of arm, thumb	Biceps, wrist extensors	Biceps, brachio-radialis
C7	2nd and 3rd fingers	Triceps, wrist flexors, finger extensors	Triceps
C8	4th and 5th fingers	Interossei, finger flexors	
L3	Hip, medial thigh	Quadriceps	Knee
L4	Hip, posterolateral thigh	Quadriceps	Knee
L5	Lateral leg, great toe	Foot and toe extensors	
S1	Back of calf, lateral foot	Plantar flexion of foot and toes	Ankle

From Adams, AC: Neurology in Primary Care. FA Davis, Philadelphia, 2000, p 80. Used with permission of Mayo Foundation for Medical Education and Research.

between these two conditions are listed in Table 4.9.

Patients who have spinal stenosis often have a flexed posture when standing and walking. The range of motion of the lumbar spine is reduced and can cause leg pain with extension of the back. Other examination findings are normal unless a nerve root is impinged.

The diagnosis of lumbar spinal stenosis can be confirmed with CT, myelography with CT, and MRI (Fig. 4.12). Nonsurgical management of spinal stenosis includes patient education, medications to control pain, and exercises and physical treatments to regain or maintain activities of daily living. Surgical consultation should be sought for patients who do not have a response to these measures. Decompressive laminectomy is the standard surgical procedure for spinal stenosis.

CERVICAL SPONDYLOSIS

Degenerative changes of the cervical spine, including cervical spondylosis, occur with increasing frequency with age. Narrowing of the spinal canal and the intervertebral foramina can compress the spinal cord and nerve roots. Cervical spondylosis can cause headache, radiculopathy, and myelopathy. Cervical spine disease can cause neck pain or refer pain to the frontal or occipital part of the head, shoulder, or the interscapular area.

The cervical nerve root most often affected by a herniated disk is C7, and the cervical nerve roots most frequently affected in cervical spondylosis are C5 and C6. Neck and arm pain caused by spondylotic changes occurs more gradually than that due to disk herniation. Patients with cervical spondylosis usually are older than those with a herniated disk.

Cervical spondylotic myelopathy is a difficult clinical problem. The patient may complain of stiff neck, arm pain, leg weakness, and easy fatigability. Neurologic examination may show spastic paraparesis with hyperactive reflexes and bilateral Babinski signs. Amyotrophic lateral sclerosis and vitamin B_{12} deficiency are important disorders in the differential diagnosis

Table 4.7. Clinical Features Suggestive of Cervical Radiculopathy

Feature	Cervical radiculopathy			
	Definite	Probable	Possible	Poor evidence
Location of pain				
Neck			•	
Scapula			•	
Shoulder			•	
Proximal arm		•		
Distal arm and hand	•			
Associated paresthesias				
Shoulder	•(C5)			
Thumb and proximal forearm	•(C6)*			
3rd Finger	•(C7)			
4th and 5th Fingers	•(C8)†			
Character of pain				
Deep, "toothache"		•		
Electric, "shooting"				•
Location of pain with Valsalva maneuver (strain is more meaningful than cough or sneeze)				
Arm	•			
Shoulder		•		
Neck			•	
Provocation (location of pain with neck movement)				
Shoulder		•		
Proximal arm		•		
Individual fingers	•			
Entire upper extremity				•

*Be sure to distinguish between cervical radiculopathy and median neuropathy.
†Be sure to distinguish between cervical radiculopathy and ulnar neuropathy.
From Adams, AC: Neurology in Primary Care. FA Davis, Philadelphia, 2000, p 83. Used with permission of Mayo Foundation for Medical Education and Research.

of cervical spondylotic myelopathy. Although cervical spondylotic myelopathy has a slow and progressive course, it can develop suddenly in an elderly patient from trauma or hyperextension of the neck.

The diagnosis of cervical spondylotic myelopathy can be made with the neurologic examination, and plain radiographs and MRI can readily identify the problem. The management of cervical spondylosis is complicated. It has been

Table 4.8. Clinical Features of Lumbar Radiculopathy

Feature	Lumbar radiculopathy			Poor evidence
	Definite	Probable	Possible	
Location of pain				
Back			•	
Superior buttock				•
Lateral buttock				•
Medial/inferior buttock		•		
Leg, above knee			•	
Leg, below knee		•		
Associated paresthesias				
Dorsum of foot, great toe	•(L5)			
Sole of foot, little toe	•(S1)			
Knee, medial calf		•(L4)		
Knee, anterior thigh		•(L3)		
Other				•
Character of pain				
Deep, "toothache"		•		
Electric, "shooting"				•
Postural effect				
Increased with sitting		•		
Onset with extension, relief with flexion	•(Spinal stenosis)			
Location of pain with Valsalva maneuver (strain is more meaningful than cough or sneeze)				
Leg	•			
Buttock		•		
Back			•	
Observations				
List to side	•			
Bent knee, symptomatic leg		•		
Motions				
Unilateral limited side flexion		•		
"Corkscrewing" forward flexion	•			
Bending symptomatic knee with forward flexion		•		
Slow flexion, slow irregular return				•

Table 4.8   (continued)

Feature	Lumbar radiculopathy			
	Definite	Probable	Possible	Poor evidence
Palpation tenderness				
Sciatic notch		•		
Popliteal fossa	•			
Spine			•	
Sacrum, gluteal attachments, trochanter				•
Skin				•
Provocation				
Leg pain with SLR		•		
Buttock pain with SLR			•	
Back pain with SLR				•
Opposite leg or buttock pain with SLR	•			
Leg or anterior thigh pain with reverse SLR		•(L3, L4)		
Buttock, back pain with reverse SLR			•(L3, L4)	
Immediate leg pain with back extension			•	
Delayed leg pain with back extension		•(Spinal stenosis)		
Buttock, leg pain with back flexion, knees flexed				•

SLR, straight leg raising test.
From Adams, AC: Neurology in Primary Care. FA Davis, Philadelphia, 2000, p 81. Used with permission of Mayo Foundation for Medical Education and Research.

estimated that 70% of women and 85% of men have cervical spondylosis by age 59 years and 93% and 97%, respectively, after 70 years. Determining whether the cervical spondylosis is symptomatic may require careful neurologic evaluation with longitudinal follow-up.

The uncertain natural history of cervical spondylotic myelopathy and the 50:50 chance of improvement with surgery complicate treatment. Surgical decompression is performed if there is evidence of progressive myelopathy. Nonsurgical measures include the use of a soft cervical collar, physiotherapy, nonsteroidal antiinflammatory drugs, and close clinical follow-up.

WHIPLASH

Whiplash is the sudden flexion and extension of the cervical spine that occurs primarily in

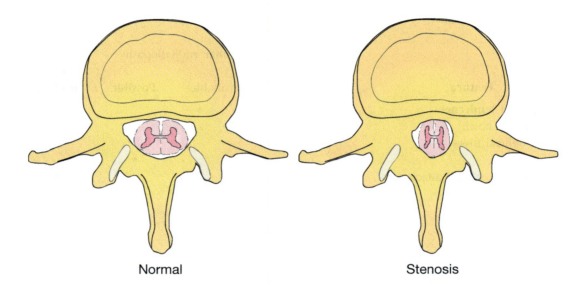

Normal   Stenosis

Fig. 4.11. Spinal stenosis.

motor vehicle accidents. Patients with whiplash may experience neck pain, headache, blurring of vision, dizziness, weakness, paresthesias, cognitive difficulty, and psychologic symptoms. Whiplash is often misunderstood because there usually are few radiographic and clinical abnormalities. Litigation issues further complicate the problem. Despite negative findings on imaging studies, injury to the zygapophyseal joints, intervertebral disks, muscles, and ligaments has been documented.

The condition of most patients with whiplash improves within the first few months after injury. Patients who have chronic symptoms are difficult to treat, and no definitive treatment has been established. Early in the treatment, mobilization is more beneficial than rest. Chronic symptoms may respond to injection of corticosteroids into the cervical zygapophyseal joints and physical therapy. Management of chronic pain is discussed in Chapter 10.

SPINAL SURGERY

The decision to perform spinal surgery should be made on the basis of specific clinical indications and in consultation with an orthopedic surgeon or neurosurgeon. The indications include compressive radiculopathy, myelopathy, and spinal instability. Acute myelopathy and cauda equina syndrome require emergency decompression surgery (Fig. 4.5). For radiculopathy with motor deficit, early surgical treatment optimizes early recovery. Other indications for spinal surgery are increasing neurologic deficit, incapacitating neurogenic claudication, motor weakness, and impaired bladder and bowel function. Surgical treatment for pain only or for patients with negative findings on imaging studies is ill advised.

Many factors influence surgical outcome. The most important is diagnostic accuracy. The patient's psychologic and social background is also important. Patients at risk for

Table 4.9. Differences Between Neurogenic and Vascular Claudication

Symptoms and signs	Neurogenic	Vascular
Pain at rest	Yes, if spine extended	No
Time to relief of symptoms with rest	5-20 min	1-2 min
Distance walked before onset of pain	Variable distance	Same distance
Vascular history	No	Yes
Leg pain with bicycling	No	Yes
Absent or reduced pedal pulses	No	Yes
Patient can continue walking after onset of pain	Yes, maybe	No

From Adams, AC: Neurology in Primary Care. FA Davis, Philadelphia, 2000, p 84. Used with permission of Mayo Foundation for Medical Education and Research.

a poor surgical outcome include those who have pending workers' compensation claims, have been on sick leave longer than 3 months, have features of nonorganic pain, or have unsatisfying jobs. Somatization, hysteria, and hypochondriasis are often demonstrated on tests such as the Minnesota Multiphasic Personality Inventory (MMPI).

The possible complications of surgery include diskitis, meningitis, cerebrospinal fluid leak, vascular injury, and neurologic deterioration. Recurrent disk herniation, scarring, and spinal instability are common postoperative complications. The more accurate the preoperative diagnosis, the better the surgical outcome and the less risk for reoperation.

PLEXOPATHY

Plexopathy is important to consider if the patient has limb pain, weakness, or numbness. Trauma, inflammation, neoplasm, ischemia, and radiation can cause plexopathy, which can also be idiopathic or inherited. The differential diagnosis of plexopathy is limited to involvement of nerve roots or multiple named nerves. The temporal profile of symptoms suggests the cause.

The brachial plexus is derived from cervical roots C5 through T1. Roots C5 and C6 form the upper trunk, C7 the middle trunk, and C8 and T1 the lower trunk (Fig. 4.13). The three trunks divide into anterior and posterior divisions. The posterior divisions come together as the posterior cord, which forms the axillary and radial nerves. The anterior

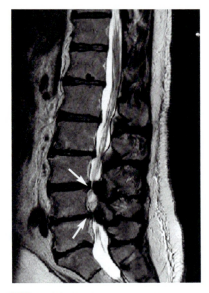

Fig. 4.12. MRI showing multilevel spinal stenosis (*arrows*). (Sagittal view.)

division of the lower trunk becomes the medial cord, which gives rise to the ulnar nerve and the C8 portion of the median nerve. The rest of the median nerve and the musculocutaneous nerve are from the lateral cord. Injuries above the clavicle affect the trunks, and injuries below the clavicle affect the cords. Trauma to the axilla affects the nerve branches.

The upper trunk of the brachial plexus is frequently traumatized in shoulder injuries such as an impact injury (called a "stinger") to the shoulder during a football game or injury from the recoil of a shotgun. Clinically, an upper trunk brachial plexopathy resembles avulsion of nerve roots C5 and C6. This plexopathy is caused by downward traction on the shoulder, as during a difficult delivery (Erb palsy). Hand strength is strong but the upper arm is weak.

The lower trunk of the brachial plexus can be affected by a cervical rib or a tumor of the lung apex (Pancoast tumor). Avulsion of the C8 and T1 nerve roots (Klumpke paralysis) is clinically similar to lesions of the lower trunk. Forceful traction of the arm upward can cause this injury, for example, when an adult pulls a child's arm. All intrinsic hand muscles are weak, and Horner syndrome can occur from injury to the sympathetic fibers in root T1. Distinguishing between root avulsion and plexus trauma is important because traumatic injuries to the plexus may be more amenable to surgical repair.

Obstetrical injury to the brachial plexus during delivery is well described. However, injury can also occur before birth. EMG studies performed soon after delivery may

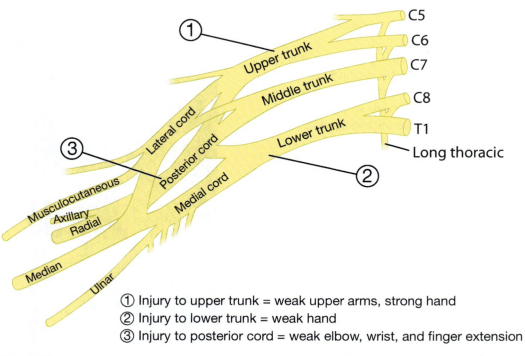

① Injury to upper trunk = weak upper arms, strong hand
② Injury to lower trunk = weak hand
③ Injury to posterior cord = weak elbow, wrist, and finger extension

Fig. 4.13. Brachial plexus. (Modified from Patten, J: Neurological Differential Diagnosis, ed 2. Springer-Verlag, London, 1996, p 297. Used with permission.)

show that brachial injury occurred before delivery. The medical-legal implications can be important.

The terms *brachial neuritis*, *Parsonage-Turner syndrome*, and *neuralgic amyotrophy* are all used to describe a presumed inflammatory condition of the brachial plexus. Evidence suggests that this is an immune-mediated condition. It has been reported to develop after vaccinations and viral illnesses. Males are affected more often than females. Shoulder pain frequently is the first symptom, followed by upper extremity weakness and numbness. The condition can be bilateral, and it usually resolves within 6 months to 1 year. Treatment is primarily supportive.

The brachial plexus is often affected by neoplasm. Also, radiation exposure can cause brachial plexopathy, from days to years after the exposure. The distinction between recurrent cancer and radiation-induced plexopathy may require clinical, electrophysiologic, and imaging studies. Plexopathy from recurrent cancer tends to be painful and to affect the lower plexus. In contrast, radiation-induced plexopathy tends to be painless and to affect the upper trunk. Myokymic discharges seen on EMG suggest radiation-induced plexopathy. MRI is sensitive for detecting tumor infiltration of the brachial plexus.

Compression of the brachial plexus and the brachial artery and vein at the thoracic outlet describes the *thoracic outlet syndrome*. Its diagnosis and management are matters of controversy. Compression is caused by an anomalous fibrous band or a cervical rib. Neurogenic thoracic outlet syndrome is extremely rare. The lower trunk of the plexus is affected and the patient should have weakness and numbness in the distribution of roots C8 and T1. In patients who do not have neurologic deficit, the hand pain may be due to compression of the brachial artery. Many physicians believe that

this condition is caused by drooping shoulders and that it responds to correcting the posture and strengthening the cervicoscapular muscles. Surgery is considered when conservative measures fail or when there is a structural anomaly such as a cervical rib.

The lumbosacral plexus is affected by the same types of conditions that affect the brachial plexus, although inflammatory conditions are less likely to affect the lumbosacral plexus. Involvement of the lumbar portion of the plexus mimics a femoral neuropathy, with weak hip flexion and knee extension. However, the two conditions can be distinguished by assessing the function of the obturator nerve (hip adduction). Weakness of hip adduction is not seen in femoral neuropathy. Abdominal surgery can often traumatize the lumbar portion of the plexus. The sacral portion of the plexus can be injured in hip surgery. Symptoms from injury to the sacral portion of the plexus may mimic sciatica.

Ischemic injury to the plexus from diabetes mellitus or other conditions that can cause a mononeuritis multiplex occurs suddenly and is extremely painful. Radiation-induced plexopathy, as mentioned above, tends to be painless. Lymphoma, leukemia, and tumors of the prostate, rectum, and cervix can affect the lumbosacral plexus. Bleeding into the iliopsoas muscle can also cause lumbosacral plexopathy.

The lateral femoral cutaneous nerve, a sensory nerve of the thigh, is a branch of L2 and L3 that innervates the skin of the lateral aspect of the thigh (Fig. 4.14). The nerve courses over the iliac crest and can be injured by seat belts, abdominal surgery, or tight clothing. Obesity and pregnancy can predispose patients to lateral femoral cutaneous neuropathy. The syndrome of pain and numbness in the distribution of this nerve is called *meralgia paresthetica*. Treatment with tricyclic antidepressants or anticonvulsants can lessen the symptoms. The reassurance of patients about this benign neuropathy is usually

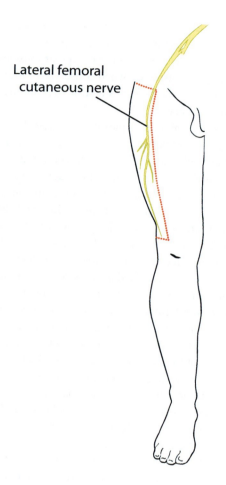

Lateral femoral
cutaneous nerve

Fig. 4.14. Distribution of lateral femoral cutaneous nerve.

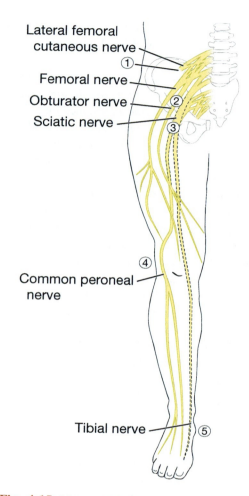

Lateral femoral
cutaneous nerve

①

Femoral nerve

Obturator nerve

②

Sciatic nerve

③

Common peroneal
nerve

④

Tibial nerve

⑤

Fig. 4.15. Nerves of the lower extremity. **1-5**, common sites of damage. **1**, Lateral femoral cutaneous nerve: compression at inguinal ligament; **2**, obturator nerve: complication of pelvic surgery; **3**, sciatic nerve: complication of hip surgery; **4**, common peroneal nerve: knee injury: "crossed-leg" palsy; **5**, tibial nerve: tarsal tunnel syndrome. (From Adams, AC: Neurology in Primary Care. FA Davis, Philadelphia, 2000, p 87. Used with permission of Mayo Foundation for Medical Education and Research.)

the most helpful treatment.

Mononeuropathies of the arm and leg can cause limb pain. The sites of common nerve injuries are shown in Figures 4.15 and 4.16. Focal neuropathies are discussed in Chapter 6.

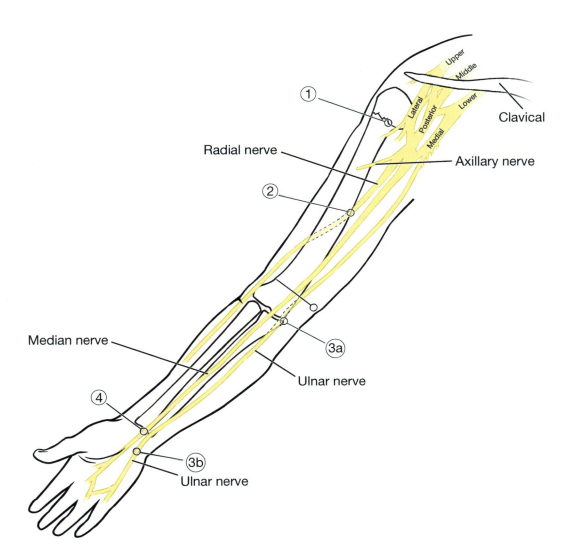

Fig. 4.16. Nerves of the upper extremity. Common sites of damage (**1-4**) and associated causes. **1**, Axillary nerve: fracture of humeral head, intramuscular injections; **2**, radial nerve: fracture of humerus, compression: "Saturday night palsy"; **3**, ulnar nerve: **a**, compression; **b**, trauma; **4**, median nerve: carpal tunnel syndrome. (From Patten, J: Neurological Differential Diagnosis, ed 2. Springer-Verlag, London, 1996, p 283. Used with permission.)

SUGGESTED READING

Atlas, SJ, and Delitto, A: Spinal stenosis: Surgical versus nonsurgical treatment. Clin Orthop Relat Res 443:198-207, 2006.

Braddom, RL: Perils and pointers in the evaluation and management of back pain. Semin Neurol 18:197-210, 1998.

Deen, HG, Jr: Diagnosis and management of lumbar disk disease. Mayo Clin Proc 71:283-287, 1996.

Deyo, RA, Diehl, AK, and Rosenthal, M: How many days of bed rest for acute low back pain? A randomized clinical trial. N Engl J Med 315:1064-1070, 1986.

Frymoyer, JW: Back pain and sciatica. N Engl J Med 318:291-300, 1988.

Greer, S, et al: Clinical inquiries: What physical exam techniques are useful to detect malingering? J Fam Pract 54:719-722, 2005.

Hadler, NM: Regional back pain. N Engl J Med 315:1090-1092, 1986.

Hagen, KB, et al: The updated Cochrane review of bed rest for low back pain and sciatica. Spine 30:542-546, 2005.

Haldeman, S: Diagnostic tests for the evaluation of back and neck pain. Neurol Clin 14:103-117, 1996.

Hazard, RG: Failed back surgery syndrome: surgical and nonsurgical approaches. Clin Orthop Relat Res 443:228-232, 2006.

Kasch, H, et al: Development in pain and neurologic complaints after whiplash: A 1-year prospective study. Neurology 60:743-749, 2003.

Khadilkar, A, et al: Transcutaneous electrical nerve stimulation for the treatment of chronic low back pain: A systematic review. Spine 30:2657-2666, 2005.

Levin, KH, Maggiano, HJ, and Wilbourn, AJ: Cervical radiculopathies: Comparison of surgical and EMG localization of single-root lesions. Neurology 46:1022-1025, 1996.

Nordin, M, Balague, F, and Cedraschi, C: Nonspecific lower-back pain: Surgical versus nonsurgical treatment. Clin Orthop Relat Res 443:156-167, 2006.

Paradiso, G, Granana, N, and Maza, E: Prenatal brachial plexus paralysis. Neurology 49:261-262, 1997.

Practice parameters: Magnetic resonance imaging in the evaluation of low back syndrome (summary statement). Report of the Quality Standards Subcommittee of the American Academy of Neurology. Neurology 44:767-770, 1994.

Rowland, LP: Surgical treatment of cervical spondylotic myelopathy: Time for a controlled trial. Neurology 42:5-13, 1992.

Samuels, MA, and Feske, SK (eds): Office Practice of Neurology, ed 2. Churchill Livingstone, Philadelphia, 2003.

Suarez, GA, et al: Immune brachial plexus neuropathy: Suggestive evidence for an inflammatory-immune pathogenesis. Neurology 46:559-561, 1996.

Thyagarajan, D, Cascino, T, and Harms, G: Magnetic resonance imaging in brachial plexopathy of cancer. Neurology 45:421-427, 1995.

Waddell, G, et al: Nonorganic physical signs in low-back pain. Spine 5:117-125, 1980.

Wolinsky, AP: The illusion of certainty. N Engl J Med 335:46-48, 1996.

CHAPTER 5

Dizziness

Patients frequently complain of "dizziness" and use this term to describe various symptoms. It can be difficult to obtain an accurate history of the symptoms, especially with the time constraints that clinicians often face. The symptom of dizziness requires taking an open-ended history. Direct questions often suggest symptoms to the patient and can lead to a wrong diagnosis. The first 10 questions to ask (or the question that should be asked 10 times) of a patient with a complaint of dizziness should be, "What do you mean by 'dizzy'?"

Dizziness has many mechanisms and causes. The diagnostic approach is simplified by categorizing dizziness into four different types. The first category is *vertigo*, that is, a sensation of movement. This type of dizziness implies a problem with the vestibular system and may be peripheral or central. The second category is *presyncope*, or the sensation of impending faint. This symptom indicates a disturbance of cardiovascular function. The third category is *dysequilibrium*, which is a disturbance of postural balance caused by a neurologic disorder. The fourth category is an *ill-defined* symptom characteristic of psychiatric disorders. It is important to remember that patients may have more than one type of dizziness. The four categories of dizziness, the mechanism associated with each type, and some common clinical examples are listed in Table 5.1.

DIAGNOSTIC APPROACH

The history is the most important aspect of the diagnostic work-up of a patient who presents with dizziness. The situation in which the patient responds, "You know, dizzy," is all too frequent and can be trying for you and the patient. It may help to ask the patient if the sensation compares with anything else he or she has experienced. Inquire about the associated symptoms, such as auditory, cardiac, neurologic, and psychiatric symptoms. Loss of hearing, tinnitus, and ear fullness may suggest involvement of the vestibulocochlear nerve (cranial nerve [CN] VIII) in the periphery. Ask about symptoms that indicate brainstem involvement, such as diplopia, dysarthria, visual disturbance, and ataxia. Medications frequently cause dizziness (thousands of drugs are associated with the complaint of dizziness and hundreds with vertigo). Some of the more

Table 5.1. Types of Dizziness and Their Mechanisms and Common Causes

Type	Mechanism	Common cause

Vertigo (sensation of movement)	Disturbance of vestibular function	Peripheral
		    Benign positional vertigo
		    Vestibular neuronitis
		    Labyrinthitis
		    Ménière disease
		Central
		    Vertebrobasilar ischemia
		    Multiple sclerosis
		    Posterior fossa tumor
		    Migraine

Presyncope (sensation of impending faint, light-headedness)	Diffuse or global cerebral ischemia	Cardiac
		    Arrhythmia
		    Vasovagal
		Orthostatic hypotension
		    Volume depletion
		    Medication effect
		    Autonomic insufficiency

Dysequilibrium (disturbance of postural balance)	Loss of vestibulospinal, proprioceptive, or cerebellar function	Ototoxicity Peripheral neuropathy Cerebellar dysfunction Drug intoxication Extrapyramidal syndrome
Ill-defined	Impaired central integration of sensory signals	Anxiety Panic disorder Hyperventilation syndrome Affective disorder

From Adams, AC: Neurology in Primary Care. FA Davis, Philadelphia, 2000, p 91. Used with permission of Mayo Foundation for Medical Education and Research.

common drugs associated with this symptom are listed in Table 5.2. The periodicity and the duration of symptoms, factors that provoke dizziness, and the circumstances associated with it are important historical details. Some of the clinical features associated with common causes of dizziness are listed in Table 5.3.

The physical examination should include measuring orthostatic blood pressure and pulse and examining the ear. Examination of the

patient's gait is a critical component of the neurologic evaluation. Patients with positional vertigo walk with very limited head movement. A wide-based ataxic gait may indicate cerebellar disease, and a slow, flexed, shuffling gait may indicate an extrapyramidal syndrome. Peripheral neuropathy should be suspected if the Romberg sign is present.

Dizziness may be stimulated by many tests. A patient may complain of dizziness if he or she

Table 5.2. **Drugs Associated With Dizziness**

Drug	Mechanism	Type of dizziness
Aminoglycoside antibiotics	Vestibular hair cell damage	Vertigo, dysequilibrium
Antihypertensives, diuretics	Postural hypotension, decreased cerebral blood flow	Presyncope
Anticonvulsants	Cerebellar toxicity	Dysequilibrium
Alcohol	CNS depression, cerebellar toxicity	Dysequilibrium, vertigo
Tranquilizers	CNS depression	Dysequilibrium
Antihistamines	CNS depression	Dysequilibrium
Tricyclic agents	CNS depression	Dysequilibrium
Methotrexate	Brainstem and cerebellar toxicity	Dysequilibrium
Anticoagulants	Hemorrhage into inner ear or brain	Vertigo
Cisplatin	Vestibular hair cell damage	Vertigo, dysequilibrium

CNS, central nervous system.
From Adams, AC: *Neurology in Primary Care.* FA Davis, Philadelphia, 2000, p 91. *Used with permission of Mayo Foundation for Medical Education and Research.*

hyperventilates for 3 minutes, changes position, or performs the Valsalva maneuver. Also, when a patient's orthostatic blood pressure and pulse are measured, the patient may complain of dizziness. If the Valsalva maneuver aggravates vertigo, the patient may have a perilymph fistula or a craniovertebral junction anomaly. This maneuver may also aggravate presyncope in patients who have cardiovascular disease.

A useful stimulation test for positional vertigo is a positioning maneuver called the *Nylen-Bárány* or *Dix-Hallpike test* (Fig. 5.1). It is performed by moving the patient from the sitting to the lying position, with the head extended back by 45 degrees. This is repeated with the head extended and turned to the right and then with the head extended and turned to the left. Examine the patient for positional nystagmus. The presence of nystagmus with this positional maneuver suggests positional vertigo.

Nystagmus is discussed further in the section on vertigo.

The laboratory evaluation of a patient who complains of dizziness may include audiometry, electronystagmography, posturography, brainstem auditory evoked responses, and neuroimaging. Auditory testing is helpful because of the close association between the auditory and vestibular systems from the level of the inner ear to the cerebral cortex. Office evaluation of hearing often includes assessing the patient's response to whisper, conversational speech, and shouting. A tuning fork can be useful in distinguishing between hearing loss due to middle ear disease (conductive) and that due to sensorineural injury. For the *Rinne test*, place the stem of a vibrating tuning fork on the patient's mastoid process until the vibrations are no longer audible to the patient, then hold the tuning fork next to the ear. Normally, the vibrations are

Table 5.3. Clinical Features of Common Causes of Dizziness

Type of dizziness	Diagnosis	Clinical features
Vertigo	Benign positional vertigo	Aggravated by certain head positions, positional nystagmus
	Vestibular neuronitis	Antecedent viral infection, spontaneous nystagmus
	Ménière disease	Fluctuating hearing loss, tinnitus
	Vertebrobasilar insufficiency	Focal neurologic signs and symptoms
Presyncope	Orthostatic hypotension	Occurs with standing, antihypertensives, peripheral neuropathy
	Vasovagal	Prolonged standing, heat
	Cardiogenic	Exertional, valvular disease, arrhythmias, angina
	Hyperventilation	Stressful situations, perioral and acral paresthesias
Dysequilibrium	Peripheral neuropathy	Trouble walking in the dark or on uneven surfaces
	Cerebellar dysfunction	Chronic and continuous
Ill-defined	Panic disorder	Provoked by stress, crowds, panic attacks
Physiologic	Motion sickness	Positive family history, migraine

From Adams, AC: Neurology in Primary Care. FA Davis, Philadelphia, 2000, p 92. Used with permission of Mayo Foundation for Medical Education and Research.

still audible when the tuning fork is held next to the ear, because air conduction is better than bone conduction. This is true, too, if the patient has sensorineural hearing loss. However, if the patient has conductive hearing loss, bone conduction is better than air conduction. Thus, the vibrations will not be heard when the tuning fork is moved from the mastoid and held next to the ear. The Rinne test is used in conjunction with the *Weber test*, in which the stem of the tuning fork is held on the vertex of the head. Normally, the vibrations are heard equally in both ears. This is also true for patients with conductive hearing loss. However, in patients with sensorineural hearing loss, the vibratory sounds are diminished in the affected ear.

Audiometry is a valuable screening test for patients who have vertigo, tinnitus, or hearing loss. In conductive hearing loss, all frequencies of sound are affected, but speech discrimination is preserved. If the cochlea or CN VIII is involved, high-frequency sounds are lost, and patients have difficulty with speech discrimination, especially if there is background noise. Consequently, they may be annoyed by loud speech. The audiograms in Figure 5.2 compare normal findings with those typical of asymmetric sensorineural hearing loss and asymmetric conductive hearing loss.

Electronystagmography is used to document a unilateral vestibular lesion and to determine whether it is peripheral or central. A

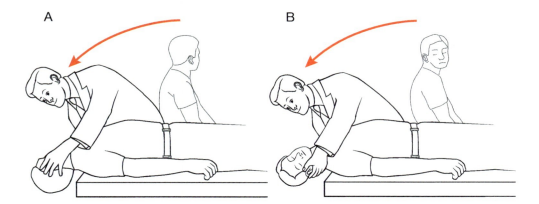

Fig. 5.1. Dix-Hallpike maneuver. *A*, The patient is brought from a sitting to a supine position, with the head turned to one side and extended about 45 degrees backward. When the patient is supine, the eyes are observed for nystagmus. *B*, The maneuver is repeated, with the head turned to the other side. (From Adams, AC: Neurology in Primary Care. FA Davis, Philadelphia, 2000, p 93. Used with permission of Mayo Foundation for Medical Education and Research.)

peripheral lesion is suggested by unidirectional spontaneous or positional nystagmus without visual fixation. Direction-changing spontaneous or positional nystagmus with fixation indicates a central lesion. If the patient is not taking any sedating medications, then abnormal saccades, abnormal smooth pursuit, and optokinetic nystagmus indicate a central lesion.

For posturography, place the patient on a platform that can be moved, so that the patient moves at the same time as the visual surroundings. This test was designed to assess the vestibular system without involving the visual and somatosensory systems. Instead of being used as a diagnostic tool, this test is better for following a patient's balance function.

Brainstem auditory evoked responses can help distinguish between nerve and cochlear lesions. The absence of all waveforms is not diagnostically useful. However, the delay of all waves indicates a conductive or cochlear problem. Delay of waves I through V indicates a CN VIII or brainstem lesion.

The clinical diagnosis should determine whether neuroimaging is required for the patient who complains of dizziness. Neuroimaging is needed for patients with cerebrovascular disease, but these conditions rarely occur with vertigo or dysequilibrium in isolation. Neuroimaging results are likely to be negative unless other neurologic symptoms or signs are present. Magnetic resonance imaging is preferred to computed tomography for evaluating the posterior fossa. However, computed tomography is valuable if an intracranial hemorrhage is suspected.

VERTIGO

Vertigo is the sensation of movement. Its presence implies a problem within the vestibular system (Fig. 5.3). The vestibular receptors are hair cells in the semicircular canals, utricle, and saccule of the inner ear. They are mechanoreceptors that detect changes in the motion and position of the head. This information is con-

Normal Audiogram

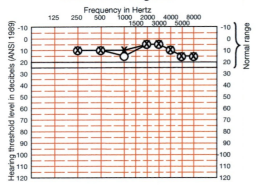

Right Conductive Hearing Loss

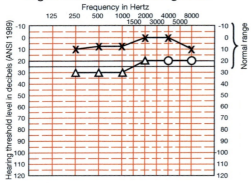

Right Sensorineural Hearing Loss

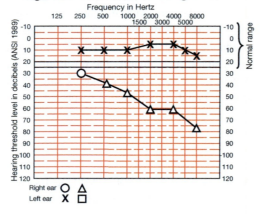

Right ear ○ △
Left ear ✗ ☐

Fig. 5.2. Audiograms. (From Adams, AC: Neurology in Primary Care. FA Davis, Philadelphia, 2000, p 94. Used with permission of Mayo Foundation for Medical Education and Research.)

veyed by CN VIII to the vestibular nuclei, which are located at the junction between the medulla and pons. Vestibular information is distributed widely to the cerebellum, the motor nuclei controlling eye and neck muscles, autonomic centers, and ventral horn cells that innervate skeletal muscles of the extremities and trunk. The cortical representation of the vestibular system is thought to involve the insula and the parietal, temporal, and frontal lobes.

If a patient has vertigo, first determine whether the problem is peripheral or central. Central disease involves disturbances of vestibular projections in the brainstem, cerebellum, or cerebral hemispheres. Some central causes of vertigo, such as cerebellar hemorrhage or infarction, require immediate intervention. Peripheral disease involves the cochlea and CN VIII in the internal auditory meatus or cerebellopontine angle.

A simple clinical test of the vestibulo-ocular reflex, called the *head thrust* or *head impulse test* (Fig. 5.4), helps determine if the patient has a peripheral or central cause of vertigo. The patient's head is held and a brief, small-amplitude, high acceleration head turn is applied to one side and then the other. The patient fixates on the examiner's nose while the examiner watches for corrective rapid eye movements (saccades). In a unilateral peripheral vestibular disorder, the eyes move with the head in one direction instead of staying fixed. A refixation saccade is seen that brings the eye back on to the target.

The patient may describe vertigo as "spinning," "falling," or "tilting" and compare the sensation to motion sickness or being drunk. Head movement and position changes often precipitate the sensation. Symptoms commonly associated with vertigo are nausea, vomiting, and oscillopsia (the subjective sensation of oscillation of viewed objects). Peripheral causes of vertigo are associated

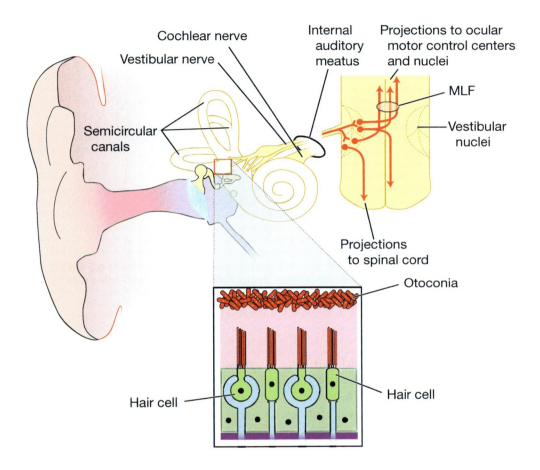

Fig. 5.3. Peripheral and central vestibular pathway. *Inset*, Enlarged view of vestibular receptors. *MLF*, medial longitudinal fasciculus. (From Adams, AC: Neurology in Primary Care. FA Davis, Philadelphia, 2000, p 95. Used with permission of Mayo Foundation for Medical Education and Research.)

with more severe nausea and vomiting than central causes are.

A patient with vertigo often has nystagmus. The presence of spontaneous or induced nystagmus is an important physical finding. Rhythmical oscillation of the eyes is called *nystagmus*. It may be horizontal, vertical, or rotatory. The direction of the fast phase designates the direction of the nystagmus. The presence of nystagmus indicates a problem involving the vestibular system, brainstem, cerebellum, or

cortical center for ocular pursuit. The features that distinguish peripheral nystagmus from central nystagmus are listed in Table 5.4.

If a patient has acute vertigo and imbalance, the most serious diagnosis to consider is cerebellar hemorrhage or infarct. Both of these conditions can cause a mass effect that causes brainstem compression and death. Prompt neuroimaging is needed if the patient has profound imbalance, direction-changing nystagmus, or focal neurologic findings. Because cerebellar

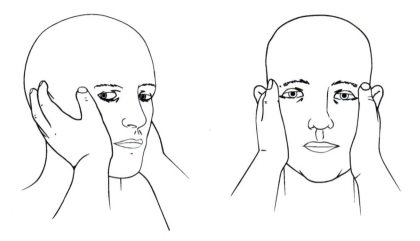

Fig. 5.4. Head thrust, or head impulse, test. The patient views a fixed target while the head is moved rapidly to one side. In cases of significant vestibulo-ocular reflex deficit, the eyes move with the head and a refixation saccade is observed that brings the eyes back on to the target.

infarcts may mimic a peripheral vestibular lesion, neuroimaging may be needed if the patient has cerebrovascular risk factors and it is difficult to evaluate his or her gait, balance, and eye movements.

The peripheral causes of vertigo include labyrinthitis, vestibular neuronitis, Ménière disease, syphilis, and drug effects (eg, aminoglycoside antibiotics). Benign positional vertigo can be due to otolithiasis and perilymph fistula. Acoustic schwannoma and meningioma cause peripheral vertigo. Severe trauma with a basilar skull fracture or vestibular concussion can cause vertigo.

Central diseases that cause vertigo include vascular disease (vertebrobasilar artery disease), migraine, and demyelinating disease (eg, multiple sclerosis). Anticonvulsant drugs, alcohol, and hypnotic agents can cause vertigo through a depressive effect on the central nervous system. Seizures rarely cause vertigo. The differences between peripheral and central vertigo are listed in Table 5.5.

Acute Vertigo

When a patient presents with acute and prolonged (more than a few hours) vertigo, the diagnostic considerations include vestibular neuritis (neuronitis), labyrinthitis, labyrinthine infarction, perilymph fistula, and brainstem and cerebellar infarction. The vertigo in vestibular neuritis develops over a period of hours, is severe for several days, and resolves within a few weeks. Often, a previous flulike illness is associated with vestibular neuritis. On physical examination, patients have spontaneous peripheral nystagmus, imbalance, and a positive head thrust test. Treatment of vestibular neuritis has been primarily symptomatic for nausea and vomiting (Table 5.6). Some advocate the use of these "vestibular sedatives" (agents listed in Table 5.6) only for severe nausea and vomiting because they suppress the ability of the nervous system to habituate and compensate for the vertigo. Corticosteroids and antiviral agents have been recommended for the treatment of vestibular neuritis. Because this condition

Table 5.4. Comparison of Peripheral and Central Nystagmus

Feature	Nystagmus	
	Peripheral	**Central**
Location of lesion	Labyrinthine or vestibular nerve	Brainstem or cerebellum
Gaze	Unidirectional	Usually changes direction
Appearance	Horizontal or rotatory	Vertical, horizontal, torsional
Fixation	Nystagmus is inhibited	Little effect
Direction change	Nystagmus increases when patient looks toward the fast phase	Change with convergence
Associated clinical features		
Nausea, vomiting	Severe	Variable
Hearing loss, ear symptoms	Common	Rare
Imbalance	Mild	Severe
Neurologic symptoms	Rare	Common

From Adams, AC: Neurology in Primary Care. FA Davis, Philadelphia, 2000, p 95. Used with permission of Mayo Foundation for Medical Education and Research.

improves spontaneously in most patients, many authorities recommend vestibular exercises and symptomatic treatment of the vertigo.

Labyrinthitis can develop over minutes to hours and can be associated with systemic, ear, or meningeal infection. The physical examination findings of these patients are comparable to those of patients who have vestibular neuritis, with the addition of unilateral hearing loss. Syphilitic labyrinthitis can lead

Table 5.5. Comparison of Peripheral and Central Vertigo

Feature	Vertigo	
	Peripheral	**Central**
Nausea and vomiting	Severe	Variable
Hearing loss, ear symptoms	Common	Rare
Imbalance	Mild	Severe
Nystagmus	Unidirectional, inhibited with fixation	Direction changing, not inhibited with fixation
Head thrust test	Positive	Negative
Neurologic symptoms	Rare	Common
Location of lesion	Labyrinthine or cranial nerve VIII	Brainstem, cerebellum

From Adams, AC: Neurology in Primary Care. FA Davis, Philadelphia, 2000, p 96. Used with permission of Mayo Foundation for Medical Education and Research.

Table 5.6. Medications for Symptomatic Treatment of Vertigo

Drug class and medication	Dosage	Relative contraindication
Antihistamines		
Dimenhydrinate (Dramamine)	50 mg orally every 4-6 hours	Prostate enlargement, asthma, glaucoma
Meclizine (Antivert)	25-50 mg orally 1-4 times daily	Prostate enlargement, asthma, glaucoma
Promethazine (Phenergan)	25 mg orally every 6 hours	History of seizures
Benzodiazepines		
Clonazepam (Klonopin)	0.5 mg orally 3 times daily	History of drug addiction
Diazepam (Valium)	2-10 mg 2-4 times daily	History of drug addiction
Lorazepam (Ativan)	1-2 mg orally 3 times daily	History of drug addiction
Anticholinergic agents		
Scopolamine (Transderm-Scop)	1 patch every 3 days	Prostate enlargement, asthma, glaucoma, liver or kidney disease
Phenothiazines		
Prochlorperazine (Compazine)	5-10 mg orally 3 times daily	Prostate enlargement, glaucoma
Butyrophenones		
Droperidol (Inapsine)	2.5 mg intramuscularly or intravenously	Cardiac disease

From Adams, AC: Neurology in Primary Care. FA Davis, Philadelphia, 2000, p 99. Used with permission of Mayo Foundation for Medical Education and Research.

to recurrent episodes of vertigo, hearing loss, and tinnitus.

Perilymph fistula is an abnormal communication between the perilymph of the inner ear and the middle ear. It should be considered if vertigo develops abruptly in association with trauma, heavy lifting or straining, coughing or sneezing, or barotrauma. Coughing or sneezing can cause severe vertigo because of the change in pressure that is transmitted directly to the inner ear. Patients with chronic otomastoiditis with cholesteatoma are at risk for this. The fistula test is positive when the Valsalva maneuver produces vertigo. Refer the patient to otolaryngology.

Labyrinthine ischemia has an abrupt onset and is usually associated with other neurologic signs and symptoms. Infarction confined to the inner ear or brainstem is usually the result of intra-arterial thrombosis of the posterior

inferior cerebellar artery, anterior inferior cerebellar artery, or superior cerebellar artery.
Isolated episodes of vertigo may represent
transient ischemic attacks and may precede
infarction of the labyrinth. This diagnosis
should be suspected if the patient has cerebrovascular risk factors and suddenly develops
hearing loss and vertigo.

Vertigo due to vertebrobasilar ischemia
is usually associated with other neurologic
symptoms. However, vertigo can be the only
symptom of vertebrobasilar ischemia and
should be suspected in a patient who has prominent cerebrovascular risk factors. Ischemia of
the vestibular system in the brainstem should
be suspected if a patient has unexplained
vomiting that seems out of proportion to the
symptoms of dizziness.

Vertebrobasilar ischemia can cause recurrent attacks of vertigo. Associated symptoms
include visual symptoms, unsteadiness, extremity numbness or weakness, dysarthria, confusion,
and drop attacks. The most common causes of
vertebrobasilar ischemia are embolism, large-
artery atherosclerosis, penetrating small-artery
disease, and arterial dissection. The diagnosis
is made on the basis of associated clinical signs
and symptoms.

Recurrent Vertigo

Patients often complain of recurrent
episodes of vertigo. The duration of the
episodes is important. Transient ischemic
attacks usually last minutes, as compared with
hours for diseases of the inner ear. The differential diagnosis of recurrent attacks of vertigo
includes vertebrobasilar ischemia, multiple
sclerosis, Ménière disease, autoimmune inner
ear disease, syphilis, and migraine.

Ménière disease is characterized by recurrent episodes of vertigo, tinnitus, and a fluctuating low-frequency hearing loss. All three of these
features may not be present initially. Sudden

falling spells, called *otolithic catastrophes*, have
been reported in this disorder. In Ménière disease, the volume of the endolymph increases,
causing distention of the endolymphatic system.
Treatment recommendations include a salt-
restricted diet, diuretics, and vestibular suppressants. Ablative surgery is performed for
intractable cases.

Autoimmune disease of the inner ear can
cause recurrent episodes of vertigo. The patient
may present with a fluctuating hearing loss,
tinnitus, and vertigo suggestive of Ménière disease. Unlike Ménière disease, autoimmune disease of the inner ear progresses rapidly over
weeks to months and involves both ears. This
disorder may involve only the inner ear or may
be part of a systemic autoimmune disease such
as polyarteritis nodosa or rheumatoid arthritis.
Inner ear disease in conjunction with interstitial keratitis is called *Cogan syndrome*. These
disorders have been treated with corticosteroids,
cytotoxic drugs, and plasmapheresis.

Syphilis, acquired or congenital, can cause
recurrent episodes of vertigo and hearing loss.
Syphilis can cause meningitis involving CN
VIII, and it can cause temporal bone osteitis
with labyrinthitis. The diagnosis is based on
positive findings on a fluorescent treponemal
antibody absorption test. The VDRL test is
positive in only 74% of cases. Treat syphilitic
ear infections with penicillin.

The association between vertigo and
migraine is strong, and patients with migraine
frequently have vertigo as part of their headache
syndrome. Motion sensitivity is reported by
more than 50% of patients with migraine.
Vertigo without headache can be a symptom of
migraine. This diagnosis should be suspected
in a patient with recurrent attacks of vertigo
who has a history of migraine or a positive
family history of migraine.

Positional vertigo is a common problem
that is often due a benign condition, such as

viral infection or head trauma. However, the cause is usually idiopathic. The mechanism of positional vertigo is attributed to lesions of the otoliths and connections of the vestibular nuclei. Under the influence of gravity, otoliths move from one position to another in the semicircular canals and cause positional vertigo.

In benign positional vertigo, patients experience vertigo with a change in head position. The onset of symptoms often occurs when patients get into or out of bed or when they extend their neck, the *top shelf syndrome*. The diagnosis can be confirmed by eliciting fatigable nystagmus during the positioning maneuver described in Figure 5.1.

Benign positional vertigo is usually caused by otolithiasis of the posterior semicircular canal. A variant involves the horizontal semicircular canal. Patients with this variant often complain that they have vertigo when they turn over in bed or when they turn their head from side to side while walking.

Benign positional vertigo can be treated effectively by procedures designed to rotate the freely moving otoliths around the semicircular canal. One of these methods is the *canalith repositioning procedure* (Fig. 5.5). After the procedure has been performed, have the patient keep the head upright for 48 hours. The maneuver is repeated as needed. The variant of benign positional vertigo also responds to a positioning maneuver—one that rotates the head in the plane of the horizontal semicircular canal.

Central causes of positional vertigo include multiple sclerosis, brainstem tumor, cerebellar tumor or atrophy, and Arnold–Chiari malformation. These conditions are usually associated with other neurologic findings. Nystagmus due to a central cause is nonfatigable.

As noted above, the treatment of vertigo is primarily symptomatic. All the medications listed in Table 5.6 can cause drowsiness, and patients should be advised accordingly. Antihistamines have moderate vestibular suppression capabilities and a minimal antiemetic effect. In comparison, benzodiazepines are more effective vestibular suppressants. The most effective antiemetic agents, such as prochlorperazine (Compazine), have little vestibular suppressant effect. Droperidol (Inapsine) is an effective antiemetic and vestibular suppressant (Table 5.6).

PRESYNCOPE

The sensation of impending faint is often described as "dizziness." This sensation implies a disturbance of cardiovascular function. The mechanism for this type of dizziness is pancerebral ischemia. Cardiac causes of presyncope or syncope include arrhythmias, valvular disease, vasovagal (reflex syncope), and carotid sinus hypersensitivity. Orthostatic hypotension, defined as a decrease in systolic blood pressure of 20 mm Hg or more, can be caused by cardiac dysfunction, decreased intravascular volume, venous pooling, or medications. Common medications that can cause orthostatic hypotension include diuretics, antihypertensive agents, antianginal agents, and tricyclic antidepressants.

Neurologic causes of orthostatic hypotension or autonomic dysfunction include disorders of the central or peripheral nervous system. Although central nervous system disorders such as pure autonomic failure, dysautonomias, or multiple system atrophy can cause orthostatic hypotension, they are relatively rare. A more common cause of autonomic dysfunction is parkinsonism or cerebrovascular disease.

Most cases of autonomic dysfunction involve disease of the peripheral nervous system. Diabetes mellitus, amyloidosis, connective tissue disease, neoplasia, human immunodeficiency virus infection, and pernicious anemia can cause autonomic neuropathy. In most developed countries, diabetes mellitus is the most

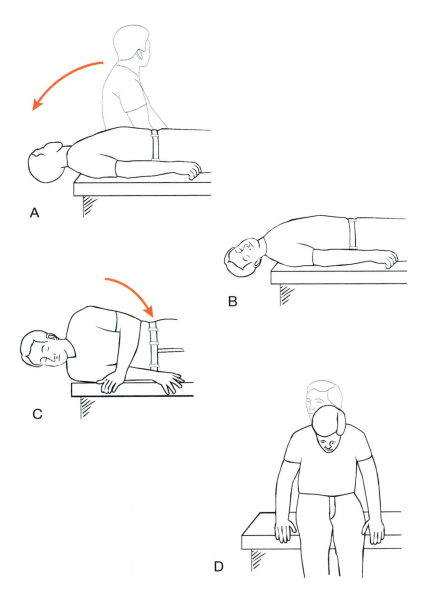

Fig. 5.5. Canalith repositioning procedure. (Modified from Dizziness. Mayo Clinic Health Letter 12:2, December 1994. Used with permission of Mayo Foundation for Medical Education and Research.)

common cause. The symptoms of orthostatic hypotension include dizziness, blurred or tunnel vision, and head and neck discomfort. The clinical features of autonomic neuropathies are protean (Table 5.7).

The management of symptomatic hypotension entails both pharmacologic and nonpharmacologic measures. Patients need to exercise care when changing positions, and they need to know that hypotension can be caused by certain

Table 5.7. Clinical Features of Autonomic Neuropathies

System	Features
Gastrointestinal	Nausea, vomiting, early satiety, postprandial bloating, epigastric pain, constipation, diarrhea (nighttime)
Genitourinary	Urinary retention, inadequate bladder emptying, overflow incontinence
Sudomotor	Anhidrosis (stocking-glove distribution), compensatory hyperhidrosis, gustatory sweating
Cardiovascular	Increased heart rate, fixed heart rate

From Adams, AC: Neurology in Primary Care. FA Davis, Philadelphia, 2000, p 100. Used with permission of Mayo Foundation for Medical Education and Research.

stimuli and situations. These include hot ambient temperatures, large meals, prolonged recumbency, isometric exercise, hyperventilation, standing motionless, alcohol consumption, and straining at stool or with voiding. Any unnecessary medications should be eliminated. Increased sodium intake, the use of elastic or compression stockings, and raising the head of the bed can help prevent hypotension.

Medications used to treat orthostatic hypotension—acetylcholinesterase inhibitor, mineralcorticoids, sympathomimetic amines, prostaglandin synthetase inhibitors, and others—are listed in Table 5.8. The most serious problem with these agents is supine hypertension.

DYSEQUILIBRIUM

Many patients who complain of dizziness describe "unsteadiness" or a concern that they might fall. Dysequilibrium is a disturbance in postural balance. Postural balance depends on visual, somatosensory, and vestibular sensory input. Dysequilibrium may result from a disorder of sensory input or the central processing of this input and the motor response. Causes of dysequilibrium are listed in Table 5.9.

Disturbance of two of the three sensory inputs is called *multisensory dysequilibrium*. An example is a patient with diabetes mellitus who has both peripheral neuropathy and retinopathy. Dysequilibrium is a major problem, especially among the elderly population, because of the risk of falling. Medications such as meclizine that can cause drowsiness and blurred vision are ill-advised for these patients.

Bilateral vestibular dysfunction also causes dysequilibrium. The diagnosis should be suspected if the patient complains of unsteadiness and oscillopsia. A history of vertigo or exposure to ototoxic drugs supports the diagnosis. Classes of ototoxic drugs include antibiotics (especially aminoglycosides), antiinflammatory, antimalarial, diuretic, and antineoplastic agents. The more common ototoxic medications are listed in Table 5.10. On examination, patients with bilateral vestibular dysfunction are unsteady but do not show any signs of cerebellar dysfunction. In addition to the causes listed in Table 5.9, idiopathic, congenital, familial, and infectious conditions can cause bilateral vestibular loss.

Patients with sensory ataxia often complain of dizziness. Peripheral neuropathies are the most common cause of sensory ataxia. Patients may report that they have increasing

Table 5.8. Pharmacologic Agents for Treating Orthostatic Hypotension

Acetylcholinesterase inhibitor
    Pyridostigmine
Mineralcorticoid
    Fludrocortisone
Sympathomimetic agents
    Clonidine
    Dextroamphetamine
    Ephedrine
    Methylphenidate
    Midodrine
    Phenylpropanolamine
    Pseudoephedrine
Prostaglandin synthetase inhibitors
    Ibuprofen
    Indomethacin
    Naproxen
Nonspecific pressor agents
    Caffeine
    Ergot derivatives
β-Adrenergic blocking agent
    Propranolol
Dopamine blocking agent
    Metoclopramide

From Adams, AC: Neurology in Primary Care. FA Davis, Philadelphia, 2000, p 100. Used with permission of Mayo Foundation for Medical Education and Research.

difficulty walking in the dark or maintaining their balance in the shower when they close their eyes. Uneven surfaces are frequently more difficult to walk on, and there is a tendency to fall. Neurologic examination shows reduced peripheral proprioception, Romberg sign, and reduced ankle reflexes. Peripheral neuropathies are discussed in Chapter 6. Myelopathies can also cause sensory ataxia.

Many neurologic disorders are associated with dysequilibrium. Cerebellar dysfunction can be the source of dizziness. The findings on physical examination of a patient with cerebellar dysfunction are those seen in acute alcohol intoxication. Familiar signs of cerebellar dysfunction are nystagmus, dysarthria, wide-based ataxic gait, intention tremor, and dysdiadochokinesia. Chronic alcohol consumption can lead to similar findings. Cerebellar symptoms in a patient with ovarian cancer or small cell carcinoma of the lung should raise the suspicion of a paraneoplastic syndrome. Many familial degenerative disorders of the cerebellum can present as dizziness. These genetic degenerative disorders progress much more slowly than do paraneoplastic syndromes.

Dysequilibrium is common in patients with Parkinson disease, parkinsonism, or gait apraxia. Apractic gait is wide-based, with slow and short steps. Patients have difficulty with starting and turning and often appear as though their feet are glued to the ground. This type of gait is called a *frontal gait*, or *lower body parkinsonism*. It is the characteristic gait of patients who have normal-pressure hydrocephalus, multiple strokes, or a frontal lobe syndrome.

ILL-DEFINED DIZZINESS

Dizziness that cannot be categorized as vertigo, presyncope, or dysequilibrium may fall into the *ill-defined group*. This category of dizziness has been called functional, psychogenic, hyperventilation syndrome, phobic postural vertigo, and psychiatric dizziness. It has been estimated that 20% to 50% of all patients who complain of dizziness have this type of dizziness. Features that characterize psychiatric dizziness have traditionally included the absence of true vertigo, replication of symptoms with hyperventilation, psychiatric symptoms preceding the

Table 5.9. Causes of Dysequilibrium

Disorders of sensory input
   Peripheral neuropathy
      Diabetes mellitus, vitamin B_{12} deficiency, hypothyroidism, syphilis
   Myelopathy
      Cervical spondylosis, subacute combined degeneration (vitamin B_{12} deficiency),
         tabes dorsalis
   Bilateral vestibular loss
      Ototoxic drugs, meningitis, autoimmune disorders, hydrocarbon solvents, bilateral
         Ménière disease, bilateral vestibular neuritis
Disorders of central processing and motor response
   Cerebellar dysfunction
      Chronic alcohol use, cerebellar degeneration, paraneoplastic syndrome
   Apractic syndromes
      Multi-infarct state, hydrocephalus, frontal lobe lesions
   Extrapyramidal syndromes
      Parkinson disease, progressive supranuclear palsy, striatonigral degeneration

From Adams, AC: Neurology in Primary Care. FA Davis, Philadelphia, 2000, p 101. Used with permission of Mayo Foundation for Medical Education and Research.

onset of dizziness, and the presence of dizziness in anxious or phobic patients.

This concept of psychiatric dizziness has several problems: 1) vertigo does not distinguish between psychiatric and otologic disorders, 2) hyperventilation can cause symptoms in many disorders, and 3) patients with psychiatric illness are not immune to otologic disorders. Furthermore, fear and anxiety are common symptoms of patients who have vestibular disease. A more restricted definition of psychiatric dizziness is dizziness that occurs in combination with other symptoms as part of a recognized psychiatric symptom cluster that is not itself related to vestibular function.

Panic disorder is the psychiatric diagnosis that includes dizziness, vertigo, or unsteady feelings as a diagnostic criterion. Patients with depressive symptoms may describe the difficulty they have with concentrating as a "dizzy"

or "swimming" feeling. Dizziness as part of a conversion disorder or malingering is rare. Dizziness and imbalance are not features of personality disorders.

Table 5.10. Ototoxic Drugs

Drug	Effect	
	Vestibulotoxic	**Cochleotoxic**
Cisplatin	High	High
Gentamicin	High	Low
Tobramycin	Moderate	Moderate
Amikacin	Low	High
Aspirin	…	Low
Furosemide	…	Low

From Adams, AC: Neurology in Primary Care. FA Davis, Philadelphia, 2000, p 101. Used with permission of Mayo Foundation for Medical Education and Research.

It is important not to confuse psychogenic overlay, or amplification of somatic concerns, with psychiatric dizziness. Many patients have a tendency to exaggerate their symptoms and complicate the diagnosis. Patients with hypochondria are prone to exaggeration. Psychogenic overlay is frequent in patients with depressive, panic, or somatoform disorders. It is important to remember that many patients experience more than one kind of dizziness.

SUGGESTED READING

Baloh, RW: Clinical practice: Vestibular neuritis. N Engl J Med 348:1027-1032, 2003.

Baloh, RW, et al: Neurotology. Continuum: Lifelong Learning in Neurology 2:9-132, 1996.

Baloh, RW, and Jacobson, KM: Neurotology. Neurol Clin 14:85-101, 1996.

Dieterich, M: Dizziness. Neurologist 10:154-164, 2004.

Fisher, CM: Vomiting out of proportion to dizziness in ischemic brainstem strokes. Neurology 46:267, 1996.

Furman, JM, and Jacob, RG: Psychiatric dizziness. Neurology 48:1161-1166, 1997.

Gizzi, M, Riley, E, and Molinari, S: The diagnostic value of imaging the patient with dizziness: A Bayesian approach. Arch Neurol 53:1299-1304, 1996.

Gomez, CR, et al: Isolated vertigo as a manifestation of vertebrobasilar ischemia. Neurology 47:94-97, 1996.

Guldin, WO, and Grusser, OJ: Is there a vestibular cortex? Trends Neurosci 21:254-259, 1998.

Halmagyi, GM: Diagnosis and management of vertigo. Clin Med 5:159-165, 2005.

Lanska, DJ, and Remler, B: Benign paroxysmal positioning vertigo: Classic descriptions, origins of the provocative positioning technique, and conceptual developments. Neurology 48:1167-1177, 1997.

Low, PA: Diabetic autonomic neuropathy. Semin Neurol 16:143-151, 1996.

Radtke, A, et al: Self-treatment of benign paroxysmal positional vertigo: Semont maneuver vs Epley procedure. Neurology 63:150-152, 2004.

Robertson, D, and Davis, TL: Recent advances in the treatment of orthostatic hypotension. Neurology 45 Suppl 5:S26-S32, 1995.

Samuels, MA, and Feske, SK: Office Practice of Neurology, ed 2. Churchill Livingstone, Philadelphia, 2003.

Savitz, SI, and Caplan, LR: Vertebrobasilar disease. N Engl J Med 352:2618-2626, 2005.

Singer, W, et al: Acetylcholinesterase inhibition in patients with orthostatic intolerance. J Clin Neurophysiol 23:476-481, 2006.

Staab, JP: Chronic dizziness: The interface between psychiatry and neuro-otology. Curr Opin Neurol 19:41-48, 2006.

Straube, A: Pharmacology of vertigo/nystagmus/oscillopsia. Curr Opin Neurol 18:11-14, 2005.

Strupp, M, et al: Methylprednisolone, valacyclovir, or the combination for vestibular neuritis. N Engl J Med 351:354-361, 2004.

CHAPTER 6

Sensory Loss and Paresthesias

Diseases of the peripheral nervous system are common. Patients often present with complaints of numbness and tingling. The many diagnostic possibilities include endocrinopathies, malignancies, infections, and metabolic, toxic, inflammatory, and genetic disorders. Considering all the potential causes of polyneuropathy is impractical. It has been estimated that a cause will not be identified, despite a thorough evaluation, in almost one-half of patients who have neuropathy (13%-22% at specialty centers). Diagnosis is essential to avoid missing a correctable neuropathy and to provide accurate prognostic information. This chapter considers the common polyneuropathies and focal neuropathies that underlie patients' complaints of sensory loss and paresthesias (ie, spontaneous abnormal sensations).

DIAGNOSTIC APPROACH

The anatomy of a peripheral nerve is shown in Figure 6.1. Disease of peripheral nerves may involve motor, sensory, and autonomic nerve fibers (axons). Motor fibers and the sensory fibers that convey vibratory and joint position sensations are large-diameter myelinated axons. Autonomic fibers are small-diameter myelinated axons, and sensory fibers that convey pain and temperature sensations are small-diameter myelinated and unmyelinated axons. The symptoms that a patient with disease of the peripheral nervous system reports and the signs that may be found on examination are summarized in Table 6.1.

In evaluating a patient who has sensory loss or paresthesias, first determine whether there is disease of the peripheral nervous system. Some of the many disorders that may mimic peripheral nerve disease are listed in Table 6.2. After establishing that the patient has disease of the peripheral nervous system, determine whether the pattern of involvement is focal, multifocal, or diffuse. Localization of the neuropathy should answer many questions. Does the process involve an individual nerve, nerve root, plexus, or several nerves? Is the neuropathy diffuse? Is the neuropathy symmetrical? Does the process affect distal or proximal aspects of the extremities? Localization is based on the clinical examination and can be supplemented by electrodiagnostic tests. Knowledge of the distribution of individual

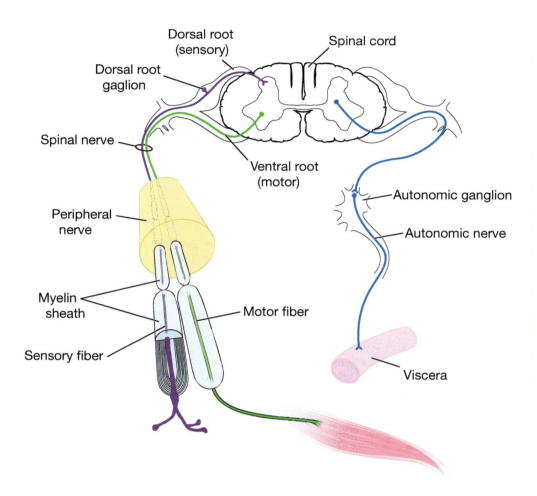

Fig. 6.1. Structure of a peripheral nerve. (Modified from Leeson, TS, and Leeson, CR: Histology, ed 4. WB Saunders, Philadelphia, 1981, p 218. Used with permission.)

nerves and patterns of sensory involvement helps to localize the problem (Fig. 6.2).

Most neuropathies are symmetrical, and the patient has distal symptoms and findings. This reflects axonal degeneration, the most common type of pathologic process, with injury to the distal ends of the longest nerves. Thus, patients report sensory loss and paresthesias in their feet. Large-fiber paresthesias are often described as "pins and needles" or an "electric sensation." These neuropathies have

the common stocking-glove pattern. The fingers usually are not affected until the "stocking" pattern is at the level of the upper calf. In rare neuropathies like porphyria and some inflammatory demyelinating neuropathies, proximal areas can be involved before distal areas. The common physical findings in a length-dependent axonal neuropathy are decreased sensation or absence of sensation distally in the lower extremities, decreased ankle reflexes or absence of ankle reflexes, Romberg sign, and difficulty

Table 6.1. General Clinical Features of Peripheral Nervous System Disease

Nerve	Historical symptoms	Physical signs
Sensory	Numbness Tingling, burning, "pins and needles" sensation Clumsiness	Sensory loss, areflexia, hypotonia, ataxia
Motor	Weakness, clumsiness, cramps, muscle twitches	Weakness, atrophy, fasciculations, areflexia, hypotonia, deformities (pes cavus, kyphoscoliosis)
Autonomic	Light-headedness, fainting, excessive sweating, heat intolerance, impotence, bowel and bladder disturbance	Orthostatic blood pressure changes, hyperhidrosis, anhidrosis, pupil abnormalities

From Adams, AC: Neurology in Primary Care. FA Davis, Philadelphia, 2000, p 105. Used with permission of Mayo Foundation for Medical Education and Research.

Table 6.2. Disorders That Mimic Peripheral Nerve Disease

Symptom/sign	Disorder	Distinguishing clinical feature
Generalized weakness	Myopathy	Normal sensation
	Myasthenia gravis	Normal sensation
	Motor neuron disease	Normal sensation
Sensory symptoms	Myelopathies	Sensory level
	Multiple sclerosis	Upper motor neuron signs
	Syringomyelia	Sensory dissociation
	Dorsal column disease (tabes dorsalis)	Sensory dissociation
Multiple symptoms	Conversion disorder, somatoform disorder	Nonanatomical features
	Malingering	Secondary gain, disability issues

From Adams, AC: Neurology in Primary Care. FA Davis, Philadelphia, 2000, p 106. Used with permission of Mayo Foundation for Medical Education and Research.

performing tandem gait. If the patient has difficulty walking on the toes and heels, suspect motor involvement. Marked weakness or inability to extend the foot may result in footdrop. Bilateral footdrop causes a high steppage gait (Fig. 6.3); thus, the foot is not scraped on the ground. Muscle bulk may be reduced in the interossei muscles of the hands or in the extensor digitorum muscles of the feet (Fig. 6.4). Anhidrotic skin, pupil abnormalities, and orthostatic changes indicate involvement of autonomic nerves.

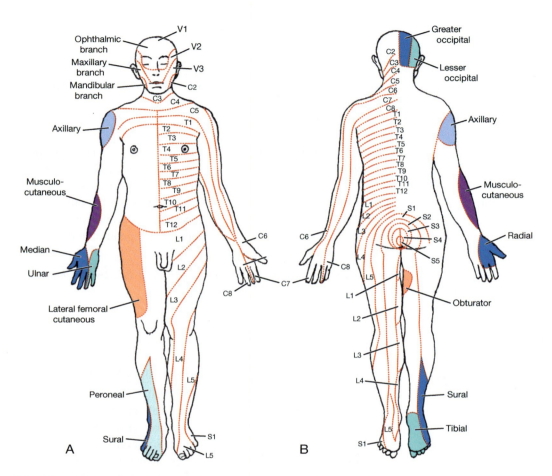

Fig. 6.2. Dermatomes and area of distribution of peripheral nerves. *A*, Anterior and *B*, posterior views. V1, V2, V3, branches of cranial nerve V. (From Adams, AC: Neurology in Primary Care. FA Davis, Philadelphia, 2000, p 21. Used with permission of Mayo Foundation for Medical Education and Research.)

Patients with small-fiber neuropathies may have few abnormal findings on neurologic examination except for reduced pain and touch sensations in the distal lower extremities. They often complain of painful burning dysesthesias. Other adjectives used to describe the paresthesias include "stinging," "coldness," and "heat." Nonpainful stimuli such as a sheet or blanket covering the feet can be painful (allodynia). The findings on electrodiagnostic tests are often normal. Important causes of small-fiber neuropathies

are diabetes mellitus, amyloidosis, human immunodeficiency virus (HIV) infection, acquired immunodeficiency syndrome (AIDS), and alcohol abuse. Small-fiber neuropathies involve the autonomic nervous system. Diabetes mellitus is the most common cause of an autonomic neuropathy. If a patient has an autonomic neuropathy but does not have diabetes, consider amyloidosis.

Asymmetry is an important finding and suggests a mononeuropathy multiplex pattern,

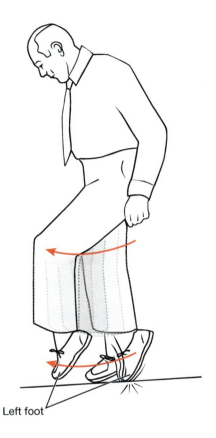

Left foot

Fig. 6.3. Steppage gait.

a superimposed radiculopathy, an entrapment mononeuropathy, or an acquired demyelinating neuropathy. The pattern of mononeuropathy multiplex is distinct from that of a length-dependent "dying back" axonal neuropathy. Individual cranial nerves and peripheral nerves are involved in an asymmetrical stepwise progression. Over time, the pattern may become confluent and difficult to distinguish from a generalized polyneuropathy. The temporal profile of symptoms is helpful in this regard. Mononeuropathy multiplex is important to recognize because many of its causes can be treated. Disorders associated with mononeuropathy multiplex include vasculitis, leprosy,

sarcoidosis, chronic inflammatory polyradiculoneuropathy, some malignancies, diabetes, and HIV infection or AIDS.

The patient's history provides the temporal course, or how the neuropathy has evolved over time. Most neuropathies are chronic and slowly progressive; thus, whether the onset is acute or subacute limits the extensive differential diagnosis. Acute inflammatory demyelinating polyradiculoneuropathy (AIDP, or Guillain-Barré syndrome) has an onset of days to weeks. A mononeuropathy multiplex pattern is suggested if the neuropathy progresses in a stepwise fashion. For example, the onset of sensory loss and weakness in the distribution of one nerve is followed by similar symptoms in the distribution of another nerve. A history of relapsing and remitting sensory symptoms suggests either autoimmune inflammatory neuropathy or an exposure or intoxication. Neuropathies that can be differentiated on the basis of their clinical course are listed in Table 6.3.

The next major distinction to make is whether the neuropathy is acquired or hereditary. This distinction may be difficult because inherited polyneuropathies begin gradually and progress very slowly. The family history may be negative or a family history of "polio" or "arthritis" may in fact represent an inherited neuropathy. The important clues to an inherited neuropathy include skeletal abnormalities of the foot (pes cavus) (Fig. 6.5) and spine (kyphoscoliosis), the absence of positive sensory phenomena, and positive findings in asymptomatic family members. Hereditary motor and sensory neuropathies include most of the inherited neuropathies and account for the many cases in which diagnosis is difficult. Understanding these disorders genetically is rapidly increasing, and many genetic tests are available. The diagnosis of inherited neuropathy is important for prognosis and genetic counseling.

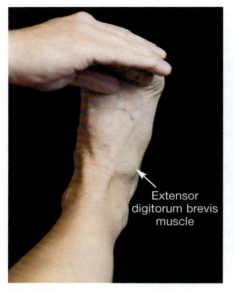
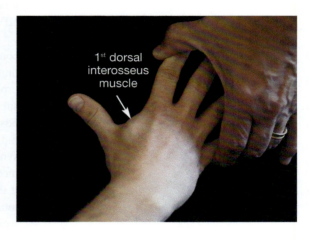

1st dorsal
interosseus
muscle

Extensor
digitorum brevis
muscle

Fig. 6.4. Topography of the extensor digitorum brevis muscle of the foot and the interosseous muscles of the hand.

Clues to systemic and other medical illnesses associated with peripheral neuropathies are provided by the general history and physical examination findings. It is important to look for historical and physical evidence of diabetes mellitus and other endocrinopathies, cancer, connective tissue disorders, infections, and deficiency states. The patient's occupational

Table 6.3. Neuropathy Differential Diagnosis by Temporal Profile

Acute (days)	Subacute (weeks to months)	Relapsing-remitting course
AIDP	CIDP	AIDP
Porphyria	Paraneoplastic syndrome	CIDP
Infarction (vasculitis)	Continued toxic exposure	Porphyria
Diabetes mellitus (diabetic radiculoplexus neuropathy)	Abnormal metabolic state	HIV/AIDS
Diphtheria	Persisting nutritional deficiency	Toxic
Toxins (thallium, arsenic)		
Tick paralysis		
Trauma		
Critical illness neuropathy		

AIDP, acute inflammatory demyelinating polyradiculoneuropathy; AIDS, acquired immunodeficiency syndrome; CIDP, chronic inflammatory demyelinating polyradiculoneuropathy; HIV, human immunodeficiency virus.
From Adams, AC: Neurology in Primary Care. FA Davis, Philadelphia, 2000, p 107. Used with permission of Mayo Foundation for Medical Education and Research.

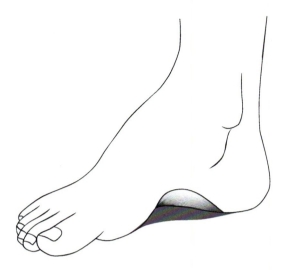

Fig. 6.5. Pes cavus. (From Adams, AC: Neurology in Primary Care. FA Davis, Philadelphia, 2000, p 108. Used with permission of Mayo Foundation for Medical Education and Research.)

and exposure history is important in narrowing the differential diagnosis of neuropathy. Alcohol is a frequent cause of toxic neuropathy. In addition, many prescription and over-the-counter medications can cause neuropathy (Table 6.4). Most of these drugs damage peripheral nerve axons. Amiodarone, chloroquine, and gold affect Schwann cells and cause a demyelinating neuropathy, and cisplatin, pyridoxine, and thalidomide injure axons.

Electrodiagnostic tests are invaluable in evaluating patients who have sensory loss and paresthesias due to disease of peripheral nerves. Electromyography and nerve conduction studies confirm the presence of a neuropathy, help localize the neuropathy (focal, multifocal, or diffuse), and predict the pathologic process (eg, demyelinating or axonal neuropathy). Electrodiagnostic tests can also provide information about the symmetry, chronicity, and severity. The important diagnostic distinction

between demyelinating and axonal neuropathies cannot be made without electrodiagnostic tests. Because most neuropathies are axonal, the presence of a demyelinating neuropathy restricts the differential diagnosis. In axonal neuropathy, the amplitude of the nerve action potential is decreased and, on needle examination, denervation potentials are found in the affected muscles. With demyelinating neuropathy, the findings include slow nerve conduction velocities, prolonged distal latencies, temporal dispersion, and prolonged F-wave latencies. Hereditary demyelinating neuropathies are characterized by uniform slowing of nerve conduction. Acquired demyelinating neuropathies show a nonuniform slowing and can be distinguished further by their temporal profile. Demyelinating neuropathies are listed in Table 6.5.

It is important to remember the limitations of electrodiagnostic tests. Electromyography and nerve conduction studies examine large myelinated fibers. Thus, the findings of these tests can be normal in a patient who has small-fiber neuropathy. Proximal sensory nerves cannot be tested, and in normal elderly subjects, lower extremity sensory responses can be reduced or absent. Remember, electrodiagnostic tests are an extension of the clinical examination and are operator-dependent.

Several laboratory tests are available for evaluating polyneuropathy. A reasonable screening evaluation for common distal symmetrical neuropathies includes a complete blood count, urinalysis, and determining the following values: fasting serum level of glucose, glycosylated hemoglobin, blood urea nitrogen, creatinine, erythrocyte sedimentation rate, vitamin B_{12}, and thyroid-stimulating hormone. Many neurologists include serum protein electrophoresis in the initial screening evaluation. Other important laboratory tests may be indicated on the basis of the patient's clinical presentation or the results of the screening evaluation. If the

Table 6.4. Common Drugs Associated With Neuropathy

Amiodarone (Cordarone)
Amitriptyline (Elavil, Endep)
Chloramphenicol (Chloromycetin)
Chloroquine (Aralen)
Cimetidine (Tagamet)
Cisplatin (Platinol)
Clioquinol (Vioform, nonprescription antidiarrheal medicine)
Colchicine and probenecid (Col-Probenecid)
Dapsone (Avlosulfon)
Didanosine (Videx)
Disulfiram (Antabuse)
Ethambutol (Myambutol)
Gold
Hydralazine (Apresoline)
Immunizations
Isoniazid (Nydrazid)
Lithium (Eskalith, Lithobid)
Metronidazole (Flagyl)
Nitrofurantoin (Furadantin, Macrodantin)
Nitrous oxide
Paclitaxel (Taxol)
Phenytoin (Dilantin)
Pyridoxine (Nestrex, Beesix)
Simvastatin (Zocor)
Tacrolimus (Prograf)
Thalidomide (Thalomid)
Vincristine (Oncovin, Vincasar PFS)
Zalcitabine (Hivid)

From Adams, AC: Neurology in Primary Care. FA Davis, Philadelphia, 2000, p 108. Used with permission of Mayo Foundation for Medical Education and Research.

Table 6.5. Demyelinating Neuropathies

Hereditary—uniform demyelination
    Hereditary sensory and motor neuropathy-I, -III, -IV
    Hereditary predisposition to pressure palsy
Acquired—nonuniform demyelination
    Acute
        Acute inflammatory demyelinating polyradiculoneuropathy
        Acute arsenic intoxication
        Dipththeria
    Subacute
        Chronic inflammatory demyelinating polyradiculoneuropathy
        Multifocal conduction block
        Osteosclerotic myeloma
        Monoclonal gammopathy of undetermined significance

From Adams, AC: Neurology in Primary Care. FA Davis, Philadelphia, 2000, p 109. Used with permission of Mayo Foundation for Medical Education and Research.

clinical examination does not provide evidence of connective tissue disease, the diagnostic yield from connective tissue laboratory tests is extremely low. Similarly, paraneoplastic antibodies are less helpful than chest radiography, breast examination, and stool guaiac testing for detecting an underlying neoplasm. The exception to this is testing for anti-Hu or anti-neuronal nuclear antibody in a patient with a sensory neuronopathy and possible small cell carcinoma of the lung.

Many tests are available that detect antibodies to glycolipids associated with peripheral nerves. Clinically useful tests include myelin-associated glycoprotein antibody (associated with chronic inflammatory demyelinating polyneuropathy) and anti-ganglioside antibody (associated with multifocal motor neuropathy with conduction block). Antibody panels are expensive and can lead to inappropriate treatment. Laboratory tests used in the evaluation of neuropathy are summarized in Table 6.6.

Nerve biopsy is valuable for a limited number of diagnostic possibilities. The rare conditions that have characteristic findings include vasculitis, amyloidosis, sarcoidosis, leprosy, and leukodystrophies. Progressive demyelinating neuropathies may require biopsy if the diagnosis is still uncertain after electrodiagnostic testing. The nerve selected for biopsy is the sural nerve. Painful dysesthesias and poor healing complicate this procedure.

DIABETIC NEUROPATHY

The term *diabetic neuropathy* describes the many disorders of the peripheral nervous system that are related to diabetes mellitus. Diabetic neuropathy is the most common neuropathy in the Western world. Because of its high incidence and significant morbidity and mortality, it deserves special attention (Table 6.7). In addition to the types of diabetic neuropathy listed in Table 6.7, neuropathies associated with the complications of diabetes include neuropathy of ketoacidosis, neuropathy of chronic renal failure, and neuropathy associated with large-vessel ischemia. Diabetic neuropathies related to treatment include insulin neuritis (acute painful sensory neuropathy after the initiation of insulin therapy) and the rare hypoglycemic neuropathy.

Diabetic Polyneuropathy

The most frequent type of diabetic neuropathy is the distal symmetrical, sensory-greater-than-motor polyneuropathy. Although this is common and frequently the cause of neurologic complications, it is prudent to use diabetic neuropathy as a diagnosis of exclusion to avoid missing other causes of neuropathy. Diabetic polyneuropathy is length-dependent and has the stocking-glove type sensory pattern. Patients may be asymptomatic or complain of paresthesias of the feet. Although this neuropathy is related to the severity and duration of diabetes, the onset of diabetes often is not known and this neuropathy may be the presenting symptom of the disease.

Diabetic polyneuropathy has a slow and insidious course, with minimal motor and variable autonomic involvement. It affects both small and large fibers, but some patients have involvement predominantly of either small or large fibers. Sensory symptoms usually develop slowly and begin in the feet and move more proximally. Upper extremity symptoms are rarely present and are more likely to be due to coexisting mononeuropathy than to the polyneuropathy. Patients complain of burning feet or "pins and needles" sensation. The symptoms tend to be more pronounced at night and can interfere with sleep. Although motor involvement is usually minimal, footdrop can occur in severe cases. A severe form of osteoarthritis of the feet (Charcot, or neuropathic, joint) may occur because of the loss of pain and proprioception sensations. Diabetic neuropathy is also a major risk factor for the development of foot ulcers. Patients with diabetic polyneuropathy often have some degree of diabetic retinopathy or nephropathy, which suggests a common pathogenesis. Other causes of neuropathy should be investigated in patients who have polyneuropathy but no retinal or renal involvement.

Infrequently, diabetic polyneuropathy can be more rapid, painful, and associated with weight loss. Some specialists consider acute painful neuropathy with weight loss separate from diabetic polyneuropathy. This illness begins with precipitous weight loss, followed by severe burning pain in the distal lower extremities. The neurologic symptoms usually subside with glycemic control and weight gain.

Treatment of diabetic polyneuropathy begins with good control of the patient's blood

Table 6.6. Laboratory Tests Used in Evaluation of Neuropathy

Test	Clinical condition detected
Glucose	Diabetes mellitus
Glycosylated hemoglobin	Diabetes mellitus
Blood urea nitrogen	Renal, metabolic
Creatinine	Renal, metabolic
Complete blood count	Hematologic, vasculitis
Erythrocyte sedimentation rate	Inflammation
Antinuclear antibody, rheumatoid factor, complement, immunoelectrophoresis, hepatitis B antigen and antibody, eosinophil count, antineutrophil cytoplasmic antibody, anti-extractable nuclear antigen, cryoglobulins	Vasculitis and other connective tissue disorders
Urinalysis	Renal, metabolic, vasculitis
Vitamin B_{12}, methylmalonic acid, homocysteine	Vitamin B_{12} deficiency
Thyrotropin-stimulating hormone	Endocrine
Serum protein electrophoresis	Hematologic, malignancy
Serum protein electrophoresis, serum and urine immunoelectrophoresis, skeletal survey, bone marrow aspiration	Amyloidosis, multiple myeloma, osteosclerotic myeloma, Waldenström macroglobulinemia, cryoglobulinemia, lymphoma, leukemia
Human immunodeficiency virus	Acquired immunodeficiency syndrome
Lyme serology	Lyme disease
Syphilis serology	Syphilis
Antineuronal nuclear antibody or anti-Hu antibody	Malignancy
Cerebrospinal fluid	Demyelinating neuropathies, vasculitis
Angiotensin-converting enzyme	Sarcoidosis
Heavy metal screen	Toxic lead, mercury, arsenic
Fat aspirate	Amyloidosis
Porphyrin, porphobilinogen deaminase, uroporphyrin synthetase	Porphyria
Myelin-associated glycoprotein antibody	Chronic inflammatory demyelinating polyradiculoneuropathy
Anti-ganglioside antibody	Multifocal motor neuropathy with conduction block
Phytanic acid	Refsum disease
Molecular genetic analysis	Hereditary motor sensory neuropathy IA, hereditary neuropathy for pressure palsy, familial amyloid polyneuropathies

From Adams, AC: *Neurology in Primary Care.* FA Davis, Philadelphia, 2000, p 110. Used with permission of Mayo Foundation for Medical Education and Research.

Table 6.7. Types of Diabetic Neuropathy, Clinical Features, Symmetry, and Presumed Underlying Pathophysiology

Type	Clinical features	Symmetry	Pathophysiology
Diabetic polyneuropathy	Stocking-glove sensory distribution Paresthesias in feet Minimal motor findings	Symmetrical	Metabolic, microvascular, hypoxic
Diabetic autonomic neuropathy	Orthostatic hypotension Pupil abnormalities Gastrointestinal, genito-urinary, and cardio-vascular signs and symptoms	Symmetrical	Metabolic, microvascular, hypoxic
Diabetic radiculoplexus neuropathies Diabetic lumbosacral radiculoplexus neuropathy Diabetic cervical radic-uloplexus neuropathy Diabetic thoracic radiculopathy	Acute to subacute painful proximal nerve involvement	Asymmetrical	Inflammatory, immune
Mononeuropathy	Carpal tunnel syndrome or median neuropathy	Asymmetrical	Compression
Cranial neuropathy	Pupil-sparing CN III palsy	Asymmetrical	Inflammatory, immune

CN, cranial nerve.
From Adams, AC: Neurology in Primary Care. FA Davis, Philadelphia, 2000, p 111. Used with permission of Mayo Foundation for Medical Education and Research.

glucose level. Glycemic control affects the development and progression of diabetic neuropathy. Proper care of the feet is extremely important to avoid foot ulcers. Patients should exercise care, particularly in the dark and on uneven surfaces, to avoid falling. Treatment has been directed mainly at symptomatic control of the pain and paresthesias (Table 6.8). The use of aldose reductase inhibitors, essential fatty acids, and antioxidants to treat neuropathy is being investigated.

Diabetic Autonomic Neuropathy

Diabetic autonomic neuropathy is also a length-dependent neuropathy, and the level of the neuropathy is correlated with the severity of somatic nerve findings. Numerous organs are affected by this neuropathy. Because the pupillary light response is abnormal, patients may complain they have trouble seeing in dim light. Decreased vagal tone causes an increase in resting heart rate. As the neuropathy becomes more severe, orthostatic hypotension may occur. Gastroparesis may cause postprandial nausea, bloating, and early satiety. Other gastrointestinal symptoms are constipation and nocturnal diarrhea. Genitourinary effects of autonomic neuropathy include decreased sensation of bladder filling, incomplete bladder emptying, impotence, and reduced vaginal secretions and lubrication. Sweating is usually decreased in a stocking-glove pattern, and severe compensatory hyperhidrosis may occur on the face and torso.

Autonomic neuropathy can be difficult to treat. The standard initial treatment of orthostatic hypotension includes a high salt diet (10-20 g daily), increased fluid intake (more

Table 6.8. Drugs for Treatment of Diabetic Neuropathic Pain

Drug	Comment
Antidepressant agents	
Amitriptyline (Elavil)—10-100 mg at bedtime	Tricyclic; anticholinergic side effects can aggravate autonomic neuropathy. Helpful for sleep
Nortriptyline (Pamelor)—10-100 mg at bedtime	Tricyclic; anticholinergic side effects can aggravate autonomic neuropathy. Helpful for sleep
Duloxetine (Cymbalta)—60 mg daily	Serotonin/norepinephrine reuptake inhibitor
Anticonvulsants	Best for paroxysmal pain
Gabapentin (Neurontin)—1,800-3,600 mg/day in 3 divided doses	
Carbamazepine (Tegretol)—200 mg 3 times daily	
Pregabalin (Lyrica)—50-100 mg 3 times daily	
Topical agent	
Capsaicin (Zostrix)—3-4 times daily	Limitations for applying to large surface area
Antiarrhythmic agent	
Mexiletine (Mexitil)—150 mg/day, increase to 10 mg/kg daily in divided doses	Cardiac arrhythmias, gastrointestinal disturbance, dizziness, tremor
Analgesic	
Tramadol (Ultram)—50-100 mg every 6 hours	Seizure risk

From Adams, AC: Neurology in Primary Care. FA Davis, Philadelphia, 2000, p 112. Used with permission of Mayo Foundation for Medical Education and Research.

than 20 oz daily), elevation of the head of the bed by 4 inches, and use of compressive stockings. The pharmacologic treatment of orthostatic hypotension is listed in Table 5.8. Gastroparesis may be helped by having patients eat small meals low in carbohydrates. Metoclopramide and cisapride may be helpful drug therapy. Diarrhea can be treated with cholestyramine, clonidine, erythromycin, or tetracycline. Constipation may respond to adequate hydration and psyllium. Laxatives may be necessary. Scheduled voiding and self-catheterization may be needed if the patient has trouble voiding. Seek urologic consultation for treating impotence.

Diabetic Radiculoplexus Neuropathies

Diabetic radiculoplexus neuropathies include diabetic lumbosacral radiculoplexus neuropathy, diabetic cervical radiculoplexus neuropathy, and diabetic thoracic radiculoneuropathy. These clinical syndromes affect the proximal nerves asymmetrically. Diabetic lumbosacral radiculoplexus neuropathy has been known by many names, including diabetic amyotrophy, Bruns-Garland syndrome, and diabetic lumbosacral plexus neuropathy. It usually involves the L2-L4 roots and tends to occur in patients with noninsulin-dependent diabetes who are older than 60 years. It is not related to the duration of the the patient's glucose intolerance. Severe pain in the back, hip, buttock, or anterior thigh may be the presenting symptom. Clinical findings include proximal and distal muscle weakness, reduced quadriceps reflex or its absence, and atrophy. The temporal course may be acute to subacute, stepwise, or progressive. Typically, improvement occurs in weeks to months. Pain is a prominent early feature and often requires treatment with narcotic analgesics. Other diagnoses to consider are intraspinal lesion, lumbar plexopathy, and femoral neuropathy. Electrodiagnostic tests and magnetic resonance imaging of the spine may be needed to exclude other serious diagnostic possibilities such as an intraspinal lesion.

Sudden stabbing pain in the chest, abdomen, or thoracic spine may represent diabetic thoracic radiculoneuropathy. Patients often attribute the pain to an intra-abdominal process or heart attack. The absence of any relation to eating, position, activity, or coughing distinguishes this pain from gastrointestinal, cardiovascular, or pulmonary disease. In most patients, diabetic thoracic radiculoneuropathy improves within several months to a year. Ischemic injury and microvasculitis are the presumed pathophysiologic mechanisms for diabetic radiculoplexus neuropathies.

Mononeuropathy

Patients with diabetes have a high incidence of mononeuropathy, both limb and cranial. Compression, or entrapment, of the median nerve (carpal tunnel syndrome) and compression of the ulnar nerve (cubital tunnel syndrome) are frequent upper extremity mononeuropathies. Decompression surgery may be necessary to maintain function, even for patients who have a compression neuropathy and polyneuropathy. The nerve frequently affected in the lower extremity is the peroneal nerve at the head of the fibula. Diabetes can cause mononeuritis multiplex.

Cranial nerves (CNs) affected by diabetes include CNs III, IV, and VI. Although CN VII is often included in this list, it is uncertain that it should be because of the high frequency of involvement of this nerve in nondiabetic patients in the general population. The most common cranial neuropathy is the pupil-sparing CN III (third nerve) palsy. A patient with this nerve palsy may complain of periorbital pain, droopy eyelid, and double vision. The affected eye is positioned down and out. Because the pupilloconstrictor fibers (parasympathetic) are located in the periphery of CN III, pupil sparing is thought to exclude a compressive lesion. Despite this clinical finding, neuroimaging is recommended to exclude other causes. Recovery usually occurs in 2 to 5 months.

NEUROPATHY OF OTHER ENDOCRINE DISORDERS

Peripheral neuropathies are not commonly associated with other endocrine disorders. Hypothyroidism and hyperthyroidism may be associated with carpal tunnel syndrome and, rarely, a distal neuropathy. Acromegaly is also associated with carpal tunnel syndrome and a distal polyneuropathy. Hyperparathyroidism can mimic motor neuron disease, with weakness, sparse sensory abnormalities, and hyperreflexia.

METABOLIC NEUROPATHIES

Many metabolic disorders are associated with neuropathy. Most metabolic neuropathies are axonal in type, associated with systemic disease, and have a length-dependent pattern. In addition to neuropathies from endocrine disease, metabolic neuropathies are caused by nutritional disorders, chronic renal failure, porphyria, and critical illness polyneuropathy.

Nutritional Disorders

Nutritional disorders in developed countries are due to chronic alcoholism, malabsorption, abnormal diet, or drug toxicity. Malabsorption of vitamin B_{12} (cyanocobalamin) is a common deficiency disorder associated with peripheral neuropathy, myelopathy, and dementia. Defective production of intrinsic factor, the vitamin B_{12} binding protein secreted by gastric parietal cells, is the most common cause. This can result from various gastrointestinal disorders or a genetic predisposition (pernicious anemia).

Pernicious anemia is frequent among African Americans and northern Europeans.

Patients may experience gradual onset of paresthesias in the hands and feet. Large-fiber sensory function is affected preferentially. The neurologic examination may show reduced vibratory and joint position sense in the feet and the Romberg sign. Reflexes may be increased or decreased depending on involvement of the spinal cord. Distal sensory loss associated with brisk reflexes indicates peripheral sensory loss and spinal cord involvement. If a patient has reduced distal sensation and extensor plantar (Babinski) reflexes, consider vitamin B_{12} deficiency. This common correctable disorder should be sought in any patient with suspected peripheral neuropathy. A low serum level of vitamin B_{12} confirms the diagnosis. Other supportive laboratory results include increased levels of homocysteine and methylmalonic acid. The Schilling test can evaluate intrinsic factor function. Treatment is 1,000 μg of cyanocobalamin intramuscularly daily for 1 week and then monthly thereafter.

Neuropathies associated with a deficiency of vitamin B_1 (beriberi), vitamin B_2, niacin (pellagra), or vitamin E are rare. Thiamine, or vitamin B_1, deficiency is associated most often with alcoholism. Pyridoxine, or vitamin B_6, deficiency is usually caused by medication, for example, isoniazid, penicillamine, hydralazine, or cycloserine. Riboflavin, or vitamin B_2, deficiency is associated with burning feet syndrome. Hypophosphatemia from hyperalimentation can cause a subacute neuropathy that resembles Guillain-Barré syndrome.

Chronic Renal Failure

Peripheral nerve involvement in chronic renal failure includes uremic polyneuropathy, carpal tunnel syndrome, and ischemic mononeuropathy. Ischemic mononeuropathy can result from the arteriovenous fistula used in hemodialysis.

Porphyria

Porphyrias, rare hereditary disorders of heme biosynthesis, are associated with polyneuropathy and primarily affect motor nerves. Involvement of the facial, bulbar, and proximal arm muscles is common. Porphyria should be considered in patients who have neuropathy and gastrointestinal or neuropsychiatric symptoms (or both).

Critical Illness

Critically ill patients in an intensive care unit often have diffuse neuromuscular weakness. Many of these patients are thought to have neuropathy of critical illness, although this diagnosis is a matter of controversy. Prolonged ventilator dependence, sepsis, and multiple organ failure are associated with this condition.

TOXIC NEUROPATHIES

Many toxins can cause peripheral neuropathy. The most common toxins are pharmaceutical and iatrogenic. Occupational neuropathy is uncommon in North America. Most often, toxins cause distal axonal neuropathies that are length-dependent symmetrical or affect motor axons (motor loss) or both. Most toxic agents show a strong dose-response relation and a consistent pattern of disease related to the dose and duration of exposure. Neuropathic symptoms coincide with or soon follow toxic exposure. After exposure has been eliminated, neuropathic signs and symptoms should improve. Persons with preexistent neuropathies are more susceptible to neurotoxins. Some of the industrial and environmental toxins that cause peripheral neuropathy are listed in Table 6.9.

Heavy metals are toxic to the nervous system, including arsenic, lead, mercury, platinum, and thallium. Most heavy metal neuropathies are accompanied by gastrointestinal and hematologic problems. Heavy metals can be stored in bone and then be slowly released, prolonging the neuropathy.

Many drugs are potentially neurotoxic (Table 6.4). Chemotherapeutic agents that cause peripheral neuropathies include paclitaxel alkaloids (Taxol), platinum agents (cisplatin), and vinca alkaloids (vincristine and vinblastine). Paclitaxel is used to treat ovarian and breast cancers. The associated neuropathy is primarily sensory. Platinum agents are also associated with a sensory neuropathy that, from substantial loss of proprioception, results in gait ataxia. Vinca alkaloids affect sensory, motor, and autonomic nerves. The adverse effects of these anticancer drugs can be exaggerated by coexisting diseases such as diabetes mellitus, renal failure, and nutritional deficits.

Nucleoside analogues such as zalcitabine, used in the treatment of AIDS, can cause an acute painful sensory neuropathy when administered at high doses. Discontinuation of the medication followed by improvement is the only way to distinguish between the toxic neuropathy and the neuropathy associated with AIDS. A progressive neuropathy can occur with nucleoside analogues at lower doses.

CONNECTIVE TISSUE DISEASE

Connective tissue diseases, or collagen-vascular disorders, are systemic illnesses frequently associated with neuropathy. Neuropathy may be the initial manifestation of an undiagnosed connective tissue disease. As with diabetes mellitus, numerous neuropathies are associated with connective tissue disease, including mononeuropathy multiplex, asymmetrical polyneuropathy, compression neuropathy, trigeminal sensory neuropathy, and sensory neuronopathy. Also,

Table 6.9. Occupational and Environmental Toxins

Toxin	Environmental/occupational use or setting
Acrylamide	Flocculators and grouting agents
Allyl chloride	Pesticides
Arsenic	Suicides and homicides—note that ingestion of seafood can increase urine levels
Carbon disulfide	Production of rayon, cellophane film
Cyanide	Cassava consumption
Ethylene oxide	Sterilization of medical equipment
Hexacarbons	Glue sniffing
Lead	Paint, battery manufacturing, moonshine whiskey
Mercury	Battery manufacturing, electronics
Methyl bromide	Fumigant, fire extinguisher, refrigerant, insecticide
Organophosphates	Insecticides, petroleum additives, flame retardants
Polychlorinated biphenyls	Industrial insulation
Thallium	Rodenticides, insecticides
Trichloroethylene	Industrial solvent
Vacor	Rodenticides

From Adams, AC: Neurology in Primary Care. FA Davis, Philadelphia, 2000, p 115. Used with permission of Mayo Foundation for Medical Education and Research.

patients with connective tissue disease may have more than one type of neuropathy.

Connective tissue diseases can be associated with vasculitic neuropathies. These require immediate diagnosis and treatment to improve outcome. Vasculitic neuropathy is caused by inflammatory occlusion of blood vessels, which leads to ischemic infarction of nerves. It can occur with any connective tissue disorder, but it generally is associated with polyarteritis nodosa and rheumatoid arthritis. A vasculitic neuropathy usually has a mononeuropathy multiplex pattern. However, an asymmetrical polyneuropathy, multifocal mononeuropathies with partial confluence, or distal sensory polyneuropathies can occur. The peroneal nerve in the lower extremity and the ulnar nerve in the upper extremity are particularly vulnerable to infarction. The first symptom may be an aching sensation in the extremity, followed by burning pain, tingling, and sensory and motor loss in the distribution of the affected nerve. The diagnosis is confirmed by identifing arteritis in a nerve biopsy specimen. For persons with known connective tissue disease who present with mononeuritis multiplex and multifocal axon loss, the diagnosis can be made with electrodiagnostic tests. Treatment is with immunosuppressive agents.

A sensory neuronopathy is unique to Sjögren syndrome. This neuropathy is the result of inflammation of dorsal root ganglia. The typical presentation is that of a middle-aged woman who has sensory symptoms, clumsiness, and ataxic gait. Large-fiber sensory loss is predominant, with loss of vibratory and joint position sense. Treatment is with immunosuppressive agents.

Many connective tissue diseases, especially systemic sclerosis and mixed connective tissue disease, are associated with trigeminal sensory neuropathy. The patient may complain of slowly progressive unilateral or bilateral facial numbness. If a patient has facial numbness and negative findings on imaging studies, consider the possibility of connective tissue disease. The various connective tissue disorders and associated neuropathies are summarized in Table 6.10.

DYSPROTEINEMIC POLYNEUROPATHY

Dysproteinemias, or plasma cell dyscrasias, are frequently associated with peripheral nerve disease. These disorders, also called *monoclonal gammopathies*, produce excessive amounts of monoclonal proteins, also called *M proteins* (the M spike seen on serum electrophoresis), or immunoglobulins that may injure a nerve directly by reacting with antigens in the myelin sheaths and axonal membranes. Nerves may also be injured by the deposition of amyloid, a by-product of M proteins, or paraproteins.

Common plasma cell dyscrasias include monoclonal gammopathy of undetermined significance, osteosclerotic myeloma, multiple myeloma, Waldenström macroglobulinemia, cryoglobulinemia, and primary systemic amyloidosis. The clinical presentation of these disorders varies, but most patients have signs and symptoms of distal neuropathy. Amyloidosis is unique because of the presence of autonomic symptoms. Serum protein electrophoresis is a reasonable screening test for these disorders. However, if the patient has an idiopathic

Table 6.10. Connective Tissue Diseases and Associated Neuropathies

Connective tissue disease	Vasculitic neuropathy	Distal symmetrical	Compressive neuropathy	Sensory neuronopathy	Trigeminal neuropathy
Polyarteritis nodosa	+++	++			+
Rheumatoid arthritis	++	+++	+++		+
Systemic lupus erythematosis	+	++	+		+
Sjögren syndrome	+	++	+	+++	++
Systemic sclerosis	+	++	+		+++
Mixed connective tissue disease	++	+			+++

+, *Common;* ++, *more common;* +++, *most common.*
From Adams, AC: Neurology in Primary Care. FA Davis, Philadelphia, 2000, p 116. Used with permission of Mayo Foundation for Medical Education and Research.

polyneuropathy, the more sensitive immuno-electrophoresis or immunofixation should be performed on serum and urine. Additional studies include bone marrow evaluation, metastatic skeletal bone survey, and biopsy of appropriate tissues.

Dysproteinemic neuropathies are important to recognize because they may precede several systemic and lymphoproliferative disorders. For example, a malignant plasma cell dyscrasia develops in 20% to 25% of patients with monoclonal gammopathy of undetermined significance. Neuropathies associated with paraproteinemia often respond to treatment (Table 6.11). Hematologic consultation is recommended.

INFECTIOUS NEUROPATHY

Several infectious diseases are associated with polyneuropathy. These include leprosy, HIV, Lyme disease, syphilis, and herpes zoster radiculitis or cranial neuritis (shingles). These are discussed further in Chapter 13.

DEMYELINATING POLYRADICULONEUROPATHIES

Acute Inflammatory Demyelinating Polyradiculoneuropathy

Acute inflammatory demyelinating polyradiculoneuropathy (AIDP), or Guillain-Barré

Table 6.11. Dysproteinemic Neuropathies

Disorder	Diagnostic criteria	Treatment options for neuropathy
Monoclonal gammopathy of undetermined significance	Monoclonal protein No malignancy or amyloid	Intravenous immunoglobulin, plasma exchange, corticosteroids
Osteosclerotic myeloma	Plasmacytoma(s) with osteosclerotic features	Resection of solitary bone lesion, focused radiation, prednisone, melphalan, cyclophosphamide
Multiple myeloma	Abnormal plasma cells in bone marrow, osteolytic lesions, monoclonal protein	None
Waldenström macroglobulinemia	IgM monoclonal protein Abnormal bone marrow	Plasma exchange, prednisone, melphalan, chlorambucil
Cryoglobulinemia	IgM or IgG	Plasma exchange, prednisone, cyclophosphamide, interferon alfa
Amyloidosis	Light chain amyloid by histology	Melphalan plus prednisone, autologous stem cell transplantation

From Adams, AC: Neurology in Primary Care. FA Davis, Philadelphia, 2000, p 117. Used with permission of Mayo Foundation for Medical Education and Research.

syndrome, is an autoimmune disease characterized by rapidly evolving symmetrical limb weakness, mild sensory signs, reduced muscle stretch reflexes or absence of these reflexes, and various autonomic signs and symptoms. AIDP is the most common cause of acute generalized weakness and can occur at any age. Most patients describe an antecedent infection, respiratory tract infection, or gastroenteritis. The most common infection may be *Campylobacter jejuni* enteritis, but other precipitants include Epstein-Barr virus, cytomegalovirus, and HIV. Sensory symptoms may be the first sign of the illness, followed by ascending muscle weakness. The diagnosis requires progressive weakness in more than one limb, with areflexia or hyporeflexia. Cranial nerve VII and the autonomic nervous system are frequently involved, with the more serious consequences being cardiac arrhythmias, hypotension, hypertension, and hyperpyrexia.

Findings on cerebrospinal fluid (CSF) analysis and the electrophysiologic features of demyelination support the diagnosis of AIDP. The CSF has an increased protein concentration and few cells (albuminocytologic dissociation). The diagnosis should be questioned if there are more than 50 cells/mm^3. The cardinal electrophysiologic findings include slowing of nerve conduction and partial or complete block of conduction in motor fibers. The results of both CSF and electrophysiologic tests may be normal for the first week of the illness. Other laboratory tests are not needed unless questionable features are noted, for example, marked asymmetry of weakness, bowel and bladder dysfunction, a sensory level, or cellular CSF. Serologic testing for HIV may be reasonable if the patient has the appropriate risk factors. The differential diagnosis for a patient with an acute neuropathy is limited (Table 6.3), and the presence of other features may dictate further evaluation.

In most patients, progressive weakness develops over 2 to 4 weeks. Patients should be hospitalized because of the potential for respiratory compromise and autonomic dysfunction. Forced vital capacity should be monitored, and the patient should receive ventilatory assistance if there is any sign of fatigue or if the forced vital capacity becomes less than 15 mL/kg. Progressive neck weakness may signal impending respiratory failure. Other supportive measures include compressive stockings and subcutaneous heparin for protection against deep venous thrombosis, physical therapy for prevention of contractures, and a means of communication if the patient is on a ventilator.

Plasma exchange and intravenous immunoglobulin are used to treat AIDP. Both treatments have been shown to be effective, and both are expensive. Intravenous immunoglobulin may be preferred for patients who are hemodynamically unstable. Plasma exchange is not available in some hospitals. High-dose intravenous immunoglobulin (10% solution given at a dose of 2 g/kg divided over 2-5 days) should be administered within 2 weeks after the onset of symptoms. Contraindications to intravenous immunoglobulin include low serum levels of immunoglobulin A, advanced renal failure, uncontrolled hypertension, and hyperosmolar state. A second set of infusions can be administered if the patient experiences a limited relapse after improvement with the initial infusion. Plasma exchange regimens involve the exchange of one plasma volume, 50 mL/kg, on five separate occasions over the course of 2 weeks. Currently, treatment with corticosteroids is not recommended.

Chronic Inflammatory Demyelinating Polyradiculoneuropathy

Chronic inflammatory demyelinating polyradiculoneuropathy (CIDP) differs from the acute disease by the temporal profile. The muscle weakness is progressive for at least 2 months, and antecedent infections and respiratory involvement are less common than with AIDP.

Several conditions are associated with a syndrome similar to CIDP, including HIV infection, monoclonal gammopathy, chronic active hepatitis, inflammatory bowel disease, connective tissue disease, bone marrow and organ transplantation, lymphoma, hereditary neuropathy, diabetes mellitus, thyrotoxicosis, nephritic syndrome, and central nervous system demyelination. The diagnostic work-up of a patient with CIDP entails looking for these systemic diseases. Treatment options include corticosteroids, intravenous immunoglobulin, plasma exchange, and other immunosuppressive agents.

FOCAL NEUROPATHIES

Four mechanisms can cause focal neuropathies or mononeuropathies: an external insult, a lesion intrinsic to the nerve, increased susceptibility to nerve injury, and internal entrapment or compression. An example of an external insult is prolonged external compression of a nerve in an unconscious patient. A nerve infarct from vasculitis is an example of an intrinsic nerve lesion. Increased susceptibility to nerve injury is seen in patients with diabetes mellitus who have minor nerve entrapment or in patients with a genetic condition such as hereditary neuropathy with liability to pressure palsies. The most common focal neuropathy is compression neuropathy of the median nerve, or carpal tunnel syndrome.

Carpal tunnel syndrome is the result of compression of the median nerve at the wrist by the volar ligament (Fig. 6.6). This most common entrapment neuropathy is associated with several conditions, including pregnancy, diabetes mellitus, hypothyroidism, acromegaly, rheumatoid arthritis, and amyloidosis. The incidence

of carpal tunnel syndrome is high among assembly line workers, keyboard operators, and those whose occupations require forceful repetitive movement of the hand. The relation of carpal tunnel syndrome to work is not clear, and some evidence suggests that nonoccupational factors such as age are important in its development.

Patients often report numbness and pain in the hand, and activity-related and nighttime paresthesias are common. Although the median nerve supplies only the palmar surface of the thumb and index and middle fingers and half of the ring finger, patients often complain of pain and numbness of the entire hand. The pain can radiate into the forearm (and, rarely, the shoulder). If pain is the most prominent symptom, it is important to consider other diagnoses. Musculoskeletal causes that may mimic carpal tunnel syndrome include tenosynovitis, arthritis, muscle strain, and overuse. Neurologic causes to consider include C6 radiculopathy, thoracic outlet syndrome, and brachial plexopathy.

Examination findings in a patient who has mild to moderate carpal tunnel syndrome may be normal. Percussion of a nerve that causes paresthesias in the distribution of that nerve (Tinel sign) indicates a partial lesion of the nerve or early regeneration. Reproduction of the symptoms with wrist flexion (Phalen maneuver) is consistent with a median neuropathy at the wrist. Reduced sensation to pinprick in the thumb and index and middle fingers and half of the ring finger, weakness, and atrophy of the thenar muscles are seen in moderate to severe carpal tunnel syndrome.

Additional neurologic findings differentiate carpal tunnel syndrome from other neurologic diseases. Patients with C6 radiculopathy complain of neck pain and may have C6 muscle weakness and reflex (biceps) loss. Patients with thoracic outlet syndrome develop C8 and T1 symptoms and neurologic deficits (interosseous and hypothenar muscle weakness) when they elevate

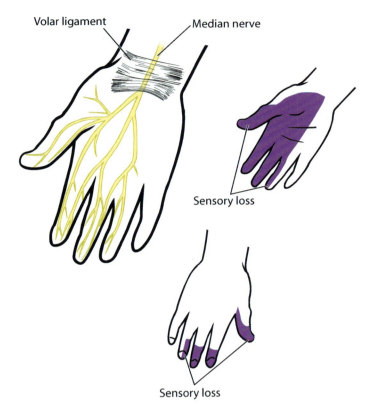

Volar ligament

Median nerve

Sensory loss

Sensory loss

Fig. 6.6. Median nerve at the wrist, and distribution of sensory loss (purple) in the hand in carpal tunnel syndrome. (From Adams, AC: Neurology in Primary Care. FA Davis, Philadelphia, 2000, p 118. Used with permission of Mayo Foundation for Medical Education and Research.)

and abduct the arm. Pronation of the wrist (pronator teres muscle) and flexion of the distal thumb joint (flexor pollicis longus muscle) test median nerve function proximal to the wrist.

Electrophysiologic tests can provide an accurate diagnosis of carpal tunnel syndrome and detect other conditions such as peripheral neuropathy, cervical radiculopathy, and ulnar neuropathy. Electromyography is useful in determining the severity of the condition and the response to treatment. Conservative treatment includes wrist splinting, avoidance of aggravating activities, nonsteroidal antiinflammatory drugs, and injection of corticosteroid under the

volar ligament. If the patient does not have a response to conservative treatment and has progressive symptoms, recommend surgery.

The ulnar nerve can be compressed at the elbow as it courses by the medial epicondyle and enters the cubital tunnel under the edge of the aponeurosis of the flexor carpi ulnaris muscle (Fig. 6.7). Numbness and paresthesias occur in the 4th and 5th digits of the hand. If the motor fibers of the ulnar nerve are affected, interosseous muscles become weak and the patient has difficulty spreading the fingers. Atrophy of the 1st dorsal interosseous muscle (the "web" between the thumb and index finger) is frequently seen. Repetitive flexion of the elbow, leaning on the elbow, prolonged bed rest, and the position of the arm during certain surgical procedures may compress the nerve at the elbow. The nerve can also be injured at the wrist (see Fig. 4.17). Cycling and using the hand in lieu of a hammer can injure the ulnar nerve at the wrist.

Radial nerve compression can cause numbness and paresthesias on the dorsum of the hand. The nerve can be injured by the incorrect use of a crutch. Prolonged compression of

the upper arm on the edge of a chair may injure the radial nerve along its course in the posterior aspect of the upper arm (spiral groove). This focal neuropathy is often called *Saturday night palsy*, for persons who wake up with hand numbness and wristdrop after a night of drinking.

Common focal neuropathies of the lower extremity include those of the lateral femoral cutaneous nerve and the peroneal nerve. It is important to differentiate these from lumbosacral radiculopathies and plexopathies. Compression of the lateral femoral cutaneous

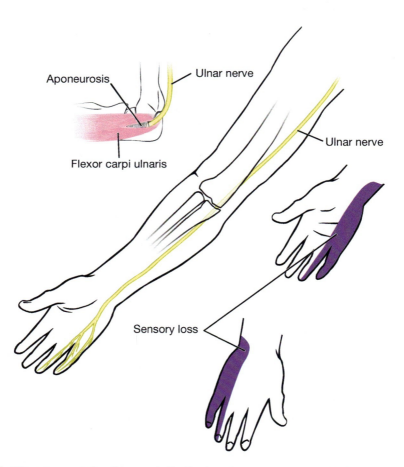

Fig. 6.7. Ulnar nerve at the elbow, and distribution of sensory loss (purple) in the hand following compression of the ulnar nerve. (Modified from Adams, AC: Neurology in Primary Care. FA Davis, Philadelphia, 2000, p 119. Used with permission of Mayo Foundation for Medical Education and Research.)

nerve, called *meralgia paresthetica*, occurs at the inguinal ligament, for example, with pregnancy, obesity, abdominal surgery, and constrictive clothing (Fig. 6.8). This neuropathy is characterized by paresthesias of the upper thigh, well-demarcated sensory loss, and no motor involvement. Symptomatic treatment and reassurance are usually effective for this focal neuropathy.

The peroneal nerve can be compressed at the head of the fibula, for example, by crossing the legs, prolonged squatting, and knee injury (Fig. 6.9). Numbness occurs in the dorsum of the foot. Footdrop results from weakness of the muscles innervated by the peroneal nerve. Both peroneal nerve and posterior tibial nerve are derived from the L5 nerve root. Thus, weakness of ankle inversion (posterior tibial nerve) can help distinguish between a peroneal neuropathy and an L5 radiculopathy.

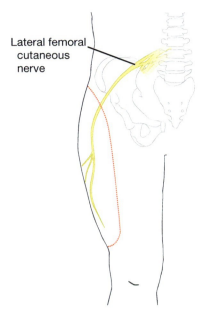

Fig. 6.8. Lateral femoral cutaneous nerve. The cutaneous distribution of the nerve is outlined in red.

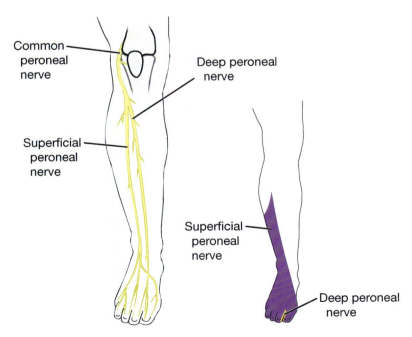

Fig. 6.9. Peroneal nerve, and the distribution of sensory loss (colored areas) in the foot and lower leg following compression of the peroneal nerve. (From Adams, AC: Neurology in Primary Care. FA Davis, Philadelphia, 2000, p 120. Used with permission of Mayo Foundation for Medical Education and Research.)

SUGGESTED READING

Amato, AA, and Collins, MP: Neuropathies associated with malignancy. Semin Neurol 18:125-144, 1998.

Barohn, RJ: Approach to peripheral neuropathy and neuronopathy. Semin Neurol 18:7-18, 1998.

Barohn, RJ, and Saperstein, DS: Guillian-Barre syndrome and chronic inflammatory demyelinating polyneuropathy. Semin Neurol 18:49-61, 1998.

Berger, AR: Toxic peripheral neuropathies. In Samuels, MA, and Feske, S (eds): Office Practice of Neurology. Churchill Livingstone, New York, 1996, pp 534-540.

Diabetes Control and Complications Trial Research Group: The effect of intensive treatment of diabetes on the development and progression of long-term complications in insulin-dependent diabetes mellitus. N Engl J Med 329:977-986, 1993.

Fuller, G: Diagnosing and managing mononeuropathies. Clin Med 4:113-117, 2004.

Kelly, JJ, Jr: Dysproteinemic polyneuropathy. In Samuels, MA, and Feske, S (eds): Office Practice of Neurology. Churchill Livingstone, New York, 1996, pp 522-528.

Kissel, JT: Autoantibody testing in the evaluation of peripheral neuropathy. Semin Neurol 18:83-94, 1998.

Li, J, et al: Hereditary neuropathy with liability to pressure palsy: The electrophysiology fits the name. Neurology 58:1769-1773, 2002.

Logigian, EL: Approach to and classification of peripheral neuropathy. In Samuels, MA, and Feske, S (eds): Office Practice of Neurology. Churchill Livingstone, New York, 1996, pp 492-497.

Low, PA, et al: Autonomic function and dysfunction. Continuum: Lifelong Learning in Neurology 4, no. 2, April 1998.

Mendell, JR, et al: Peripheral neuropathy. Continuum: Lifelong Learning in Neurology 1, no. 1, December 1994.

Mendell, JR, and Sahenk, Z: Clinical practice: Painful sensory neuropathy. N Engl J Med 348:1243-1255, 2003.

Nathan, PA, et al: Natural history of median nerve sensory conduction in industry: Relationship to symptoms and carpal tunnel syndrome in 558 hands over 11 years. Muscle Nerve 21:711-721, 1998.

Olney, RK: Neuropathies associated with connective tissue disease. Semin Neurol 18:63-72, 1998.

Partanen, J, et al: Natural history of peripheral neuropathy in patients with non-insulin-dependent diabetes mellitus. N Engl J Med 333:89-94, 1995.

Poncelet, AN: An algorithm for the evaluation of peripheral neuropathy. Am Fam Physician 57:755-764, 1998.

Ropper, AH, and Gorson, KC: Neuropathies associated with paraproteinemia. N Engl J Med 338:1601-1607, 1998.

Rowbotham, MC, et al: Oral opioid therapy for chronic peripheral and central neuropathic pain. N Engl J Med 348:1223-1232, 2003.

Sinnreich, M, Taylor, BV, and Dyck, PJ: Diabetic neuropathies: Classification, clinical features, and pathophysiological basis. Neurologist 11:63-79, 2005.

Vinik, A: Clinical review: Use of antiepileptic drugs in the treatment of chronic painful diabetic neuropathy. J Clin Endocrinol Metab 90:4936-4945, 2005 Aug. Epub 2005 May 17.

Weinberg, DH: Metabolic neuropathy. In Samuels, MA, and Feske, S (eds): Office Practice of Neurology. Churchill Livingstone, New York, 1996, pp 510-516.

Wilbourn, A, and Shields, RW, Jr: Diabetic neuropathy. In Samuels, MA, and Feske, S (eds): Office Practice of Neurology. Churchill Livingstone, New York, 1996, pp 506-510.

CHAPTER 7

Weakness

Weakness is a common complaint. Most patients use the term "weakness" to imply fatigue, general illness, or myalgias. Determining whether a patient has actual neuromuscular weakness can be a diagnostic challenge. Disease of the motor system can occur at all levels of the nervous system. This chapter considers disorders of the lower motor neuron, including disorders of muscle, the neuromuscular junction, and motor nerves.

DIAGNOSTIC APPROACH

The history of a patient who complains of weakness is crucial. The first question should be how the weakness has affected the person's activities. This information will help distinguish between neuromuscular weakness and generalized fatigue or malaise. The pattern of weakness provides diagnostic information (see Table 1.5). For example, proximal muscle weakness is suggested if the patient reports trouble getting up from a chair, difficulty going up or down stairs, and trouble working with the arms above the head. Proximal weakness is the usual pattern of weakness that occurs with myopathy. Distal weakness is indicated if the patient reports difficulty buttoning clothing or opening jars or complains of tripping because of footdrop. Distal weakness is the pattern of weakness that occurs most often with neuropathy. The absence of sensory symptoms limits the differential diagnosis of distal weakness. Disorders such as motor neuropathy, myotonic dystrophy, and inclusion body myositis can cause distal weakness.

The hallmark of disorders of the neuromuscular junction is *fatigable weakness*. Patients with myasthenia gravis report increasing weakness and fatigue as the day progresses. Because the extraocular muscles are frequently involved, patients often complain of double vision and ptosis. Trouble swallowing, chewing (bulbar muscles), and breathing are the most serious problems of neuromuscular junction disorders.

Amyotrophic lateral sclerosis (ALS, Lou Gehrig disease) is the prototypic disorder of motor neurons. Patients with a disorder of motor neurons report gradual onset of painless weakness. The pattern can be proximal or distal. Many patients may report "jumping muscles," that is, fasciculations. Sensory symptoms are absent, but muscle cramps are frequently reported.

It is important to obtain a family history from a patient who presents with neuromuscular disease. After you have determined that the patient has a neuromuscular problem, determine next whether it is acquired or inherited. A thorough family history may avoid an extensive neuromuscular evaluation if there is evidence of an inherited neuromuscular disorder in the family. It may not be sufficient to ask the patient if family members had weakness or difficulty walking. For example, if myotonic dystrophy is suspected, you may need to ask if any member of the family had frontal balding or early cataracts.

MOTOR EXAMINATION

The motor examination is described in Chapter 1. Test proximal muscle strength by asking the patient to squat, to get up from a chair, or to sit up from the supine position without using the hands. Assess neck flexion strength if you suspect the patient has proximal muscle weakness. Normally, neck flexion should not be overcome by the examiner. Assess distal strength by the strength of the grip and by having the patient stand on toes and heels. To eliminate any problem with balance, support the patient. Perform repetitive muscle testing if the patient has a history of fatigable weakness. Asking the patient to maintain upward gaze for several minutes may provoke extraocular muscle weakness. Another way to elicit muscle fatigue is to have the patient perform repeated squats or sit-ups. The patient's gait may show weakness. Bilateral pelvic abductor weakness produces a characteristic waddling gait, and footdrop causes a high steppage gait.

In lower motor neuron disorders, muscle tone is normal or decreased. Muscle bulk is also normal to reduced (see Table 1.4). Pseudohypertrophy occurs in some muscular dystrophies

such as Duchenne muscular dystrophy. Children with this disease may have prominent calf muscles, deltoid muscles, and forearm muscles (Fig. 7.1). The patient needs to be undressed for muscle bulk to be assessed adequately and for fasciculations to be detected. Fasciculations may be elicited by gently tapping the area over the muscle. In the absence of weakness, fasciculations are normal.

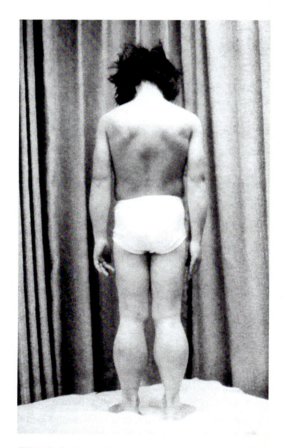

Fig. 7.1. Pseudohypertrophy. (From Darras, BT, Menache, CC, and Kunkel, LM: Dystrophinopathies. In Jones, HR, Jr, De Vivo, DC, and Darras, BT [eds]: Neuromuscular Disorders of Infancy, Childhood, and Adolescence: A Clinician's Approach. Butterworth Heinemann, Philadelphia, 2003, pp 649-699. Used with permission.)

Sensory examination findings are normal in disorders of muscle, the neuromuscular junction, or motor nerves. However, a patient may have both lower motor neuron disease and sensory neuropathy. (This is possible because of the high frequency of diabetes mellitus in the general population.) In these patients, weakness will seem out of proportion to the sensory loss. Muscle stretch reflexes are decreased or absent in lower motor neuron disease. In amyotrophic lateral sclerosis, reflexes may be increased because of the involvement of upper motor neurons.

Many systemic diseases are associated with neuromuscular weakness. Thus, patients should be evaluated for signs and symptoms of connective tissue disease, toxicity, nutritional disorders, and malignancies.

The diagnostic evaluation of a patient who has neuromuscular weakness depends on the clinical presentation. Electromyography (EMG), muscle biopsy, and measurement of creatine kinase levels are indispensable in evaluating neuromuscular weakness. Muscle degeneration causes the release of creatine kinase into the blood, increasing the plasma level of this enzyme. To avoid the artifactual increase in creatine kinase caused by needle injury to the muscle, the level of this enzyme should be determined before EMG is performed.

Electromyography

The EMG features of myopathies include short-duration, low-amplitude polyphasic motor unit potentials. In addition to these features, inflammatory myopathies have increased spontaneous activity. Defects in neuromuscular transmission can be demonstrated by repetitive stimulation. The EMG findings in motor neuron disease include large, polyphasic, varying motor unit potentials with fibrillation potentials. Demonstrating these EMG features in two muscles of each limb innervated by a different nerve and root confirms the diagnosis of motor neuron disease.

Muscle Biopsy

Muscle biopsy is a safe diagnostic procedure that can provide a definitive diagnosis in many neuromuscular disorders. Indications for biopsy include suspected inflammatory muscle disease, suspected vasculitis or collagen vascular disease, congenital or metabolic myopathy, and progressive muscular atrophy. The muscle selected for biopsy should have mild to moderate weakness. Biopsy should not be performed on a muscle that has been injured by previous trauma, injections, or EMG needles (within 4-6 weeks after EMG). The deltoid muscle is usually avoided because it is frequently used for intramuscular injections. Common muscles used for biopsy include the biceps, triceps, and quadriceps. The extensor carpi radialis and anterior tibialis are selected for biopsy of distal muscles. The pathologist needs to know which muscle is biopsied because of the variation in fiber type in different muscles. The specimen should be prepared for light and electron microscopy and histochemical stains. The clinical, EMG, and muscle biopsy findings of neuropathies and myopathies are compared in Figure 7.2.

MYOPATHIES

Disorders of muscle, called *myopathies*, are a heterogeneous group that can be due to impairment of muscle channels, structure, or metabolism. Myopathies can be classified into hereditary and acquired disorders. The hereditary myopathies include muscular dystrophies, myotonias, channelopathies, congenital myopathies, and mitochondrial myopathies. Acquired myopathies include inflammatory, endocrine, drug-induced, and toxic myopathies and myopathies associated with other systemic illness.

Finding	Neuropathy	Myopathy
Weakness	Distal>proximal	Proximal>distal
Atrophy	Yes	No (unless severe)
Reflexes	Lost early	Preserved or lost late
Fasciculation	Yes	No
EMG		
Nerve conduction	Abnormal	Normal
Fibrillation potentials	Yes	No (yes in inflammatory myopathy)
Motor unit potentials		
Normal	Large and long	Short and small

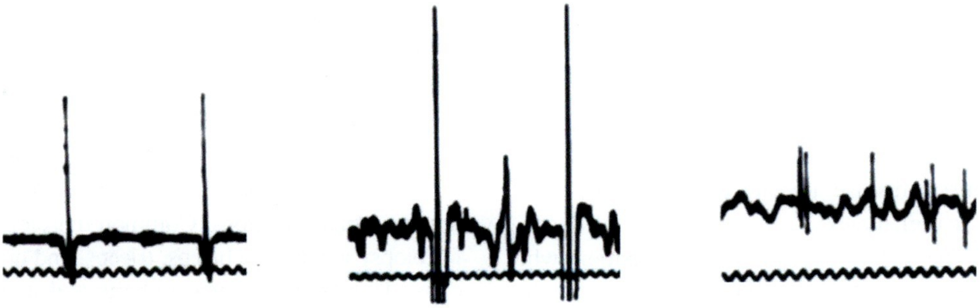

Muscle biopsy		
Normal	Group atrophy, fiber-type grouping	Atrophy or necrosis, internal nuclei, fiber splitting, inclusions

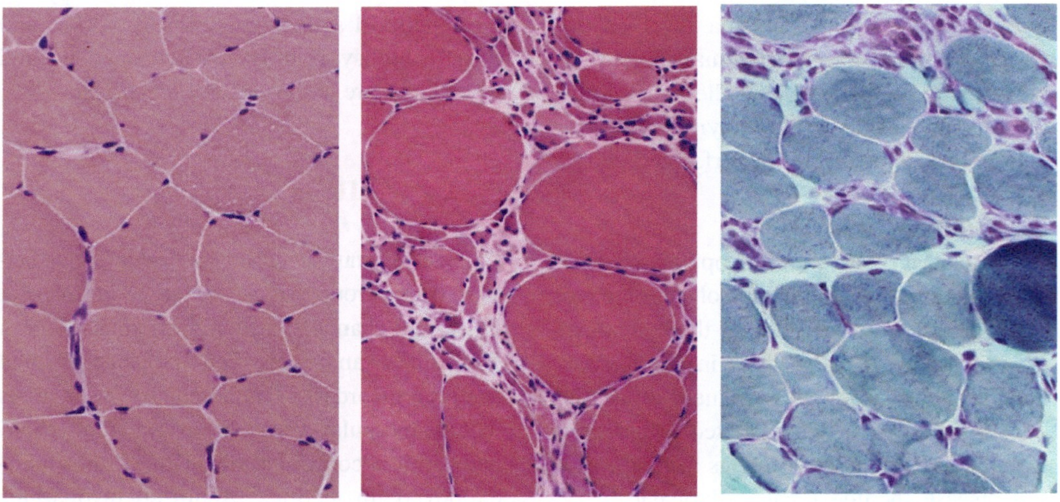

H&E	H&E	Trichrome

Fig. 7.2. Summary of clinical, electromyographic (EMG), and muscle biopsy findings in neuropathy and myopathy.

Muscular Dystrophies

Muscular dystrophies comprise a group of inherited myopathic disorders characterized by progressive muscular weakness and loss of muscle bulk. Most of the genes and defects associated with muscular dystrophies have been identified and provide accurate diagnostic tests for these disorders. The different forms of muscular dystrophy can be distinguished by mode of inheritance, distribution of muscles involved, speed of progression, and genetic defect (Table 7.1).

Duchenne muscular dystrophy is the most common form of muscular dystrophy. Its clinical features include early onset (before 5 years of age), proximal muscle weakness, gait and posture abnormalities, pseudohypertrophy, and usually cognitive impairment. Becker muscular dystrophy is clinically similar to Duchenne muscular dystrophy but has a slower rate of disease progression. Patients with Duchenne muscular dystrophy usually are confined to a wheelchair before the age of 13 years; for those with Becker muscular dystrophy, wheelchair confinement is usually after age 16 years. Both Duchenne and Becker muscular dystrophies are considered dystrophinopathies because of the dystrophin gene (chromosome Xp21). The protein product of this gene, dystrophin, appears to stabilize a glycoprotein complex in membranes and protect it from degradation. Dystrophin deficiency is thought to initiate the degenerative changes in muscle.

Muscular dystrophies should be considered multisystem disorders, and special attention should be given to the patient's cardiopulmonary status. The treatment and management of the muscular dystrophies depend on accurate diagnosis, and all patients should receive appropriate genetic counseling based on a precise diagnosis.

For Duchenne muscular dystrophy, corticosteroids have been shown to improve strength and function. Physiotherapy should be used to maintain mobility and to prevent and treat contractures. For scoliosis and contracture, orthopedic consultation may be needed. Monitoring for cardiomyopathy should begin at about age 10 years, and the patient should have follow-up once or twice annually. Pulmonary consultation is recommended twice annually at age 12 years, when vital capacity is less than 80% predicted, or when a patient is confined to a wheelchair.

Myotonic Dystrophy

Myotonic dystrophy is an autosomally dominant inherited neuromuscular disorder associated with various systemic complications. Patients with myotonic dystrophy often seek medical attention because of these systemic symptoms instead of neuromuscular complications. Patients with myotonic dystrophy type 1 have ptosis and facial and distal limb weakness. They often interpret the myotonia (the slow relaxation of muscle contraction) as "muscle stiffness" and do not complain of it. Myotonia can be demonstrated by asking patients to clench their hands tightly and then release. Patients with myotonia have a delayed release. These patients also have characteristic facial features, with facial weakness, ptosis, and, in men, frontal balding (Fig. 7.3).

The more serious systemic problems that occur in myotonic dystrophy include cardiac conduction defects and arrhythmias and aspiration pneumonia from involvement of the esophagus and diaphragm. These problems increase the risk of perioperative morbidity. Cataracts, atrophic testicles, diabetes mellitus, hypersomnia, and mild mental deterioration also occur with myotonic dystrophy.

The diagnosis of myotonic dystrophy had been made on the basis of clinical findings and a positive family history. Currently, genetic testing is available for accurate diagnosis. The EMG findings include myopathic changes and

Table 7.1. Muscular Dystrophies

Muscular dystrophy	Inheritance	Gene location	Clinical note
Becker	X-linked recessive	Xp21	Like Duchenne but clinically milder, wheelchair confinement after age 16 years
Congenital	Autosomal recessive	Gene location for each type	Infants with hypotonia and weakness at birth
Distal	Autosomal dominant	Gene location for each type	Heterogeneous group of disorders
	Autosomal recessive		Distal weakness progressing to involve proximal muscles
Duchenne	X-linked recessive	Xp21	Onset before age 5 years Pelvic girdle weakness Rapid progression Pseudohypertrophy
Emery-Dreifuss	X-linked recessive	Xq28	Humeroperoneal distribution of weakness
	Autosomal dominant	1q21	Monitor cardiac status even if asymptomatic
Facioscapulohumeral	Autosomal dominant	4q35	Shoulder girdle and face weakness Slow progression
Limb-girdle 1A to 1E	Autosomal dominant	Gene location for each type 1A–1E	Pelvic and shoulder girdle weakness
Limb-girdle 2A to 2J	Autosomal recessive	Gene location for each type 2A–2J	Pelvic and shoulder girdle weakness
Myotonic			
Type 1	Autosomal dominant, variable penetrance	19q13.3	Myotonia, facial and distal weakness, frontal balding in males, cataracts, cardiac conduction defects
Type 2	Autosomal dominant	3q13.3–q24	Myotonia, cataracts, proximal weakness
Oculopharyngeal	Autosomal dominant	14q11	Dysphagia, ocular weakness, lack of myotonia

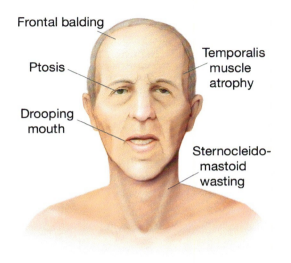

Frontal balding

Ptosis

Temporalis muscle atrophy

Drooping mouth

Sternocleido-mastoid wasting

Fig. 7.3. Facial appearance in myotonic dystrophy.

myotonic discharges. The pattern of abnormalities seen on muscle biopsy can distinguish this disorder from other myopathies and neuropathies. The gene for myotonic dystrophy type 1 is located on chromosome 19q13.3 and is an amplified trinucleotide CTG repeat. The myotonic dystrophy type 2 gene maps to chromosome 3q13.3-q24. Patients with myotonic dystrophy type 2 have more proximal weakness than those with type 1.

The treatment of myotonic dystrophy is primarily symptomatic. Physical medicine and rehabilitation may provide the most benefit. Myotonia can be treated with several medications that stabilize membranes. These include acetazolamide, carbamazepine, gabapentin, mexiletine, phenytoin, procainamide, and quinidine. However, the patient usually is disturbed more by the weakness than the myotonia. Extreme caution must be used with regard to potential cardiac effects of any medication. As with the muscular dystrophies, genetic counseling is recommended. Modafinil may provide symptomatic relief for hypersomnia, but excessive daytime sleepiness may be due to respiratory problems

and should be investigated. Close cardiac surveillance should be maintained because of the patients' high risk of arrhythmias and sudden death. Placement of a cardiac pacemaker may be necessary.

Inflammatory Myopathies

Inflammatory myopathies include dermatomyositis, polymyositis, and inclusion body myositis. Although these disorders are characterized by muscle weakness and inflammatory infiltrates within the skeletal muscle, they are distinct clinically, histologically, and pathogenically (Table 7.2).

Dermatomyositis

Dermatomyositis occurs in children or adults, with a female predominance. The temporal profile of weakness can be variable, but most often the weakness develops over several weeks. Inflammation of oropharyngeal and esophageal muscles can cause dysphagia. The skin changes consist of a blue-to-violet discoloration of the upper eyelids (heliotrope rash), with edema and papular, erythematous, scaly lesions over the knuckles (Fig. 7.4). A sunsensitive flat erythematous rash can appear on the face, neck, and anterior chest. The rash may precede the proximal muscle weakness and, in some cases, follow the weakness by several months, complicating the diagnosis.

It is important to be aware of the many associated manifestations of dermatomyositis, including pericarditis, myocarditis, congestive heart failure, and interstitial lung disease. Dermatomyositis may occur alone or in association with scleroderma or mixed connective tissue disease. An overlap syndrome has also been described in which patients have features of dermatomyositis and scleroderma or mixed connective tissue disease.

Dermatomyositis is associated with an increased risk of malignancy. Because this risk

Table 7.2. Clinical and Laboratory Features of Idiopathic Inflammatory Myopathies

Disorder	Polymyositis	Dermatomyositis	Inclusion body myositis
Pattern of weakness	Proximal > distal	Proximal > distal	Proximal = distal
Age at onset	Adult	Childhood and adult	Elderly
Sex	Female > male	Female > male	Male > female
Rash	No	Yes	No
Serum creatine kinase level	Increased (up to 50 times normal)	Normal to increased (up to 50 times normal)	Normal or mildly increased (< 10 times normal)
Pathogenesis	T-cell–mediated disorder	Humorally mediated microangiopathy	Unknown
Responsive to immunosuppressive therapy	Yes	Yes	None or minimal
Common associated conditions	Myocarditis, other connective tissue disease	Myocarditis, interstitial lung disease, malignancy, vasculitis, other connective tissue disease	Sensory neuropathy, paraproteinemia, autoimmune disorders (Sjögren syndrome, sarcoidosis, thrombocytopenia)

Modified from Amato, AA, and Barohn, RJ: Idiopathic inflammatory myopathies. Neurol Clin 15:615-648, 1997. Used with permission.

is greater for patients older than 40 years, cancer screening is recommended annually for a minimum of 3 years. Recommended studies include a complete blood count, routine blood chemistry panel, urinalysis, stool specimen for occult blood, and chest, abdominal, and pelvic computed tomographic scans. For women, mammography is recommended in addition to pelvic and breast examinations. Prostate and testicular evaluations should be performed in men. Colonoscopy is recommended for patients with gastrointestinal symptoms and for those older than 50 years.

Polymyositis

The diagnosis of polymyositis is based on the exclusion of other neuromuscular conditions. Exclusion criteria include the presence of a rash, a positive family history of neuromuscular disease, eye and facial involvement, exposure to myotoxic drugs, and endocrinopathies. Muscle biopsy findings can exclude inclusion body myositis and other neuromuscular disorders.

Polymyositis tends to occur in adults and usually progresses over weeks to months. Often, it is associated with several autoimmune diseases such as Crohn disease, vasculitis, primary biliary cirrhosis, discoid lupus, and adult celiac disease. No definitive association has been shown between polymyositis and malignant conditions.

Inclusion Body Myositis

Inclusion body myositis is unique among the inflammatory myopathies in that it can involve distal muscles early in the course and it is refractory to immunosuppressant therapy. The typical clinical presentation of inclusion body myositis is early weakness and atrophy of the quadriceps muscle, volar forearm muscles (wrist and finger flexors), and ankle dorsiflexors. A familial association has been shown in some cases. Connective tissue diseases have been associated with inclusion body myositis, but an association with malignant conditions has not been proved.

Treatment

Prednisone is effective treatment for dermatomyositis and polymyositis. The starting dose is 1.0 to 1.5 mg/kg, up to 100 mg daily, given as a one-time dose in the morning. The high dose is continued until the serum level of creatine kinase normalizes and muscle strength improves. Depending on the patient's clinical response and the creatine kinase level, the dose can be tapered. If the creatine kinase level remains normal, the dose can be tapered by 25% every 3 to 4 weeks. An increase in the creatine kinase level before an increase in muscle weakness is evidence of a relapse. By 6 to 12 months, most patients receive a maintenance dose (10 mg/day or 10-20 mg every other day).

Prolonged use of corticosteroids can complicate therapy by causing myopathy. Increasing weakness may indicate increasing disease activity or a steroid-induced myopathy. The creatine kinase level does not increase in steroid-induced myopathy. The creatine kinase level, EMG findings, and the patient's response

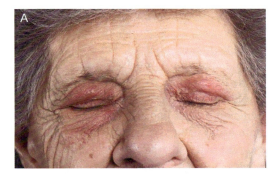

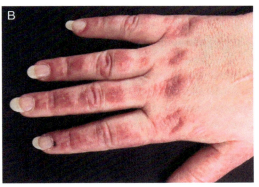

Fig. 7.4. Dermatomyositis. *A*, Heliotrope rash on upper eyelids; *B*, Gottron sign (symmetric, nonscaling, violaceous erythematous macules or plaques on dorsal surface of the fingers).

to a change in dose help determine whether the weakness is due to disease or to treatment.

Other complications of prolonged corticosteroid use should be followed closely. The patient's weight, blood pressure, and serum glucose and potassium levels should be monitored. Many authorities recommend baseline bone density scans and follow-up for the increased risk of osteoporosis. Treatment with vitamin D and calcium supplementation or bisphosphonate may be indicated. Common side effects of prednisone therapy include hypertension, fluid and weight gain, hyperglycemia, hypokalemia, cataracts, gastric irritation, osteoporosis, aseptic necrosis of the femoral head, and infection.

Other immunosuppressant therapy, such as methotrexate, azathioprine, cyclophosphamide, mycophenolate mofetil, and intravenous immunoglobulin, is used for disease resistant to corticosteroids or for patients who have intolerable adverse effects. Methotrexate, a common second-line agent, is associated with pulmonary fibrosis, which limits its use in patients with interstitial lung disease. It is important to remember that azathioprine may take up to 18 months to become effective. Physical therapy is important to prevent disuse atrophy and joint contractures.

Metabolic Myopathies

Metabolic myopathies are disorders that result from insufficient energy production. They include disorders of metabolism in glycogen, lipids, purine nucleotides, and mitochondria. The clinical features of metabolic myopathies in older children and adults include exercise intolerance, weakness, and myoglobinuria. Glycogen storage disorders and lipid metabolism disorders are summarized in Tables 7.3 and 7.4, respectively.

The only disorder of nucleotide metabolism in muscle is myoadenylate deaminase deficiency. Patients with this disorder complain of muscle pain with exertion and fatigue. Complicating this diagnosis is that many patients are asymptomatic.

Mitochondrial myopathies are a complex group of disorders with defects in mitochondria. In addition to myopathy, these disorders have many other systemic problems. Kearns-Sayre syndrome (progressive external ophthalmoparesis, pigmentary retinopathy, and heart block), myoclonic epilepsy and ragged red fibers (MERRF), and mitochondrial encephalomyopathy, lactic acidosis, and strokelike episodes (MELAS) syndrome are three examples of mitochondrial myopathies.

Muscle Channelopathies

Disorders caused by mutations in cell membrane ion channels have been designated channelopathies. These are rare disorders and include nondystrophic myotonias and periodic paralyses (Table 7.5).

Myopathies Associated With Drugs and Toxins

Many drugs can cause muscle injury. Myotoxic injury is important to recognize to decrease further damage to the muscle. If a patient has muscle weakness, review all the medications the patient is taking to discover possible myotoxic effects. The mechanism of muscle injury varies with the toxin. D-Penicillamine and procainamide can cause inflammatory myopathy. Diuretics, laxatives, and alcohol can cause hypokalemia, which in turn produces muscle weakness and injury. The majority of toxic substances, for example, lipid-lowering agents, cause a necrotizing myopathy. Patients may present with acute or subacute muscle pain and proximal weakness. The serum level of creatine kinase is increased. If muscle necrosis is severe, myoglobinuria can occur. Many of the drugs that can cause myopathy are listed in Table 7.6.

Muscle injury is also associated with illicit drug use. Because heroin impairs consciousness, it can lead to pressure-induced damage of skeletal muscles. Cocaine, amphetamines, and phencyclidine can cause myoglobinuria as a result of agitation, convulsions, and catatonic muscular rigidity. Weakness develops in chronic glue sniffers because of metabolic derangements associated with exposure to toluene.

Nutritional deficiencies can cause muscle weakness. The myopathy seen in alcoholics may have a nutritional component. Vitamin E deficiency, which can cause peripheral neuropathy, can also cause muscle weakness. This

Table 7.3. Summary of Glycogen Storage Disorders

Type	Enzyme and gene (chromosome)	Clinical features
II, Pompe disease	Acid maltase, *GAA* (17q21-23)	Infants: hypotonia Adults: proximal or distal weakness, dementia, UMN and LMN involvement, incontinence
III, Cori-Forbes disease	Debrancher, *AGL* (1p21)	Infants: hypotonia Adults: proximal or distal weakness, dementia, UMN and LMN involvement, incontinence
IV, Andersen disease	Branching, *GBE1* (3p12)	Infants: generalized weakness Adults: proximal or distal weakness
V, McArdle disease	Myophosphorylase, *PYGM* (11q13)	Infants: profound weakness Adults: exercise intolerance, cramps, fatigue
VII, Tarui disease	Phosphofructokinase *PFKM* (12q13)	Childhood: cramps, fatigue, exercise intolerance
VIII	Phosphorylase *b* kinase, *PHBK* (16q12-q13)	Infancy to adult: exercise intolerance, myoglobinuria, weakness
IX	Phosphoglycerate kinase, *PGK* (Xq13)	Childhood: cramps, myoglobinuria, exercise intolerance, rare weakness, central nervous system dysfunction, hemolytic anemia, X-linked
X	Phosphoglycerate mutase, *PGAM-M* (7p13-p12.3)	Childhood or adolescence: exercise intolerance, cramps, myoglobinuria
XI	Lactate dehydrogenase, *LDHA* (11p15.4)	Childhood to adulthood: exercise intolerance, cramps, myoglobinuria

LMN, lower motor neuron; UMN, upper motor neuron.
Modified from Walsh, RJ: Metabolic myopathies. Continuum: Lifelong Learning in Neurology 12:76-120, 2006. Used with permission.

Table 7.4. Summary of Lipid Metabolism Disorders

Disorder	Clinical features
Primary muscle carnitine deficiency	Proximal weakness and atrophy Treatment: L-Carnitine 　Adults: 2-6 g/day 　Children: 100 mg/kg
Primary systemic carnitine deficiency	Systemic features, encephalopathy, cardiomyopathy, impaired fatty acid oxidation
Carnitine palmitoyltransferase II deficiency	Adult: recurrent myoglobinuria, muscle pain and cramping after exercise
Very long-chain acyl-CoA dehydrogenase deficiency	Mild before age 2 years without cardiomyopathy Severe with cardiomyopathy
Long-chain acyl-CoA dehydrogenase deficiency	Failure to thrive
Medium-chain acyl-CoA dehydrogenase deficiency	Failure to thrive, lethargy, vomiting, coma
Short-chain acyl-CoA dehydrogenase deficiency	Failure to thrive and metabolic acidosis
3-OH long-chain acyl-CoA dehydrogenase deficiency	Failure to thrive

CoA, coenzyme A.

deficiency occurs in patients with lipid malabsorption syndromes such as cystic fibrosis and cholestatic liver disease. Excessive consumption of vitamin E causes muscle injury. Vitamin D deficiency is associated with muscle weakness. Osteomalacia responds to treatment with vitamin D.

Endocrine Myopathies

Muscle dysfunction frequently accompanies endocrine disorders because muscle function depends on hormonal balance. Both hormonal excess and deficiency are associated with muscle weakness. Patients with hyperthyroidism frequently have proximal muscle weakness in the course of the illness, and a small percentage

have muscle weakness as the initial complaint. The serum level of creatine kinase is not usually increased in hyperthyroidism, but it is in hypothyroidism. Patients with hypothyroidism frequently report muscle weakness, cramps, pain, and stiffness. Myopathic changes on EMG and nonspecific histologic changes in muscle are seen in both hyperthyroidism and hypothyroidism. The muscle weakness resolves with treatment of the thyroid condition.

Hyperparathyroidism can cause proximal muscle weakness and, infrequently, bulbar weakness. Muscle stretch reflexes may be brisk, unlike in other myopathies. The underlying cause of the myopathy may be related to vitamin D deficiency, hypercalcemia, phosphate

Table 7.5. Muscle Channelopathies

Disorder	Ion channel	Clinical features	Drug therapy
Myotonia congenita	Chloride	Moderate to severe myotonia	Mexiletine
Paramyotonia congenita	Sodium	Moderate myotonia	Mexiletine
Hyperkalemic periodic paralysis	Sodium	Episodes of weakness triggered by cold and by rest after exercise	Thiazide diuretics, carbonic anhydrase inhibitors
Hypokalemic periodic paralysis	Calcium Sodium	Episodes of weakness triggered by rest after exercise and by high carbohydrate meals	Carbonic anhydrase inhibitors, potassium chloride, potassium-sparing diuretics
Thyrotoxic periodic paralysis	Unknown	Episodic weakness triggered by rest after exercise and by high carbohydrate meals	β-Blockers, antithyroid treatments, potassium chloride, potassium-sparing diuretics
Andersen-Tawil syndrome	Potassium	Episodic weakness triggered by rest after exercise and by menses	Carbonic anhydrase inhibitors

deficiency, or neurogenic influences. Hypoparathyroidism and the associated hypocalcemia can cause tetany (a condition marked by intermittent tonic muscle contractions).

Myopathy associated with corticosteroid excess is described above. The same type of pattern is seen in Cushing syndrome. Adrenocortical deficiency (Addison disease) is also associated with muscle weakness, fatigue, and cramping. Attacks of periodic paralysis can occur in this disorder because of hyperkalemia. Hyperaldosteronism and associated hypokalemia also can cause attacks of periodic paralysis. Muscle weakness is frequently a feature of hyperaldosteronism.

Acromegaly, due to excess growth hormone, is associated with proximal muscle weakness, wasting, and hypotonia. The myopathy resolves with normalization of growth hormone levels.

The absence of growth hormone affects muscle. Muscle fails to develop properly without growth hormone, as in children with pituitary failure. Thyroid deficiency and adrenocortical hormone deficiency in pituitary failure also impair muscle function.

DISORDERS OF THE NEUROMUSCULAR JUNCTION

The cardinal feature of neuromuscular junction dysfunction is fatigable weakness. Myasthenia gravis is the most common disorder of the neuromuscular junction. It is an autoimmune disease in which sensitized T-helper cells mediate an IgG-directed attack on nicotinic acetylcholine receptors on muscle cells. Other neuromuscular junction disorders include

Table 7.6. Myotoxic Agents

Toxin (brand name)	Use or setting
Alcohol	Abuse
Aminocaproic acid	Antihemorrhagic agent
Amiodarone (Cordarone)	Antiarrhythmic agent
Amphotericin B (Abelcet)	Antifungal agent
Atorvastatin (Lipitor)	Antihyperlipidemic
Chloroquine (Aralen)	Antimalarial agent
Cimetidine (Tagamet)	Histamine antagonist (ulcer/reflux)
Clofibrate (Atromid-S)	Antihyperlipidemic
Colchicine and probenecid (ColBenemid)	Uricosuric agent (gout)
Contaminated tryptophan	Dietary supplement
Cyclosporine (Neoral)	Immunosuppressant
Gemfibrozil (Lopid)	Hypertriglyceridemia
Ipecac syrup	Emetic agent
Labetalol (Normodyne)	Antihypertensive agent
Lovastatin (Mevacor)	Antihyperlipidemic
Organophosphates	Insecticide exposure
Penicillamine (Cuprimine)	Heavy metal antagonist (rheumatoid arthritis)
Pravastatin (Pravachol)	Antihyperlipidemic
Prednisone (Deltasone)	Immunosuppressant
Procainamide (Pronestyl)	Antiarrhythmic
Rosuvastatin (Crestor)	Antihyperlipidemic
Simvastatin (Zocor)	Antihyperlipidemic
Toluene	Solvent exposure (glue sniffing)
Vincristine (Oncovin)	Antineoplastic agent
Vitamin E	Excessive self-medication
Zidovudine (Retrovir)	Antiviral agent

Modified from Adams, AC: Neurology in Primary Care. FA Davis, Philadelphia, 2000, p 129. Used with permission of Mayo Foundation for Medical Education and Research.

Lambert-Eaton myasthenic syndrome and botulism. Also, many drugs and toxins can impair neuromuscular transmission.

Myasthenia Gravis

Myasthenia gravis is an acquired disorder of neuromuscular transmission caused by the binding of pathogenic autoantibodies to postsynaptic nicotinic acetylcholine receptors (AChRs) located in the membrane of skeletal muscle end plates. Approximately 10% of patients with generalized myasthenia gravis have serum antibodies directed at the muscle-specific receptor tyrosine kinase (MuSK), an intrinsic protein of the end-plate membrane. Patients with disease classified as seronegative myasthenia gravis often have antibodies directed at MuSK. The loss of the cation channel protein required to activate the muscle action potential causes the fatigable weakness.

The muscles most often affected are bulbar muscles (used in speaking, chewing, and swallowing), extraocular muscles, and proximal limb muscles. Thus, patients complain of ptosis, diplopia, dysarthria, dysphagia, and fatigable weakness. The symptoms are least noticeable first thing in the morning after the patient has rested and are worse at the end of the day. In contrast, patients with depression complain of fatigue that is worse at the beginning of the day.

Ophthalmoplegia, with ptosis and diplopia, is a common sign in myasthenia gravis. However, the pupil is not affected in this disease (although it is affected in most diseases involving cranial nerve III). Extraocular muscle weakness can be provoked by having the patient look upward for several minutes. The muscles of mastication may be affected and cause difficulty with chewing. This should not be confused with jaw claudication that occurs in temporal arteritis.

Diagnostic Tests for Myasthenia Gravis

If myasthenia gravis is suspected, testing is needed to confirm the diagnosis. Antibodies to AChRs are found in the blood of more than 75% of patients with generalized myasthenia. The presence of AChR antibodies supports the diagnosis of autoimmune myasthenia gravis, and quantification of the antibodies provides a baseline for future comparisons. These antibodies are not found in congenital myasthenia gravis. Other disorders that may be seropositive for AChR antibodies are Lambert-Eaton myasthenic syndrome, paraneoplastic autoimmune neurologic disorders, and autoimmune liver disease. Other antibodies associated with myasthenia gravis are listed in Table 7.7. The detection of AChR antibodies confirms the diagnosis of myasthenia gravis.

Electrophysiologic tests to confirm the diagnosis of myasthenia gravis include repetitive nerve stimulation and single fiber EMG. Repetitive nerve stimulation fatigues the neuromuscular junction by depleting the nerve endings of acetylcholine. A decremental response in the compound muscle action potential of 10% or more is seen in patients with myasthenia gravis (Fig. 7.5). Single fiber EMG, a technique for recording from individual muscle fibers, is extremely sensitive in detecting a defect in neuromuscular transmission, even in clinically unaffected muscles. The single fiber EMG electrode is inserted into voluntary activated muscle to record action potentials from two or more muscle fibers of the same motor unit, and the variation of the interpotential interval during consecutive discharges is measured. In disorders of neuromuscular transmission, variability is marked (abnormal jitter). Single fiber EMG requires a skilled electromyographer, special equipment, and a cooperative patient.

Intravenous injection of edrophonium (the Tensilon test) has been used in diagnosing myasthenia gravis. Edrophonium, a short-acting cholinesterase inhibitor, must be administered with care because of potential serious reactions, including bradycardia and bronchospasm. The test should be considered only if definite muscle weakness is observed, for example, ptosis. The decision to perform this test should be made only on the basis of physical signs, not subjective symptoms.

Other diagnostic tests that are frequently performed if myasthenia gravis is suspected are thyroid function tests, antinuclear antibody test, antistriated muscle antibody test, and chest computed tomography or magnetic resonance imaging. Thyroid function tests are useful because autoimmune thyroid disease occurs in approximately 10% of patients with myasthenia gravis. The antinuclear antibody test may indicate other autoimmune disorders; lupus erythematosus is associated with a false-positive AChR antibody test. Chest imaging is important because of the high incidence of thymic hyperplasia and thymoma in myasthenia gravis. A positive anti-striated muscle antibody test suggests lymphoma.

Treatment

The treatment of myasthenia gravis includes cholinesterase inhibitors, immunosuppressant drugs, immune-directed therapy (plasmapheresis and intravenous immunoglobulin), and thymectomy. Pyridostigmine (Mestinon), a cholinesterase inhibitor, is frequently the initial therapy for symptomatic relief. Most patients with myasthenia gravis require additional medication. The adverse effects of pyridostigmine are signs of acetylcholine excess and include muscle cramps, diarrhea, and an increase in oral secretions. The increase in oral secretions may pose a difficulty for patients with weakness of pharyngeal and respiratory muscles.

Because excessive anticholinesterase therapy can cause increasing weakness, patients should be instructed not to increase the dose of medication without medical direction. Acute weakness is a medical emergency, and the patient should be hospitalized in an intensive care unit and respiratory function monitored. With the patient in the hospital, stop all treatment with anticholinesterase agents to determine whether increased weakness is due to cholinergic excess or to exacerbation of the disease. Any concurrent infections and electrolyte abnormalities need to be corrected. The patient should be intubated if the respiratory status declines (vital capacity, 15 mL/kg or less) or there is risk of aspiration. Plasmapheresis or intravenous administration of a high dose of immunoglobulin will rapidly improve the patient's condition.

When symptomatic treatment with pyridostigmine is not effective, then treatment with immunosuppressant drugs is required. Immunosuppressant therapy includes corticosteroids (prednisone), azathioprine (Imuran), cyclophosphamide (Cytoxan), and mycophenolate mofetil (CellCept).

Table 7.7. Antibodies Associated With Neuromuscular Transmission Disorders

Antibody	Comment
Myasthenia gravis	
Acetylcholine receptor (AChR) antibodies	Serologic marker for myasthenia gravis
AChR binding	Low sensitivity but related to severity
AChR blocking	High titers in severe disease and thymoma
AChR modulating	
Striational antibody	Antibody to striated muscle, associated with thymoma
Titin antibody	Antibody to muscle protein, associated with thymoma
Ryanodine receptor	Antibody to a calcium release channel in the sarcoplasmic reticulum
Muscle-specific receptor tyrosine kinase	Positive in about 40% of patients with negative AChR, more common in women
Lambert-Eaton myasthenic syndrome	
Antibodies to voltage-gated calcium channel	Located on presynaptic terminal

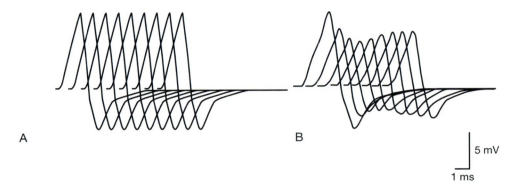

A   B

5 mV

1 ms

Fig. 7.5. Repetitive nerve stimulation. *A*, Normal; *B*, in myasthenia gravis. Responses were obtained with repetitive stimulation of the ulnar nerve at 3 Hz, recording from the abductor digiti minimi muscle. The maximal decrement in *B* (30%) occurs after the fourth stimulation, producing the classic "U-shaped," or "saddle-shaped," envelope pattern. (From Meriggioli, MN, Howard, JF, Jr, and Harper CM: Neuromuscular Junction Disorders: Diagnosis and Treatment. Marcel Dekker, New York, 2004, p 73. Used with permission.)

Prednisone is effective therapy for myasthenia gravis, but care needs to be exercised because the patient's condition may worsen clinically 1 to 2 weeks after therapy is initiated, requiring hospitalization. The initial dose of prednisone is 1 mg/kg daily in three divided doses. The patient usually notices improvement after 6 weeks of treatment. This dose is maintained until remission (approximately 3 months), after which the dose can be tapered. The tapering should be modified according to the patient's response, but every-other-day dosing should be attempted to reduce adverse effects. The side effects of corticosteroids include weight gain, hypertension, diabetes mellitus, depression, insomnia, glaucoma, osteoporosis, cataracts, ulcer, myopathy, opportunistic infections, and avascular necrosis of the femoral head.

The side effects of long-term corticosteroid treatment are often the reason to try other immunosuppressant therapy. Azathioprine is effective, but the time to onset of improvement is slow. The initial dose is 1 mg/kg, with a gradual increase to 2 to 3 mg/kg. Nausea and vomiting are common side effects. The potential for serious hematologic effects requires weekly monitoring during the first month of therapy, bimonthly for the second and third months, and monthly thereafter. Cyclophosphamide has been helpful for patients who are unable to tolerate corticosteroids. However, cyclophosphamide has a high risk of serious side effects. Mycophenolate mofetil, another steroid-sparing immunosuppressant, has also been shown to be effective in the treatment of myasthenia gravis.

Plasmapheresis and intravenous immunoglobulin can produce a rapid improvement in myasthenia gravis, but the improvement is of short duration. These therapies are most useful for myasthenic crises or preoperative management.

Thymectomy improves the condition in the majority of patients, and it is often recommended even if there is no thymoma or thymic hyperplasia. Thymectomy is indicated for all patients with thymoma and those younger than 60 years who have generalized myasthenia gravis. It also should be considered for older patients on an individual basis. Young adults with early myasthenia gravis tend to have the best results, with high rates of remission.

Factors That Exacerbate Myasthenia Gravis

It is important to be aware of factors that exacerbate myasthenic weakness. These include major physical stress, fever, pregnancy, and heat. Also, many antibiotics exacerbate the condition, for example, aminoglycosides, fluoroquinolone antibiotics, erythromycin, clindamycin, polymyxin B, and tetracycline. Other medications that can exacerbate it include phenytoin, lithium, β-blockers, calcium channel blockers, quinine, antiarrhythmic agents, sedatives, and muscle relaxants. Except for penicillamine, which is contraindicated, these medications can be administered when necessary. However, be aware of the potential effect, and be prepared to manage an exacerbation of weakness.

Lambert-Eaton Myasthenic Syndrome

Lambert-Eaton myasthenic syndrome (LEMS) is a rare autoimmune disorder characterized by fluctuating muscle weakness, autonomic dysfunction, and hyporeflexia. It is often associated with small cell carcinoma of the lung and has been reported in other malignancies. A primary autoimmune nonparaneoplastic form of LEMS has also been reported. Patients may have trouble walking or have symptoms of proximal muscle weakness. Unlike myasthenia gravis, some improvement may be noted with exercise. Autonomic symptoms include dry mouth and, in men, erectile dysfunction. Vague numbness in the thighs is often reported.

LEMS is caused by antibodies to presynaptic voltage-gated calcium channels in motor and autonomic nerve terminals that disrupt the influx of calcium and decrease the release of acetylcholine. A decremental response occurs with repetitive nerve stimulation, similar to that in myasthenia gravis. However, after a brief period of exercise, facilitation of the compound action potential is seen. An underlying malignancy should be sought and treated. Pyridostigmine, 3,4-diaminopyridine, and various immunosuppressant regimens have been used to treat LEMS.

Botulism

Botulism is caused by the exotoxin of *Clostridium botulinum*. The four types of botulism that have been described are infant, foodborne, wound, and from an undetermined source. The toxin binds to autonomic and motor nerve terminals and blocks the presynaptic release of acetylcholine. Symptoms include progressive muscle weakness that begins in the extraocular or pharyngeal muscles and then affects other muscles. Gastrointestinal symptoms are prominent. Dilated unreactive pupils and dry mucous membranes indicate autonomic involvement. An antitoxin is available, and treatment should be initiated as soon as the diagnosis is made.

Medications

Neuromuscular junction problems can be caused or unmasked by several medications. Medications that exacerbate myasthenia gravis impair neuromuscular transmission through a direct effect. Medications such as penicillamine, chloroquine, and trimethadione cause neuromuscular dysfunction by producing an immune response. Many poisons, snake venom, and some spider bites also have an effect on neuromuscular junctions.

MOTOR NEURON DISEASE

There are several types of motor neuron disease. The most common disorder is *amyotrophic lateral sclerosis* (ALS), or Lou Gehrig disease. This is a progressive disease that involves both upper and lower motor neurons. *Progressive bulbar palsy* affects primarily the bulbar muscles; it is characterized by speech and swallowing dysfunction and may be the initial manifestation of motor neuron disease. *Spinal muscular atrophy* is a motor neuron disease of predominantly lower motor neurons. Several inherited disorders, categorized by age at onset, are included in the category of spinal muscular atrophy (Table 7.8). *Primary lateral sclerosis* is a disorder of upper motor neuron dysfunction. Spinal muscular atrophy and primary lateral sclerosis are both rare forms of motor neuron disease.

If both upper and lower motor neurons are involved, the differential diagnosis is limited. Cervical spondylosis can cause weakness, atrophy, and fasciculations in the upper extremities because of nerve root involvement and hyperreflexia in the lower extremities because of spinal cord compression. Hyperthyroidism causes muscle wasting and weight loss and may resemble ALS. If lower motor neurons are predominantly involved, inclusion body myositis and multifocal motor neuropathy should be considered. Multifocal motor neuropathy responds to immunosuppressive therapy. Lymphoma (through its remote effect), radiation exposure, hyperparathyroidism, and adult-onset hexosaminidase A deficiency can mimic ALS. Diagnostic tests used to confirm and to exclude other causes of ALS are summarized in Table 7.9.

A multidisciplinary approach should be taken in treating ALS. Although the prognosis is poor, much can be done to care for patients. Active participants in this care should include neurologists; nurses; physical, occupational, and speech therapists; dieticians; home health aides; mental health workers; and other medical specialists. Currently, riluzole, an inhibitor of glutamate metabolism, is the only medicine available that slows the progression of the disease. Tertiary medical centers should be contacted about the availability of other drug treatments being assessed in clinical trials.

Table 7.8. Classification of Spinal Muscular Atrophy

Type	Clinical feature or age at onset
0	Arthrogryposis
I, acute Werdnig-Hoffmann disease	Acute infantile form
II, chronic Werdnig-Hoffmann disease	Intermediate
III, Kugelberg-Welander syndrome	Mild
IV	Adult

Poliomyelitis and Postpolio Syndrome

Poliomyelitis, or polio, was a common disorder of motor neurons until vaccination became available. Patients who had poliomyelitis in early life are at risk for postpolio syndrome. The clinical features of this syndrome include fatigue, myalgias, arthralgias, weakness, cold intolerance, sleep apnea syndrome, and depression. The cause has not been established; two suggestions are that 1) it is caused by a gradual loss of motor units as a result of aging or 2) it is due to increased metabolic demand on reinnervated muscle fibers. Treatment guidelines for postpolio syndrome include assessment for the treatment of sleep apnea, depression, pulmonary function, and any other medical disorder. Patients should avoid exhausting activities and maintain their ideal weight. Individualized physical therapy, with stretching, range of motion, and nonfatiguing exercises, is helpful. Joint and muscle pain can be reduced with heat, massage, and antiinflammatory medication.

West Nile Virus

Although poliomyelitis essentially has been eliminated in developed countries, West Nile virus can cause a similar clinical syndrome, with the two conditions sharing many clinical, laboratory, and pathologic features. According to several reports, an acute flaccid paralysis syndrome is associated with West Nile virus infection.

Cramps and Fasciculations

Muscle cramps and fasciculations are often considered manifestations of motor neuron disease, and, although they can represent serious disease, most often patients need only to be reassured that these are normal phenomena. Fasciculations are the visible spontaneous contractions of muscle fibers and the only sign of lower motor neuron dysfunction in the presence of weakness. A cramp is a painful muscle spasm, which usually occurs in the muscles of the calf and feet. Dehydration from exercise, diuretics, or hemodialysis is frequently associated with muscle cramps. Metabolic abnormalities associated with muscle cramps include hyponatremia, hypomagnesemia, hypocalcemia, and hypoglycemia. Other conditions associated with muscle cramps are thyroid disease, adrenal insufficiency, and pregnancy. Medications that can cause cramps include albuterol, clofibrate, cyclosporine, labetalol, nifedipine, and terbutaline. The neurologic causes of cramps are motor neuron disease and peripheral neuropathy. Familial cramp syndrome is rare.

The treatment of cramps involves eliminating any underlying metabolic or medical condition that could be associated with them. Quinine sulfate, 260 mg at bedtime, has been prescribed to prevent and treat painful muscle spasms, but it has several adverse effects.

Table 7.9. Diagnostic Tests for Amyotrophic Lateral Sclerosis (ALS)

Test	Finding in ALS	Other diagnoses the test excludes
Electromyography	Large, polyphasic motor unit potentials with fibrillation potentials	Multifocal motor neuropathy Inclusion body myositis Myasthenia gravis
Cervical cord imaging	Normal or asymptomatic degenerative changes	Cervical spondylosis with spinal cord compression
Creatine kinase	<1,000 IU/L	Inclusion body myositis
Muscle biopsy	Neurogenic changes	Inclusion body myositis
Anti-GM$_1$ ganglioside antibody	Negative	Multifocal motor neuropathy
Serum protein electrophoresis	Normal	Lymphoma Multifocal motor neuropathy
Thyroid-stimulating hormone	Normal	Hyperthyroidism
Blood levels of calcium, phosphorus, alkaline phosphatase	Normal	Hyperparathyroidism
Hexosaminidase A	Normal	Hexosaminidase A deficiency

From Adams, AC: Neurology in Primary Care. FA Davis, Philadelphia, 2000, p 133. Used with permission of Mayo Foundation for Medical Education and Research.

Carbamazepine, clonazepam, gabapentin, phenytoin, and verapamil have also been used to treat this painful condition.

SUGGESTED READING

Amato, AA, and Barohn, RJ: Idiopathic inflammatory myopathies. Neurol Clin 15:615-648, 1997.

Bushby, K, and Straub, V: Nonmolecular treatment for muscular dystrophies. Curr Opin Neurol 18:511-518, 2005.

Dalakas, MC: Polymyositis, dermatomyositis and inclusion-body myositis. N Engl J Med 325:1487-1498, 1991.

Darras, BT: Muscular dystrophies. Continuum: Lifelong Learning in Neurology 12:33-75, 2006.

Engel, AG: The muscle biopsy. In Engel, AG, and Franzini-Armstrong, C (eds): Myology: Basic and Clinical. Vol 1, ed 2. McGraw-Hill, New York, 1994, pp 822-831.

Engel, AG, Hohlfeld, R, and Banker, BQ: The polymyositis and dermatomyositis syndromes. In Engel, AG, and Franzini-Armstrong, C (eds): Myology: Basic and Clinical. Vol 2, ed 2. McGraw-Hill, New York, 1994, pp 1335-1383.

Gordon, PH, et al: The natural history of primary lateral sclerosis. Neurology 66:647-653, 2006.

Gupta, A, et al: Adult botulism type F in the United States, 1981-2002. Neurology 65:1694-1700, 2005.

Harper, PS, and Rüdel, R: Myotonic dystrophy. In Engel, AG, and Franzini-Armstrong, C (eds): Myology: Basic and Clinical. Vol 2, ed 2. McGraw-Hill, New York, 1994, pp 1192-1219

Hopkins, LC: Clinical features of myasthenia gravis. Neurol Clin 12:243-261, 1994.

Jones, HR, Jr: Lambert-Eaton myasthenic syndrome. In Samuels, MA, and Feske, S (eds): Office Practice of Neurology. Churchill Livingstone, New York, 1996, pp 567-571.

Kaminski, HJ, and Ruff, RL: Endocrine myopathies (hyper- and hypofunction of adrenal, thyroid, pituitary, and parathyroid glands and iatrogenic corticosteroid myopathy). In Engel, AG, and Franzini-Armstrong, C (eds): Myology: Basic and Clinical. Vol 2, ed 2. McGraw-Hill, New York, 1994, pp 1726-1753.

Massey, JM: Treatment of acquired myasthenia gravis. Neurology 48 Suppl 5:S46-S51, 1997.

Meriggioli, MN, and Sanders, DB: Advances in the diagnosis of neuromuscular junction disorders. Am J Phys Med Rehabil 84:627-638, 2005.

Mitsumoto, H, et al: Motor neuron disease. Continuum: Lifelong Learning in Neurology 3:8-127, 1997.

Pickett, J: Toxic and metabolic disorders of the neuromuscular junction. In Samuels, MA, and Feske, S (eds): Office Practice of Neurology. Churchill Livingstone, New York, 1996, pp 571-577.

Preston, DC: Myasthenia gravis. In Samuels, MA, and Feske, S (eds): Office Practice of Neurology. Churchill Livingstone, New York, 1996, pp 562-567.

Richman, DP, and Agius, MA: Treatment of autoimmune myasthenia gravis. Neurology 61:1652-1661, 2003.

Sejvar, JJ: West Nile virus and "poliomyelitis." Neurology 63:206-207, 2004.

Shaw, PJ: Molecular and cellular pathways of neurodegeneration in motor neurone disease. J Neurol Neurosurg Psychiatry 76:1046-1057, 2005.

Simmons, Z: Management strategies for patients with amyotrophic lateral sclerosis from diagnosis through death. Neurologist 11:257-270, 2005.

Victor, M, and Sieb, JP: Myopathies due to drugs, toxins, and nutritional deficiency. In Engel, AB, and Franzini-Armstrong, C (eds): Myology: Basic and Clinical. Vol 2, ed 2. McGraw-Hill, New York, 1994, pp 1697-1725.

Walsh, RJ: Metabolic myopathies. Continuum: Lifelong Learning in Neurology 12:76-120, 2006.

CHAPTER 8

Cognitive Loss

This chapter discusses memory loss, dementia, and other cognitive dysfunction. *Dementia* is defined as significant loss of cognitive function involving multiple cognitive areas and the absence of clouded consciousness. Memory, the ability to learn new information or to recall previously learned information, is impaired. The diagnostic criteria for dementia include at least one of the following: language disturbance (aphasia), impaired ability to perform motor activities despite intact motor function (apraxia), failure to recognize or to identify objects despite intact sensory function (agnosia), personality change, constructional difficulties, and a disturbance in executive functioning. Executive functioning includes planning, organizing, sequencing, and abstracting. The loss of intellectual abilities needs to be sufficiently severe to interfere with social or occupational functions.

The most common cause of dementia is Alzheimer disease (Table 8.1). Accurate diagnosis is important because reversible causes of dementia must be excluded and because of the treatment options available. Early diagnosis is advantageous not only for treatment but also so the patient can be more involved in making important decisions (eg, living arrangements and financial affairs) before the disease progresses to the point when this is not possible. Family members can be educated about the disease process, and proactive measures can be taken with regard to financial affairs, legal matters, driving, living arrangements, and safety. The inherited nature of some dementing illnesses makes the correct diagnosis of dementia important to family members.

The incidence and prevalence of dementia increase with age, with the prevalence doubling every 5 years. One percent of persons 65 years old have dementia, compared with 50% of those older than 90 years. As the population ages, prompt recognition and intervention will become increasingly important. Failure to diagnose dementia correctly has been attributed to lack of attention to cognitive functioning in routine medical examinations and to misperceptions about the normal aging process.

DIAGNOSTIC APPROACH

From 50% to 75% of patients with dementia have Alzheimer disease. When a patient complains of cognitive impairment, the initial focus

Table 8.1. Causes of Dementia

Degenerative
  Alzheimer disease
  Parkinson disease
  Frontotemporal dementia
  Pick disease
  Huntington disease
  Progressive supranuclear palsy
  Dementia with Lewy bodies
  Multiple system atrophy
  Olivopontocerebellar degeneration
  Focal cortical degeneration
  Corticobasal degeneration
  Wilson disease
  Hallervorden-Spatz disease
Vascular
  Multi-infarct dementia
  Binswanger disease
  Amyloid dementia
  Vasculitis
  Specific vascular syndrome (thalamic,
    inferotemporal, bifrontal)
  Diffuse hypoxic and/or ischemic injury
  Mitochondrial disease
  CADASIL
Trauma
  Subdural hematoma
  Postconcussion syndrome
  Dementia pugilistica
  Anoxic brain injury
Inflammation and infection
  HIV dementia, opportunistic organisms
  Chronic meningitis (tuberculosis,
    cryptococcosis, cysticercosis)
  Syphilis
  Lyme encephalopathy
  Creutzfeldt-Jakob disease
  Post-herpes simplex encephalitis
  Progressive multifocal leukoen-
    cephalopathy
  Sarcoidosis

  Whipple disease of the brain
  Subacute sclerosing panencephalitis
Neoplastic
  Primary brain tumors
  Metastatic tumors
  Lymphoma
  Paraneoplastic limbic encephalitis
Drugs or toxins
  Medications: β-blockers, neuroleptics,
    antidepressants, anticonvulsants,
    histamine receptor blockers, dopamine
    blockade
  Alcohol abuse
  Recreational drug abuse
  Lead
  Mercury
  Arsenic
Psychiatric
  Depression
  Personality disorder
  Anxiety disorder
Metabolic
  Thyroid disease
  Vitamin B_{12} deficiency (pernicious anemia)
  Vitamin B_1 (thiamine) deficiency
    (Wernicke-Korsakoff syndrome)
  Uremia and dialysis dementia
  Chronic hepatic encephalopathy
  Chronic hypoglycemic encephalopathy
  Chronic hypercapnia and/or hypoxemia
  Chronic hypercalcemia or electrolyte
    imbalance
  Addison disease
  Cushing disease
  Hartnup disease
Autoimmune
  Systemic lupus erythematosus
  Polyarteritis nodosa
  Temporal arteritis
  Isolated angiitis of the central nervous
    system
  Wegener granulomatosis

Table 8.1   (continued)

Demyelinating
  Multiple sclerosis
  Adrenoleukodystrophy
  Metachromatic leukodystrophy
Obstructive
  Normal-pressure hydrocephalus
  Obstructive hydrocephalus

CADASIL, cerebral autosomal dominant arteriopathy
  with subcortical infarcts and leukoencephalopathy;
  HIV, human immunodeficiency virus.
From Adams, AC: Neurology in Primary Care. FA
  Davis, Philadelphia, 2000, p 137. Used with per-
  mission of Mayo Foundation for Medical
  Education and Research.

is to determine whether the symptoms suggest dementia, delirium, or depression. The characteristic feature of a patient with delirium or an acute confusional state is inattention and an impaired and fluctuating level of consciousness. This is uncommon in an outpatient setting.

History

The history of a patient with memory loss or cognitive dysfunction is critical. However, the patient may not be able to provide sufficient information, and a corroborative history is needed from family or friends or both. It is more meaningful when a relative complains that the patient has impaired memory than when the patient complains of memory difficulty. Studies have shown that when a family member complains that the patient's memory is impaired, the likely diagnosis is dementia; however, when the patient complains of memory difficulty, it is likely depression, not dementia.

The history should document the temporal profile of the symptoms, including the onset, duration, and progression. A gradual onset and slow insidious progression of symptoms characterize degenerative dementias such as Alzheimer

disease. Information about any changes in the patient's activities, and when these changes occurred and why, may help to clarify the onset of symptoms (eg, the patient's spouse starts managing the checkbook because the patient has been forgetting or making errors). Inquiry about instrumental activities of daily living is useful. These include questions about money management, meal preparation, shopping, traveling, housework, using the telephone, and taking medications. In a hospital setting, a patient with an unrecognized mild dementia may appear to have an acute onset of dementia. A change in familiar surroundings, medications, anesthesia, and a greater risk for an acute confusional state in demented patients are all factors for the "sudden" onset of dementia.

Vascular, traumatic, and toxic causes of dementia can have an acute onset. The onset of multi-infarct dementia can be sudden, with a stepwise deterioration in the patient's mental status. The progression of symptoms is important. Viral and prion diseases (eg, Creutzfeldt-Jakob disease) are rapidly progressive illnesses that occur over several months. Is the problem one of memory loss or memory lapse? Transient symptoms may suggest partial seizure activity, transient global amnesia, or complicated migraine.

It is common for patients and family members to attribute memory and cognitive decline to normal aging. The distinction between mild dementia and normal cognitive aging can be difficult to make. Complicating this is the marked increase in the incidence of dementia with advancing age. Cognitive functions that decline with age include sustained attention, mental flexibility, response speed, and visual memory recall. Preserved function includes immediate attention, vocabulary, temporal orientation, and certain visuospatial skills. A normal 90-year-old person is able to live independently.

Any history of personality changes is significant. Depression can complicate the diagnosis of dementia. Depression is frequently associated with degenerative dementias, and severe depression can mimic dementia. On mental status examination, patients with depression show diminished attention, memory impairment, apathy, and social withdrawal. Historical points that may lead to the diagnosis of depression include a previous history or family history of depression, sleep difficulty, and vegetative signs of depression. The onset of symptoms may follow a major event such as the death of a spouse. Cognitive testing in depression demonstrates impaired attention and performance variability. Patients frequently respond to questions with "I don't know." Some features that distinguish between dementia and depression are listed in Table 8.2.

In addition to depression, prominent changes in personality early in the course of a dementing illness may suggest a frontal lobe process, for example, a tumor, frontotemporal dementia, or Pick disease. Any change in behavior needs to be interpreted with respect to the patient's previous personality, occupation, and standing in the community. Previous psychiatric illness, such as bipolar affective disorder or schizophrenia, is relevant.

The medical history may suggest the cause of dementia. A history of vascular disease and vascular risk factors are consistent with multi-infarct dementia. A history of thyroidectomy suggests hypothyroidism, and a history of gastrectomy suggests vitamin B_{12} deficiency. Historical information about head trauma, exposure to toxins, systemic illness, risk factors for human immunodeficiency virus (HIV) infection, and alcohol intake and smoking habits is important. Information also needs to be obtained about what medications the patient is taking, because medications frequently impair cognitive function. Some of the agents that can cause cognitive side effects are β-blockers, antidepressants, psychotropic drugs, anticonvulsants, H_2-receptor blockers, and dopamine blockers.

The family history is important. Evidence indicates that mutations in at least four genes can cause Alzheimer disease. Other inherited degenerative dementias include Huntington disease, Pick disease, frontotemporal lobe dementia, Parkinson disease, and prion disease. A positive family history for dementia is a major risk factor for dementia.

Table 8.2. Comparison of the Features of Depression and Dementia

Depression	Dementia
Patient complains of memory problem	Patient minimizes memory problem
Relatives concerned about depression	Relatives concerned about memory problem
Vegetative symptoms, anxiety	No or few symptoms of depression
Subacute onset of cognitive symptoms; symptoms follow traumatic event	Insidious onset of cognitive symptoms
History of depression is common	History of depression is less common
Orientation intact	Orientation impaired
Concentration impaired	Recent memory impaired
Variable results on mental status testing	Consistent results on mental status testing
Poor effort on testing	Good effort on testing
Aphasia and apraxia absent	Aphasia and apraxia present

From Adams, AC: Neurology in Primary Care. FA Davis, Philadelphia, 2000, p 139. Used with permission of Mayo Foundation for Medical Education and Research.

Neurologic Examination

When examining a patient who has memory loss, look carefully for neurologic signs. Evidence of any focal neurologic deficit may indicate previous stroke. Abnormal gait is usually seen in Parkinson disease, normal-pressure hydrocephalus, and vascular dementias. If there is evidence of peripheral neuropathy, investigate whether the patient abuses alcohol or has vitamin B_{12} deficiency, hypothyroidism, or an infectious or inflammatory condition (Table 8.1).

Mental Status Examination

The mental status examination is crucial in the evaluation of memory loss and cognitive impairment. A mild cognitive deficit may not be noticed during superficial conversation or when the history is being taken for an unrelated problem. Major deficits in the history or non sequiturs are reasons to perform a more thorough cognitive evaluation. The mental status examination should determine whether dementia is present. Also, it should establish a baseline status that can be followed at subsequent evaluations. Comprehensive neuropsychometric testing should be performed if the results of mental status screening are equivocal.

Before testing mental status, it is important to be aware of the patient's mood and motivation. Depression has a marked effect on mental status functioning. Poor motivation also affects performance on tests of cognition. Areas of cognitive function that should be tested are attention, recent and remote memory, language, praxis, visuospatial relationships, judgment, and calculations.

The short screening tests for cognitive impairment such as the Mini-Mental State Examination (MMSE) and the "Kokmen," or Short Test of Mental Status (Fig. 8.1), are useful, despite the criticism that they are time consuming and insensitive to mild dementia. However, these standardized tests are in widespread use, and the normal values for age and education are known. The results must be interpreted in the context of the patient's age and education. A score of 23 or less on the MMSE or a score of 29 or less on the Kokmen (Short Test of Mental Status) suggests cognitive impairment. These tests are screening tests only. False-positive results can be obtained if the patient has depression and false-negative results if the patient has high intelligence and mild dementia. Mental status screening tests are valuable for longitudinal screening and should help in making decisions about additional testing.

Understanding cortical anatomy and organization is helpful in interpreting the mental status examination and in understanding abnormalities in patients with cognitive and behavioral disorders (Fig. 8.2). The frontal lobe of the brain is involved in executive functions, including attention, planning, evaluating, making decisions, executing motor acts, avoiding distraction, and social skills. The posterior portion of the cerebral hemisphere is receptive, with involvement in sensation, perception, recognition, knowledge, and naming. The right and left hemispheres are distinct. The left hemisphere of the brain can be considered the "symbolic" hemisphere, with the functions of language and calculation. The right hemisphere is considered holistic and emotional, with the function of visuospatial orientation. The parietal lobe can be considered the "where" portion (eg, spatial relationships) of the cerebral hemisphere and the temporal lobe the "what" portion (eg, naming objects) (Fig. 8.3).

The first component of the mental status examination that is tested is attention. Inattention can degrade all other cognitive function. Disruption in attention is the defining feature of an acute confusional state. Attention can be tested in several ways, including the use of digit span, as in the Kokmen, or spelling "world"

A

		Maximum points
1. Orientation	Name, address, current location (bldg), city, state, date (day), month, year	8
2. Attention/ Immediate recall	a. Digit span (present 1/second: record longest correct span) 2-9-6-8-3, 5-7-1-9-4-6, 2-1-5-9-3-6-2	7
	b. Four unrelated words Learn: "apple, Mr. Johnson, charity, tunnel" (# of trials needed to learn all four: ____)	4
3. Calculation	5 × 13, 65 - 7, 58 ÷ 2, 29 + 11	4
4. Abstraction	Similarities orange/banana, dog/horse, table/bookcase	3
5. Construction	Draw clock face showing 11:20	4

Copy

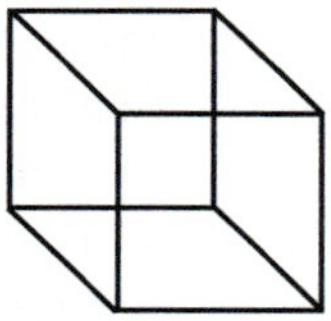

6. Information	President: first President Define an island; # weeks/year	4
7. Recall	The four words "apple, Mr. Johnson, charity, tunnel"	4
TOTAL SCORE		38
	Subtract 1, 2, or 3 if there was more than 1 trial required to learn the four words.	
FINAL SCORE		38

Fig. 8.1. Short Test of Mental Status, or the "Kokmen." *A*, Test; *B*, instructions. (From Kokmen, E, Naessens, JM, and Offord, KP: A short test of mental status: Description and preliminary results. Mayo Clin Proc 62:281-288, 1987. Used with permission of Mayo Foundation for Medical Education and Research.)

backwards as on the MMSE. Problems with attention may indicate diffuse brain dysfunction, as in a toxic encephalopathy, or frontal lobe dysfunction, as in frontotemporal dementia. Tests of language, including reading and writing, evaluate left hemisphere function. Calculations, right-left orientation, and finger recognition ("show me your left index finger") test left parietal lobe function or the symbolic "where" aspect of the brain. Visuospatial orientation (the function of

B

Instructions for administering and scoring the Short Test of Mental Status

Orientation.   Ask the patient to give his/her full name(1), home address(2), current location, ie, building(3), city(4), and state(5); and the current date, either the day of the week or the date of the month(6), the month(7), and the year(8). Each correct response is worth 1 point; maximum score is 8.

Attention.   Tell the patient, "I shall now give you a span of numbers. Please pay close attention to these numbers and repeat them in the same order that I gave you as soon as I finish giving you the series of numbers." Start with a series of 5 digits. If the patient can perform correctly, go to 6 digits and eventually to 7. If the patient cannot perform 5 digits, go to a series of 4 and, if need be, to 3 digits. One trial in each digit series is all that is needed. The patient must give the series in the exact order. Record the best performance of the patient. The maximum in this subtest is 7.

Learning.   Tell the patient, "I shall now give you 4 words. I would like you to learn them, keep them in mind, and repeat them to me from time to time when I ask you. You may repeat them in any order." Then give the 4 words. At the end of this, ask the patient to repeat the 4 words. If the patient can repeat the 4 words, record the number of trials required to learn 4 words as 1, and tell the patient to remember these words because you are going to ask them to repeat the words later. If the patient cannot recall 4 words, repeat the 4 words yourself, and ask the patient to go through the trial again. Try 4 times and if the patient is unable to repeat all 4 words at the end of the fourth trial, record the maximum attained number as the learning score and the maximum number of trials (up to 4). The maximum possible learning score is 4, and the maximum number of trials is 4.

Calculation (arithmetic).   Ask the patient to perform the following calculations: 5×13, 65–7, 58÷2, 29+11. Each correct response is worth 1 point. Maximum points are 4.

Abstraction (similarities).   Tell the patient, "Please tell me how the following two things are similar or alike: "orange/banana", "horse/dog", and "table/bookcase." Only abstract similarities are worth 1 point. The maximum for this subtest is 3. Inability to see any similarity or concrete similarities such as "You peel both orange and banana" or "Horse and dog both have four legs" obtain 0 points. Maximum points are 3.

Information.   Ask the patient to name the current United States President, the first President of the United States, and the number of weeks in a year as well as asking him/her to define an island. Correct answers are worth 1 point; the maximum score for this subtest is 4.

Construction.   On a blank piece of paper, ask the patient to draw the face of a clock showing 20 minutes after 11. Any correct depiction of this should obtain 2 points. Less than perfect diagrams should obtain 1 point. On the same sheet of paper, now ask the patient to copy the cube (as shown). If the patient's copy reflects three-dimensionality, the copy should obtain 2 points. If three-dimensionality is not reflected, the patient may obtain 1 or 0 points depending on the completeness of the diagram. The maximum score of the construction subtest is 4.

Recall.   Ask the patient to repeat the 4 words he/she was asked to remember. Do not provide cues or choices. Each correctly recalled word is worth 1 point. The maximum score of this subtest is 4.

Total Score   is the addition of all the points the patient obtained. To achieve the **final score**, subtract 1, 2, or 3 from the total score if the patient required 2, 3, or 4 trials to learn the 4 unrelated words in the learning subtest. The maximum total and final score is 38.

A

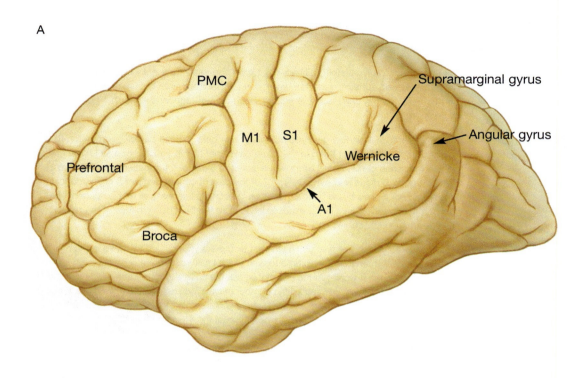

B

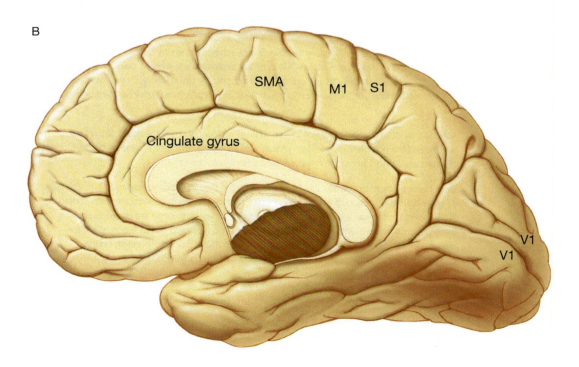

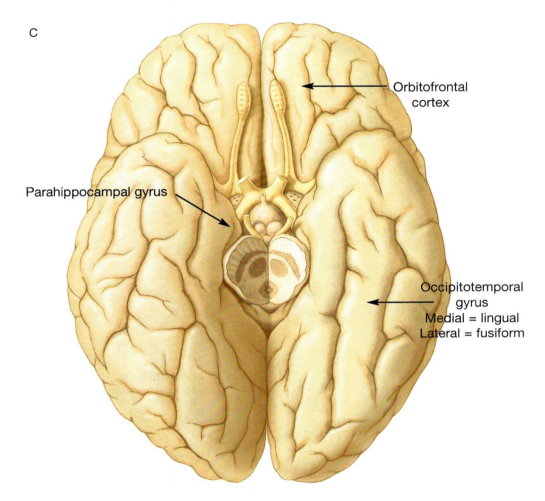

C

Orbitofrontal cortex

Parahippocampal gyrus

Occipitotemporal gyrus
Medial = lingual
Lateral = fusiform

Fig. 8.2. Cortical anatomy. *A*, Lateral aspect of the left hemisphere of the brain. *B*, Medial aspect of the right hemisphere. *C*, Ventral aspect of the brain (with brainstem detached at midbrain). A1, primary auditory cortex; M1, primary motor cortex; PMC, premotor cortex; S1, primary somatosensory cortex; SMA, supplementary motor cortex; V1, primary visual cortex.

the right parietal lobe) can be tested by asking the patient to draw a cube or clock as in the Kokmen. Testing memory and the "localization" of memory is more complicated. Working memory (eg, remembering a telephone number for a short time) is a function primarily of the frontal lobes. The ability to learn, store, and retrieve information (ie, declarative memory) involves the medial temporal lobes and limbic structures. On both the MMSE and the Kokmen, recall is used to test declarative memory. Remote memories are represented widely throughout the cerebral hemispheres (association cortex) and are the memories most resistant to pathologic change. The functional areas of the cerebral cortex are shown in Figure 8.4.

The evaluation of mental status depends on the patient's use of language. Memory complaints

Anterior: executive
Attention, planning, evaluation, decision, motor execution, avoiding distraction, social skills

Posterior: receptive
Sensation, perception, recognition, naming, knowledge

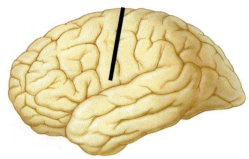

Left brain: symbolic
Language, calculations

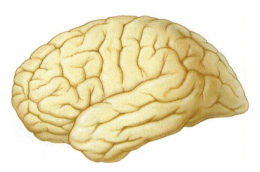

Right brain: holistic
Visuospatial orientation, prosody

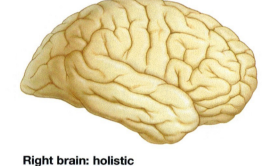

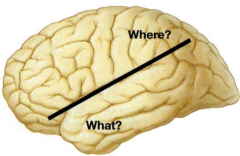

Where?

What?

Fig. 8.3. Cortical organization.

may actually represent aphasia or a language problem. Pay attention to the patient's speech during the interview. Fluency of speech is usually normal if the patient uses sentences with seven or more words. Phonemic ("the sky is glue") or paraphasic ("the sky is cheese") errors indicate a language problem. The MMSE assesses language by having the patient name objects, repeat a phrase, and read and write a sentence. To test for comprehension, ask the patient to perform a three-stage command, for example, "Look up, raise your hand, and point to the door." A test that can be used for a more thorough evaluation of languages is shown in Figure 8.5.

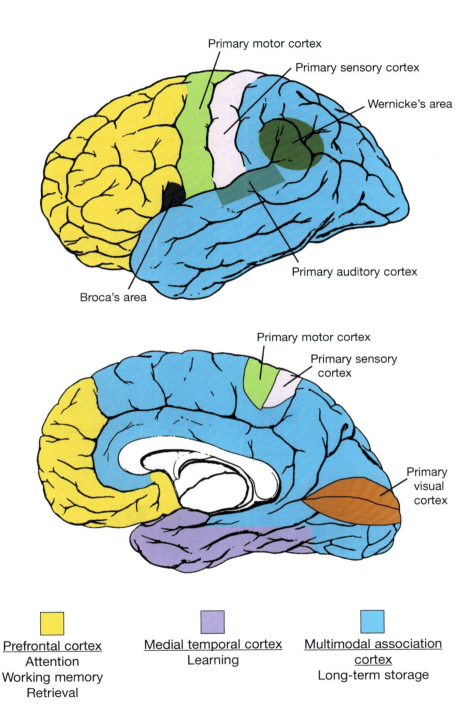

Fig. 8.4. Functional areas of the cerebral cortex. (From Adams, AC: Neurology in Primary Care. FA Davis, Philadelphia, 2000, p 142. Used with permission of Mayo Foundation for Medical Education and Research.)

A. Spoken language comprehension (no stimulus repetitions allowed) (4 points)

1. Touch your chin.
2. Touch your right ear with your left thumb.
3. Before touching your nose, point to the floor.
4. Close your eyes after you point to your chin and the ceiling.

B. Reading comprehension (Have patient read sentences on card 2 aloud and follow the direction; scoring based on comprehension, not accuracy of reading aloud.) (4 points)

1. Touch your nose.
2. Touch your right ear with your left thumb.
3. Before touching your chin, point to the ceiling.
4. Open your mouth after you point to your chin and the floor.

C. Naming (Name each item in figure; no credit for inaccurate responses, self-corrected errors, or delays >3 seconds before responding) (4 points)

1. Helicopter
2. Toothbrush
3. Bus
4. Wheelchair

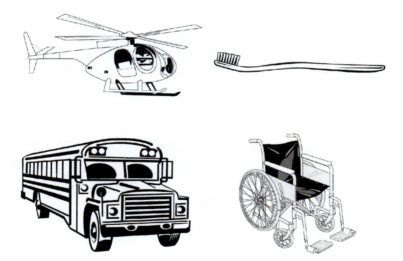

D. Repetition (Repeat each sentence. All words must be included and accurate for credit.) (4 points)

1. Please sit down.
2. What time will the bus pick you up?
3. No ifs, ands, or buts.
4. The judge sentenced the criminal.

E. Narrative picture description (Show figure and ask patient to "tell me what's happening in this picture;" award 1 point for each of the following)[*] (4 points)

1. Normal rate (ie, no significant delays or hesitation; do not penalize for dysarthria)
2. Normal word retrieval (no semantic errors or circumlocution)
3. Normal sentence length (mean = 5+ words) and prosody
4. Normal grammar and syntax

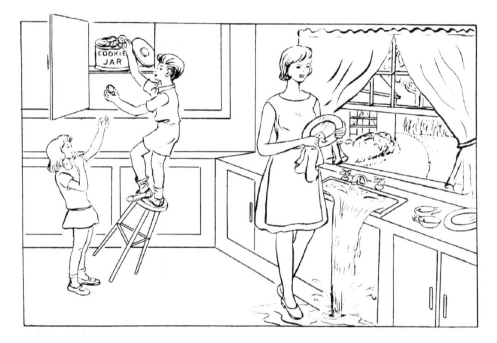

([*]If no points earned for items 3 and 4, rate as <u>nonfluent</u>; if both points earned for items 3 and 4, rate as <u>fluent</u>.)

F. Writing—On a plain neurologic examination half-sheet, ask patient to write (print or cursive) each of the following (no points for spelling, word, or grammatical errors; no penalties for legible distortions): (4 points)

1. Man
2. Watch
3. Some water is not good to drink
4. Ask patient to "Write a sentence about something you enjoy doing."

Total score = /24

Fig. 8.5. Language Screen Examination. (Figures with item **C** courtesy of Bradley F. Boeve, MD, and Joseph R. Duffy, PhD. Used with permission of Mayo Foundation for Medical Education and Research. Picture with item **E** from Goodglass, H, Kaplan, E, and Barresi, B: Boston Diagnostic Aphasia Examination. ed 3. Lippincott Williams & Wilkins, Philadelphia, 2001. Used with permission.)

Further neuropsychologic testing may be indicated if the results of the initial evaluation are borderline or suggestive of dementia. Neuropsychologic tests are helpful in identifying dementia in highly intelligent persons who may have normal results on mental status screening evaluations. In addition, these tests may be needed for patients with limited educational background or for mentally retarded persons, because of the limitations of mental status screening tests. Neuropsychologic tests are recommended for distinguishing between dementia and depression, in determining competency for legal purposes, and for determining disability. As with screening tests, a baseline study with follow-up evaluation may be necessary to make the diagnosis of dementia.

Laboratory Investigation

The laboratory work-up in the evaluation of dementia is dictated by the findings of the history and physical examination. Laboratory tests are performed to exclude metabolic and structural causes of dementia that may be amenable to specific treatment. The routine tests recommended by the American Academy of Neurology include a complete blood count; serum level of electrolytes (including calcium), glucose, blood urea nitrogen, creatinine, vitamin B_{12}, free thyroid index, and thyroid-stimulating hormone; and liver function tests. For the initial evaluation of patients with dementia, structural neuroimaging with either noncontrast computed tomography (CT) or magnetic resonance imaging (MRI) is appropriate. Optional studies include the syphilis serologic test, erythrocyte sedimentation rate, serum folate level, HIV test, chest radiography, urinalysis, 24-hour urine collection for heavy metals, toxicology screen, neuropsychologic testing, cerebrospinal fluid (CSF) analysis, electroencephalography (EEG), positron emission tomography (PET), and single-photon emission computed tomography (SPECT).

CSF analysis is recommended in the evaluation of dementia if a central nervous system infection, metastatic cancer, or central nervous system vasculitis is a possibility. Consider CSF analysis if there are atypical features such as the onset of symptoms before age 55 years or rapid progression of symptoms. The CSF 14-3-3 protein assay is useful for confirming the diagnosis of Creutzfeldt-Jakob disease. Be aware that acute neurologic conditions such as stroke, viral encephalitis, and paraneoplastic disorders can give false-positive results on this immunoassay. Before performing a lumbar puncture for CSF analysis, review the indications and contraindication for the procedure (see Chapter 2).

Removal of CSF is therapeutic for patients who have normal-pressure hydrocephalus. The clinical features of normal-pressure hydrocephalus include dementia, gait disturbance, and incontinence. Brain imaging studies show ventricular enlargement out of proportion to cortical atrophy. Ventricular shunting may be reasonable to consider if the patient's gait improves after CSF has been removed (see below).

EEG may have some value in investigating possible dementia. Patients who have cognitive impairment and seizures should have EEG. This test may be valuable in distinguishing between delirium and dementia or in evaluating any patient who has a fluctuating level of consciousness. EEG may be helpful in distinguishing between dementia and depression. If a patient has depression, one would expect the EEG to be normal, compared with a slow pattern likely to be seen if the patient has dementia. The EEG of a patient who has a rapid decline in cognitive function over a 3-month period or less and early neurologic findings may suggest prion disease. Creutzfeldt-Jakob disease often shows characteristic sharp waves on EEG (Fig. 8.6).

Neuroimaging is reasonable at least once in the evaluation of patients with dementia. CT

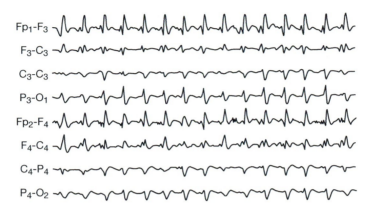

Fp₁-F₃
F₃-C₃
C₃-C₃
P₃-O₁
Fp₂-F₄
F₄-C₄
C₄-P₄
P₄-O₂

Fig. 8.6. Electroencephalogram of a 48-year-old patient with Creutzfeldt-Jakob disease showing generalized triphasic waves. (From Westmoreland, BF: Clinical EEG Manual. Available from: http://mayoweb .mayo.edu/man-neuroeeg/index.html#13. Used with permission.)

can detect all the potentially treatable causes of dementia, including tumor, subdural hematoma, hydrocephalus, and stroke. MRI is more sensitive for detecting vascular and demyelinating disease, and it often shows nonspecific white matter changes. The term used to describe periventricular white matter abnormalities is *leukoaraiosis* (Fig. 8.7). It is observed commonly in MRI scans of elderly patients and is thought to reflect vascular brain injury. Leukoaraiosis, or white matter hyperintensities, is also seen in multiple sclerosis, in certain infections, and after cardiac arrest. Leukoaraiosis is recognized as a risk factor for dementia. On CT, leukoaraiosis appears as areas of low attentuation in the periventricular region.

The role of MRI in the evaluation of dementia is likely to expand in the future. It has been shown that quantitative measurements of brain structures and size made with MRI have some predictive value in the diagnosis of Alzheimer disease. MRI is superior to CT in demonstrating atrophy. Atrophy of the cerebral cortex, hippocampi, and cerebellum evolves with age. It is important not to overinterpret atrophy seen on MRI scans of patients older than 80 years and

not to underinterpret the findings in patients younger than 65. Both coronal and axial images are useful in the evaluation of dementing disorders. Coronal images are better for showing temporal atrophy, and axial images are better for showing focal atrophy of the frontal, parietal, and occipital lobes (Fig. 8.8).

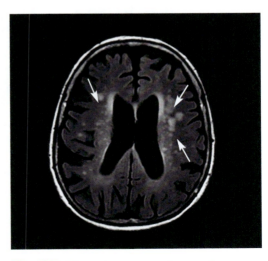

Fig. 8.7. Magnetic resonance image of leukoaraiosis (*arrows*) in a patient with Alzeimer disease.

PET and SPECT, which measure glucose metabolism and regional blood flow, respectively, may also be used in the evaluation of dementia. In patients with Alzheimer disease, glucose metabolism and cerebral blood flow are decreased in the temporopatietal region compared with those of normal controls. Although cerebral blood flow patterns are not specific for a given disease, they may be useful for distinguishing Alzheimer disease from vascular or frontotemporal dementia. However, the clinical usefulness of these tests has not been

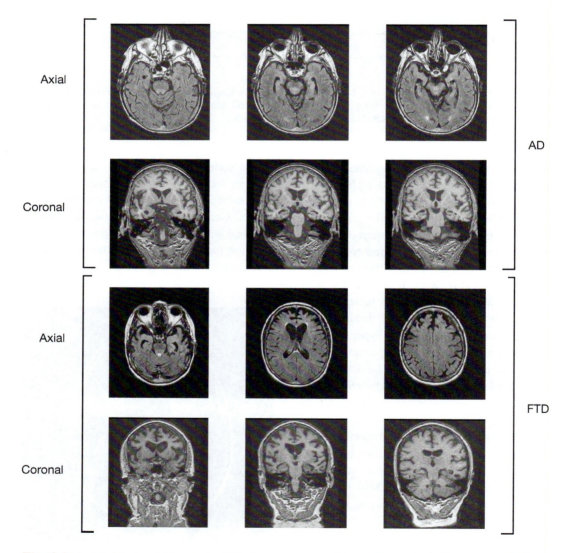

Fig. 8.8. Axial and coronal images in Alzheimer dementia (AD) and frontotemporal dementia (FTD). Coronal images show hippocampal and temporal cortical atrophy better than axial images. However, axial images show focal frontal, parietal, and occipital cortical atrophy better than coronal images.

established. The indications for optional laboratory tests used in the evaluation of memory loss are summarized in Table 8.3. The laboratory tests for dementia and the rationale for each one are summarized in Table 8.4.

MILD COGNITIVE IMPAIRMENT

The term *mild cognitive impairment* (MCI) is used to define the condition of elderly persons who have impaired memory but not dementia

Table 8.3. Indications for Diagnostic Tests in Evaluation of Dementia

Indication	Test
Routine dementia screen	Complete blood count
	Electrolytes, including calcium; glucose; BUN; creatinine
	Liver function tests
	Thyroid function tests
	Vitamin B$_{12}$
	Head CT or MRI
Clinical suspicion of infection	Syphilis serology
CNS infection CNS vasculitis Metastatic cancer Rapidly progressive dementia Early age at symptom onset	CSF analysis
Normal-pressure hydrocephalus	Lumbar puncture
Dementia versus delirium Dementia versus depression Seizures	EEG
Suspicious or borderline mental status screening test results Dementia versus depression Legal competency determination Baseline	Neuropsychologic tests

BUN, blood urea nitrogen; CNS, central nervous system; CSF, cerebrospinal fluid; CT, computed tomography; EEG, electroencephalography; MRI, magnetic resonance imaging.
Modified from Adams, AC: Neurology in Primary Care. FA Davis, Philadelphia, 2000, p 144. Used with permission of Mayo Foundation for Medical Education and Research.

Table 8.4. Laboratory Tests for Differential Diagnosis of Dementia

Test	Evaluation for
Complete blood count	Anemia, infection
Electrolytes, including calcium; glucose	Metabolic dysfunction
Glucose	Endocrine dysfunction
BUN, creatinine	Renal dysfunction
Liver function tests	Liver dysfunction
Thyroid function	Hypothyroidism
Vitamin B_{12}	Vitamin B_{12} deficiency
Syphilis serology	Syphilis
CT/MRI scan	Vascular disease, mass lesion, hydrocephalus, demyelinating disease, focal and diffuse atrophy
CSF analysis	Chronic meningitis, syphilis, vasculitis, meningeal carcinomatosis
EEG	Seizures, Creutzfeldt-Jakob disease, metabolic disturbances
Heavy metal screen	Lead, mercury, arsenic intoxication
Erythrocyte sedimentation rate	Inflammatory disease
Antinuclear antibody	Inflammatory disease
Anti-extractable nuclear antibodies	Inflammatory disease
HIV	HIV dementia
Chest radiography	Cardiopulmonary disease, lung tumor
ECG	Cardiopulmonary disease
SPECT	Focal cortical atrophy, frontotemporal dementia, Pick disease
Long-chain fatty acids	Adrenoleukodystrophy
Arylsulfatase A	Metachromatic leukodystrophy
Ceruloplasmin, copper level	Wilson disease
Angiography	Arteritis
Cerebral biopsy	Inflammatory or infectious disease
Paraneoplastic antibodies	Cancer

BUN, blood urea nitrogen; CSF, cerebrospinal fluid; CT, computed tomography; ECG, electrocardiography; EEG, electroencephalography; HIV, human immunodeficiency virus; MRI, magnetic resonance imaging; SPECT, single-photon emission computed tomography.
From Adams, AC: Neurology in Primary Care. FA Davis, Philadelphia, 2000, p 145. Used with permission of Mayo Foundation for Medical Education and Research.

or disability. The concept of MCI was developed with the assumption that there is a cognitive continuum between normal cognitive function and Alzheimer disease. Patients in whom a degenerative dementia develops undergo a transition phase of mild impairment. Among patients with MCI, the rate of progression to Alzheimer disease is high. This point emphasizes the importance of diagnosis and therapeutic intervention at an early stage, namely MCI.

The criteria for identification of MCI include the following: complaints of impaired cognition made by the patient or family, the report by the patient or informant of a decline in cognitive function during the past year relative to previous abilities, clinical evidence of memory or other cognitive impairment, absence of major repercussions on daily life, and absence of dementia.

Subtypes of MCI have been described. Patients with prominent memory impairment have *amnestic MCI*. Patients with impairment in more than one cognitive domain have *multiple-domain MCI*. Patients who have cognitive impairment in a single domain other than memory have *single nonmemory domain MCI*. For example, this may include executive function or language. This subtype of MCI may progress to frontotemporal dementia or primary progressive aphasia. Each clinical subtype can have various causes, including vascular, metabolic, traumatic, and degenerative causes.

As noted above, the rate of progression of MCI to dementia is high. Poor performance on cued memory tasks may be a clinical indicator of those at higher risk for progression to Alzheimer disease. Hippocampal atrophy has also been reported to be predictive of a more rapid progression to Alzheimer disease. This rate is variable, but 10% to 15% annually is the range reported, as compared with the 1% to 2% annually for normal older adults. This emphasizes the importance of early recognition and treatment. Currently, MCI is treated with cholinesterase inhibitors, although no consensus has been established about treatment.

ALZHEIMER DISEASE

Alzheimer disease is the most common form of dementia. The definitive diagnosis is made at autopsy, with the demonstration of neuronal loss, neurofibrillary tangles, neuritic plaques, and amyloid angiopathy. However, autopsy studies have confirmed that the clinical diagnosis of Alzheimer disease has a high rate of accuracy.

The criteria used most often for the diagnosis of Alzheimer disease include those of the *Diagnostic and Statistical Manual, 4th Edition, Text Revision* and those of the National Institute of Neurological and Communicative Disorders and Stroke and the Alzheimer's Disease and Related Disorders Association (Table 8.5).

Alzheimer disease is a complex and heterogeneous disorder, and many genes have been identified with its development. It has been divided on the basis of genetic studies into *early-onset disease* (before age 60 years) and *late-onset disease*. Genes associated with the early-onset form include the amyloid β-protein precursor on chromosome 21, presenilin 1 on chromosome 14, and presenilin 2 on chromosome 1. The genetic risk factor identified with the late-onset form is apolipoprotein E-4 (*APOE-4*). *APOE* is on chromosome 19, with three alleles (2, 3, and 4). *APOE*4* is a susceptibility gene; it does not cause the disease but may modulate the age at onset and increase the probability of the disease developing. Apolipoprotein is a plasma protein produced in the brain by astrocytes. It is involved with cholesterol transport and is found in neuritic plaques, neurofibrillary tangles, and vascular amyloid. Apolipoprotein binds strongly to amyloid protein. A patient with dementia who has the *APOE*4* genotype is more likely to have Alzheimer disease than any other dementing illness. *APOE* genotyping has been suggested as a predictive test for Alzheimer disease, but the genotype is not necessary or sufficient for the diagnosis. Currently, *APOE*4* testing is not recommended for diagnosing or predicting Alzheimer disease. Testing for amyloid β-protein precursor, presenilin 1, and presenilin

Table 8.5. Criteria for Clinical Diagnosis of Alzheimer Disease

I. DMS IV-TR criteria
- The development of multiple cognitive deficits manifested by both memory impairment and one or more of the following:
  - Aphasia
  - Apraxia
  - Agnosia
  - and disturbances in executive functioning
- The cognitive deficits represent a decline from previous functioning and cause significant impairment in social or occupational functioning
- The course is characterized by gradual onset and continuing decline
- The cognitive deficits are not due to other central nervous system, systemic, or substance-induced conditions that cause progressive deficits in memory and cognition
- The disturbance is not better accounted for by another psychiatric disorder

II. NINDS-ADRDA criteria
- Definite Alzheimer disease
  - Meets the criteria for probable Alzheimer disease and has histopathologic evidence of Alzheimer disease by autopsy or biopsy
- Probable Alzheimer disease
  - Dementia established by clinical and neuropsychologic examination and involves
    - a) Progressive deficits in two or more areas of cognition, including memory
    - b) Onset between ages of 40 and 90 years, and
    - c) Absence of systemic or other brain diseases capable of producing a dementia syndrome, including delirium
- Possible Alzheimer disease
  - A dementia syndrome with an atypical onset, presentation, or progression and without a known etiology
  - Any comorbid diseases capable of producing dementia are not believed to be the cause
- Unlikely Alzheimer disease
  - A dementia syndrome with any of the following: sudden onset, focal neurologic signs, or seizures or gait disturbance early in the course of the illness

DMS IV-TR, Diagnostic and Statistical Manual of Mental Disorders, ed 4, text revision; NINDS-ADRDA, National Institute of Neurological and Communicative Disorders and Stroke—Alzheimer's Disease and Related Disorder Association.

Modified from American Psychiatric Association: Diagnostic and Statistical Manual of Mental Disorders, ed 4, text revision. American Psychiatric Association, Washington DC, 2000, p 157. Used with permission.

From The National Institute of Neurological and Communicative Disorders and Stroke—Alzheimer's Disease and Related Disorder Association (NINDS-ADRDA) Criteria for Alzheimer's Disease. Available from: http://alzheimers.about.com/od/diagnosisissues/a/criteria_diagno.htm. Used with permission.

2 may be appropriate in families with an autosomal dominant pattern of inheritance of dementia. Appropriate genetic counseling should be part of genetic testing.

When the risk of developing Alzheimer disease is discussed with family members, emphasize that it is an age-related disease. Although the risk of developing the disorder increases with age, patients in whom it develops live a substantial portion of their lives without the disease. The risk of the disease in the population with a negative family history is about 8% per decade starting at age 70 years. In persons with a first-degree family member with the disorder, the risk doubles. The age at onset of dementia is also correlated in families. Despite all this, the chances are greater that first-degree relatives will not develop the disease.

Many risk factors have been identified for Alzheimer disease. Primary risk factors are age, positive family history, and, for persons older than 80 years, female sex. Other primary risk factors include the cerebrovascular risk factors of hypertension, diabetes mellitus, obesity, and hypercholesterolemia. Possible risk factors for Alzheimer disease include head injury, low educational attainment, hyperhomocysteinemia, folate deficiency, hyperinsulinemia, depression, and low thyroid-stimulating hormone levels (but within the normal range). The increased risk associated with head injury is thought to be related to an increase in amyloid deposition, neuronal injury, and synaptic disruption.

Factors that may help prevent or delay the onset of Alzheimer disease are being investigated for potential therapies. Possible protective factors include regular consumption of fish and omega 3 fatty acids, high educational attainment, regular exercise, moderate alcohol consumption, nonsteroidal antiinflammatory medications, folate, and vitamins C, E, B_6, and B_{12} supplementation.

Epidemiologic reports suggested estrogen replacement therapy in postmenopausal women may reduce the occurrence of Alzheimer disease, but randomized, placebo-controlled trials did not show benefit. The Women's Health Initiative study of estrogen and medroxyprogesterone showed an increased risk of dementia. Currently, estrogen is not recommended for the treatment and prevention of Alzheimer disease.

The diagnosis of Alzheimer disease is understandably devastating to the patient and family. The diagnosis is a "family" diagnosis because of the major effect the disease will have on the patient's caregiver. The patient and caregiver need to know that the disease is progressive and that cognition and function will decline continuously. Changes in the patient's behavior and personality are common and part of the dementing process. Although there is no cure for the disease, many of the common symptoms can be treated. The clinician often needs to attend to the caregiver as much as to the patient. In addition to the medical management of the disease, clinicians have an important part in addressing issues of living arrangements, legal matters, and whether the patient should drive a motor vehicle.

The strategy in the treatment of Alzheimer disease is to improve the patient's quality of life and to maximize function. Several pharmacologic treatments are based on the neurodegenerative mechanisms involved in the disease. For example, the observation of a cholinergic deficit in the cerebral cortex of patients with Alzheimer disease led to the development of the first cholinesterase inhibitor, tacrine. Clinical studies have demonstrated that cholinesterase inhibitors have a modest benefit in treating the clinical symptoms of mild-to-moderate Alzheimer disease. Three cholinesterase inhibitors have been approved by the US Food and Drug Administration for the treatment of mild-to-moderate dementia (Table 8.6).

Table 8.6. Symptomatic Treatment of Dementia

Symptom	Nonpharmacologic therapy	Pharmacologic therapy, dose	Adverse effects
Cognitive impairment	Compensatory strategies: notes, pillbox, calendar, signs	**Cholinesterase inhibitors** Donepezil (Aricept), 5 mg daily, may increase to 10 mg daily in 4 weeks	Nausea, diarrhea, insomnia
		Galantamine (Reminyl, Razadyne), 4 mg twice daily (with food) for 4 weeks, may increase if tolerated every 4 weeks to maximum 32 mg daily	Nausea, diarrhea, insomnia
		Rivastigmine (Exelon), 1.5 mg twice daily (with food), may increase every 2 weeks to maximum 6 mg twice daily	Nausea, diarrhea, insomnia
		Tacrine (Cognex), 10 mg four times daily for 4 weeks, may increase every 4 weeks to maximum 40 mg four times daily	Liver toxicity, must be monitored, in limited use
		N-methyl-D-aspartate antagonist Memantine (Namenda), 5 mg once daily; increase dose at minimum 1-week intervals in 5-mg increments to 5 mg twice daily to target dose of 20 mg/day	Dizziness, constipation, headache, hypertension

Table 8.6 (continued)

Symptom	Nonpharmacologic therapy	Pharmacologic therapy, dose	Adverse effects
Agitation, hallucinations, delusions	Redirect patient, reassure patient and caregiver	Haloperidol (Haldol), 0.25 mg daily	Parkinsonism, tardive dyskinesia, postural hypotension
		Risperidone (Risperdal), 0.5 mg twice daily	Nausea, insomnia, parkinsonism
		Quetiapine (Seroquel), 25 mg twice daily	Hypotension, somnolence
Depression	Modify environment, music, reduce demands on patient	Sertraline (Zoloft), 50 mg daily	Nausea, diarrhea, insomnia
		Paroxetine (Paxil), 10 mg every morning	Somnolence, insomnia
Insomnia	Improve sleep hygiene, eliminate or limit naps, daytime exercise, avoid caffeine and night-lights	Trazodone (Desyrel), 25 mg at bedtime	Oversedation, hypotension
Anxiety, agitation	Reassurance, lessen demands on memory, reduce noise	Lorazepam (Ativan), 0.5 mg 1-2 times daily	Sedation, confusion, falls, dependency

Modified from Adams, AC: Neurology in Primary Care. FA Davis, Philadelphia, 2000, p 148. Used with permission of Mayo Foundation for Medical Education and Research.

Common side effects include nausea, vomiting, and diarrhea. These effects may be reduced by introducing the medication at the lowest dose and gradually increasing it.

Overstimulation of *N*-methyl-D-aspartate (NMDA) receptors by glutamate has been implicated in dementia and other neurodegenerative disorders. On the basis of this, memantine, an NMDA receptor antagonist, has been used to treat moderate-to-severe Alzheimer disease. Memantine therapy has been associated with a decreased rate in the deterioration of global, cognitive, and functional measures. Behavioral improvement has also been noted, particularly for agitation. Memantine and cholinesterase inhibitors are often used together because of their different mechanisms of action.

Antioxidant agents are being investigated for treating Alzheimer disease. Free radicals, byproducts of oxidative metabolism, damage cell membranes and tissues. According to the oxidative stress hypothesis of neuronal death, antioxidants should prevent cytotoxic injury. Selegiline, a monoamine oxidase inhibitor, may act as an antioxidant and reduce neuronal damage. It also may improve cognitive deficits by increasing levels of catecholamines. Vitamin E (α-tocopherol), another antioxidant, is being investigated for preventing or slowing the progression of Alzheimer disease. Despite the theoretical value of these agents, the evidence is not sufficient to make recommendations about treatment.

Epidemiologic studies have suggested that nonsteroidal antiinflammatory drugs, statins, and estrogen may have a preventative effect in Alzheimer disease, but these findings were not confirmed by prospective trials. An herbal remedy extracted from the leaves of the ginkgo tree, *Ginkgo biloba*, is claimed to be effective in treating memory deficits. Its mechanism of action is not known, but it may be an antioxidant. Although a randomized trial reported the extract had a slight positive effect on dementia, several flaws have been cited in the study, limiting its usefulness. Although ginkgo has platelet-inhibiting effects, bleeding is not a common side effect. Reported adverse effects include mild gastrointestinal symptoms, headache, and allergic reactions. The purity and potency of the extract are not known. Currently, no recommendation can be made about ginkgo.

Dementia-related behavioral symptoms are common. Problems include sleep disruption, agitation, depression, hallucinations, and delusions. Before treatment is initiated with a psychoactive drug, the specific behavior needs to be documented and its cause or contributing factors investigated. Some of the causes of abnormal behavior are pain, depression, medication effect, infection, physical limitations, and hospitalization. Intervention may not be needed if safety is not an issue, if the patient is not distressed, or if the living situation is not compromised. Often, nonpharmacologic approaches can be used.

When psychoactive drugs are prescribed, they should be prescribed on a scheduled basis instead of an "as needed" basis. One drug should be prescribed and started at a very low dose and the dose slowly increased until the desired therapeutic effect occurs. Monitor the patient's condition regularly to assess response and adverse effects to the medication. Attempt periodic discontinuation of the treatment. Some pharmacologic and nonpharmacologic options for symptomatic treatment of dementia are summarized in Table 8.6.

DEMENTIA WITH LEWY BODIES

Dementia with Lewy bodies is a distinct clinical and neuropathologic dementia syndrome. It is the second most common dementing disorder, accounting for 15% to 25% of all cases of dementia. Lewy bodies are eosinophilic neuronal inclusion bodies; when present in subcortical nuclei, they are a pathologic hallmark of idiopathic Parkinson disease. These inclusion bodies occur in the brainstem and cerebral cortex of patients who have dementia with Lewy bodies.

Similar to Alzheimer disease, the clinical criteria for the diagnosis of dementia with Lewy bodies include progressive cognitive decline that interferes with normal social and occupational functions. Memory may not be impaired in the early stages but is involved as the disease progresses. Prominent deficits are apparent on tests of attention and executive and visuospatial ability. The core features of dementia with Lewy bodies are fluctuating cognition with pronounced variation in attention and alertness, recurrent visual hallucinations that are particularly well-formed and detailed, and spontaneous motor features of parkinsonism (ie, bradykinesia, resting tremor, rigidity, and loss of postural reflexes). Suggestive features include rapid eye movement (REM) sleep behavior disorder and severe neuroleptic sensitivity. Neuroleptic hypersensitivity is very important in the management of this disease. Other clinical features that support the diagnosis are repeated falls, syncope, delusions, transient loss of consciousness, and hallucinations (auditory, olfactory, or tactile). Although no diagnostic tests are available for dementia with Lewy bodies, low dopamine transporter uptake in basal ganglia seen with PET or SPECT is a suggestive feature of the disease. Supportive features include relative preservation of medial temporal lobe structures as seen with MRI or CT scans, generalized hypometabolism on SPECT and PET perfusion scans with reduced occipital activity, and prominent slow wave activity on EEG with temporal lobe transient sharp waves. The criteria for the clinical diagnosis of dementia with Lewy bodies from the third report of the Dementia With Lewy Bodies Consortium are summarized in Table 8.7.

The differential diagnosis of dementia with Lewy bodies includes Alzheimer disease and Parkinson disease. All three disorders occur with higher frequency in older age groups. Both dementia with Lewy bodies and Parkinson disease show a male predominance. Unlike Alzheimer disease and Parkinson disease, dementia with Lewy bodies can have an abrupt onset and a fluctuating and rapid progression, a feature that may cause this disease to be confused with delirium. Visual hallucinations and other psychotic symptoms are prominent features of dementia with Lewy bodies, and although hallucinations occur in Alzheimer disease, they are usually a late feature. The timing of the dementia is used to differentiate dementia with Lewy bodies from Parkinson disease dementia. Dementia with Lewy bodies should be diagnosed when dementia occurs before or concurrently with parkinsonism. The term *Parkinson disease dementia* should be used to describe dementia that occurs in the context of well-established (1 year) Parkinson disease. The clinical features of these three disorders are summarized in Table 8.8.

The treatment of dementia with Lewy bodies is the same as for Alzheimer disease (Table 8.6). Cholinesterase inhibitors are reasonable for symptomatic treatment of the

Table 8.7. Criteria for the Clinical Diagnosis of Dementia With Lewy Bodies

Central feature
 Dementia—defined as progressive cognitive decline of sufficient magnitude to interfere with social or occupational function
Core features
 Fluctuating cognition
 Recurrent visual hallucinations
 Parkinsonism
Suggestive features
 REM sleep behavior disorder
 Neuroleptic sensitivity
Supportive features
 Repeated falls and syncope
 Autonomic dysfunction
 Depression
 Systematized delusions
 Hallucinations in other modalities

REM, rapid eye movement.

Table 8.8.   Comparison of the Clinical Features of Dementia With Lewy Bodies, Alzheimer Disease, and Parkinson Disease

Clinical feature	Dementia with Lewy bodies	Alzheimer disease	Parkinson disease
Initial symptom	Confusional state	Memory impairment	Tremor, bradykinesia, rigidity
Onset	Abrupt or insidious	Insidious	Insidious
Progression	Fluctuating, rapid	Gradual	Gradual
Sex distribution	Male > female	Female > male	Male > female
Prominent feature	Visual hallucinations	Dementia	Tremor, bradykinesia, rigidity

From Adams, AC: Neurology in Primary Care. FA Davis, Philadelphia, 2000, p 149. Used with permission of Mayo Foundation for Medical Education and Research.

patient's cognitive impairment and some neuropsychiatric symptoms. The parkinsonism can be treated with carbidopa/levodopa, but care needs to be taken to avoid exacerbating psychiatric symptoms. Because irreversible parkinsonism developed after treatment with neuroleptics, the recommendation was made to avoid these agents. Neuroleptic sensitivity can occur with atypical neuroleptics such as risperidone, olanzapine, clozapine, and quetiapine. They can be given at low dose but may be of limited benefit. The management of orthostatic hypotension (see Table 5.8) and sleep disorders (see Tables 9.11–9.13) are discussed in other chapters.

VASCULAR DEMENTIA

Vascular disease is an important cause of dementia. Vascular dementia includes dementia that results from multi-infarct, strategic infarct, small-vessel disease, hypoperfusion, or hemorrhage. Among its features is a temporal relation between the clinical characteristics of dementia and cerebrovascular disease. Evidence of cerebrovascular disease can be demonstrated by

history (sudden-onset dementia, fluctuating course), clinical examination, and brain imaging (MRI or CT). The temporal relation between a stroke and the onset of dementia is probably the best predictor of vascular dementia.

Vascular dementia is heterogeneous. Multi-infarct dementia is the most frequent subtype. The dementia results from multiple, bilateral cortical and subcortical infarcts. Multi-infarct dementia occurs more often in men than in women. Hypertension and peripheral vascular disease are often associated with this dementia. The cognitive and neurologic findings vary depending on the location of the infarcts; however, gait disturbances, urinary incontinence, and pseudobulbar palsy are common. Pseudobulbar palsy is a syndrome characterized by emotional incontinence and slow, strained speech.

Vascular dementia can also result from a single infarct in a functionally important cortical or subcortical area. For example, a thalamic infarct can produce disturbances in attention, memory, language, and abstract thinking. An infarct in the left angular gyrus or left frontal lobe can impair memory. Infarcts of the caudate nuclei or right parietal lobe can also impair cognition. If dementia occurs acutely, consider the diagnosis of vascular dementia due to a strategic single infarct.

Another cause of vascular dementia is small-vessel disease. Hypertension and diabetes mellitus are frequently associated with small-vessel cerebrovascular disease. Chronic ischemia due to hypertension and arteriolar sclerosis produces central white matter demyelination, with leukoaraiosis seen on brain imaging studies (Fig. 8.7). Diffuse brain ischemia due to cardiac arrest or severe hypotension can also cause vascular dementia.

Chronic subdural hematomas, subarachnoid hemorrhage, and cerebral hemorrhage all can impair cognition. The term *hemorrhagic dementia* has been used for this subtype of vascular dementia.

Vascular dementia is treated by reducing cerebrovascular risk factors and preventing additional strokes (see Chapter 11). Also, consider treatment with cholinesterase inhibitors for patients who have either vascular or degenerative dementia. Treatment of the symptoms of vascular dementia is the same as that for Alzheimer disease (Table 8.6).

NORMAL-PRESSURE HYDROCEPHALUS

Normal-pressure hydrocephalus is characterized by the triad of dementia, gait disturbance, and urinary incontinence. It is important to recognize this disorder early in its course because it potentially can be treated with shunting. The cause of most cases of normal-pressure hydrocephalus is not known, but it can be caused by disorders that interfere with CSF absorption, for example, subarachnoid hemorrhage, meningitis, and trauma.

Despite normal CSF pressure, as determined with lumbar puncture, normal-pressure hydrocephalus causes enlargement of the lateral ventricles and, thus, compression of adjacent structures. The dementia in this condition is thought to be caused by compression of the cerebral cortex, and it is difficult to distinguish from the dementia of Alzheimer disease. The radiographic feature of this disorder is enlarged ventricles disproportionate to cortical atrophy (Fig. 8.9).

The gait disorder in normal-pressure hydrocephalus is characterized by slow short steps, reduced step height, and a widened base. It is often described by the terms *magnetic* and *lower half Parkinson*. "Magnetic" refers to the shuffling nature of the steps. As in Parkinson disease, the patient may have a slow and stiff gait and the tendency to move en bloc. However, the arm swing is normal, unlike the reduced arm swing in Parkinson disease. The incontinence in normal-pressure hydrocephalus results from an uninhibited bladder (see Table 4.4).

The earlier the diagnosis of normal-pressure hydrocephalus is made, the greater the chance of reducing the symptoms with a shunt. A useful test to determine the potential benefit from shunting is to remove 30 to 50 mL of CSF and see if the clinical symptoms improve.

FRONTOTEMPORAL DEMENTIA

The term *frontotemporal dementia* includes focal degenerative dementias of the frontal and temporal lobes. The clinical features include behavioral and language problems. Frontotemporal dementia, previously called Pick disease, has three anatomical variants: the frontal variant, temporal variant (also called semantic dementia), and left frontal-predominant variant (also called progressive nonfluent aphasia).

Patients with frontotemporal dementia may become disinhibited and exhibit inappropriate

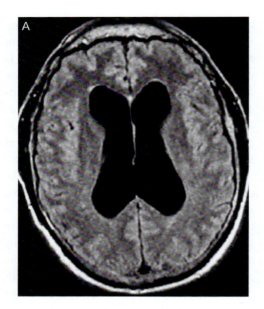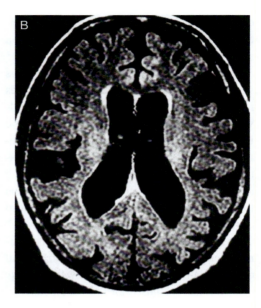

Fig. 8.9. Magnetic resonance images of normal-pressure hydrocephalus (*A*) and Alzheimer disease (*B*).

social behavior, which reflects the involvement of orbitofrontal cortex. Other frontal lobe behavioral abnormalities may include apathy, lack of motivation, and little response to stimuli. The predominant clinical feature in the temporal variant of frontotemporal dementia is impaired understanding of word meaning or object identity (agnosia) or both. This reflects pronounced degeneration of the left temporal lobe. A disorder of expressive language is the dominant clinical feature of patients with predominant left frontal lobe degeneration. The features of the three subtypes as developed by an international collaborative on frontotemporal dementia are summarized in Table 8.9.

Table 8.9. Frontotemporal Dementia (FTD) Variants

Frontal variant	Temporal variant (semantic dementia)	Left frontal-predominant (progressive nonfluent aphasia)

Core diagnostic features
Insidious onset and gradual progression
Early decline in social interpersonal conduct
Early impairment in regulation of personal conduct
Early emotional blunting
Early loss of insight
Supportive diagnostic features
Behavioral disorder
1. Decline in personal hygiene and grooming
2. Mental rigidity and inflexibility
3. Distractibility and impersistence
4. Hyperorality and dietary changes
5. Perseverative and stereotyped behavior
6. Utilization behavior
Speech and language
1. Altered speech output
  a. Aspontaneity and economy of speech
  b. Press of speech
2. Stereotype of speech
3. Echolalia
4. Perseveration
5. Mutism
Physical signs
1. Primitive reflexes
2. Incontinence
3. Akinesia, rigidity, and tremor
4. Low and labile blood pressure
	Core diagnostic features
	Insidious onset and gradual progression
	Language disorder characterized by—
	1. Progressive, fluent, empty spontaneous speech
	2. Loss of word meaning, manifest by impaired naming and comprehension
	3. Semantic paraphasias
	  and/or
	Perceptual disorder characterized by—
	1. Prosopagnosia (impaired recognition of identity of familiar faces)
	  and/or
	2. Associative agnosia (impaired recognition of object identity)
	Preserved perceptual matching and drawing reproduction
	Preserved single-word repetition
	Preserved ability to read aloud and write dictation orthographically regular words
	Supportive diagnostic features
	Speech and language
	1. Press of speech
	2. Idiosyncratic word usage
	3. Absence of phonemic paraphasias
	4. Surface dyslexia and dysgraphia
	5. Preserved calculation
		Core diagnostic features
		Insidious onset and gradual progression
		Nonfluent spontaneous speech with at least one of the following: agrammatism, phonemic paraphasias, anomia
		Supportive diagnostic features
		Speech and language
		1. Stuttering or oral apraxia
		2. Impaired repetition
		3. Alexia, agraphia
		4. Early preservation of word meaning
		5. Late mutism
		Behavior
		1. Early preservation of social skills
		2. Late behavioral changes similar to frontal variant
		Physical signs—late contralateral primitive reflexes, akinesia, rigidity, and tremor

Table 8.9   (continued)

Frontal variant	Temporal variant (semantic dementia)	Left frontal-predominant (progressive nonfluent aphasia)
Investigations 1. Neuropsychology—significant impairment on frontal lobe tests in absence of severe amnesia, or perceptuospatial disorder 2. EEG—normal on conventional EEG despite clinically evident dementia 3. Brain imaging (structural and/or functional)—predominant frontal and/or anterior temporal abnormality	**Supportive diagnostic features (cont'd)** *Behavior* 1. Loss of sympathy and empathy 2. Narrowed preoccupations 3. Parsimony *Physical signs*—absent or late primitive reflexes, akinesia, rigidity, and tremor **Investigations** 1. Neuropsychology— • Profound semantic loss, manifest in failure of word comprehension and naming and/or face and object recognition • Preserved phonology and syntax, and elementary perceptual processing, spatial skills, and day-to-day memorizing 2. EEG—normal 3. Brain imaging (structural and/or functional)—predominant anterior temporal abnormality (symmetrical or asymmetrical)	**Investigations** 1. Neuropsychology—nonfluent aphasia in the absence of severe amnesia or perceptuospatial disorder 2. EEG—normal or minor asymmetrical slowing 3. Brain imaging (structural and/or functional)—asymmetrical abnormality predominantly affecting dominant (usually left) hemisphere

EEG, electroencephalography.
From Neary D, et al: Frontotemporal lobar degeneration: A consensus on clinical diagnostic criteria. Neurology 51:1546-1554, 1998. Used with permission.

SUGGESTED READING

American Psychiatric Association: Diagnostic and Statistical Manual of Mental Disorders, ed 4, text revision. American Psychiatric Association, Washington DC, 2000.

Basile, AM, et al, LADIS Study Group: Age, hypertension, and lacunar stroke are the major determinants of the severity of age-related white matter changes. The LADIS (Leukoaraiosis and Disability in the Elderly) Study. Cerebrovasc Dis 21:315-322, 2006. Epub 2006 Feb 14.

Bastos Leite, AJ, Scheltens, P, and Barkhof, F: Pathological aging of the brain: An overview. Top Magn Reson Imaging 15:369-389, 2004.

Boxer, AL, and Miller, BL: Clinical features of frontotemporal dementia. Alzheimer Dis Assoc Disord 19 Suppl 1:S3-S6, 2005.

Bullock, R: Efficacy and safety of memantine in moderate-to-severe Alzheimer disease: The evidence to date. Alzheimer Dis Assoc Disord 20:23-29, 2006.

Cummings, JL: Alzheimer's disease. N Engl J Med 351:56-67, 2004.

Desai, AK, and Grossberg, GT: Diagnosis and treatment of Alzheimer's disease. Neurology 64 Suppl 3:S34-S39, 2005.

Doody, RS, et al: Practice parameter: Management of dementia (an evidence-based review). Report of the Quality Standards Subcommittee of the American Academy of Neurology. Neurology 56:1154-1166, 2001.

Drachman, DA: Aging of the brain, entropy, and Alzheimer disease. Neurology 67:1340-1352, 2006.

Goldman, JS, et al: Frontotemporal dementia: Genetics and genetic counseling dilemmas. Neurologist 10:227-234, 2004.

Huey, ED, Putnam, KT, and Grafman, J: A systematic review of neurottransmitter deficits and treatments in frontotemporal dementia. Neurology 66:17-22, 2006.

Kawas, CH: Clinical practice: Early Alzheimer's disease. N Engl J Med 349:1056-1063, 2003.

Knopman, DS: Dementia and cerebrovascular disease. Mayo Clin Proc 81:223-230, 2006.

Knopman, DS, et al, Report of the Quality Standards Subcommittee of the American Academy of Neurology: Practice parameter: Diagnosis of dementia (an evidence-based review). Neurology 56:1143-1153, 2001.

McGirt, MG, et al: Diagnosis, treatment, and analysis of long-term outcomes in idiopathic normal-pressure hydrocephalus. Neurosurgery 57:699-705, 2005.

McKeith, IG, et al: Diagnosis and management of dementia with Lewy bodies: Third report of the DLB Consortium. Neurology 65:1863-1872, 2005. Epub 2005 Oct. Erratum in: Neurology 65:1992, 2005.

McKhann, G, et al: Clinical diagnosis of Alzheimer's disease: Report of the NINCDS-ADRDA Work Group under the auspices of Department of Health and Human Services Task Force on Alzheimer's Disease. Neurology 34:939-944, 1984.

Morris, JC: Dementia update 2005. Alzheimer Dis Assoc Disord 19:100-117, 2005.

Neary, D, et al: Frontotemporal lobar degeneration: A consensus on clinical diagnostic criteria. Neurology 51:1546-1554, 1998.

Panza, F, et al: Current epidemiology of mild cognitive impairment and other predementia syndromes. Am J Geriatr Psychiatry 13:633-644, 2005.

Petersen, RC: Mild cognitive impairment as a diagnostic entity. J Intern Med 256:183-194, 2004.

Petersen, RC, et al, Report of the Quality Standards Subcommittee of the American Academy of Neurology: Practice parameter: Early detection of dementia: Mild cognitive impairment (an evidence-based review).Neurology 56:1133-1142, 2001.

Portet, F, et al, MCI Working Group of the European Consortium on Alzheimer's Disease (EADC): Mild cognitive impairment (MCI) in medical practice: A critical review of the concept and new diagnostic procedure: Report of the MCI Working Group of the European Consortium on Alzheimer's Disease. J Neurol Neurosurg Psychiatry 77:714-718, 2006. Epub 2006 Mar 20.

Ridha, B, and Josephs, KA: Young-onset dementia: A practical approach to diagnosis. Neurologist 12:2-13, 2006.

Schneider, LS, et al, CATIE-AD Study Group: Effectiveness of atypical antipsychotic drugs in patients with Alzheimer's disease. N Engl J Med 355:1525-1538, 2006.

Shumaker, SA, et al, WHIMS Investigators. Estrogen plus progestin and the incidence of dementia and mild cognitive impairment in postmenopausal women: The Women's Health Initiative Memory Study: A randomized controlled trial. JAMA 289:2651-2662, 2003.

Sink, KM, Holden, KF, and Yaffe, K: Pharmacological treatment of neuropsychiatric symptoms of dementia: A reveiw of the evidence. JAMA 293:596-608, 2005.

Winblad, B, et al, Report of the International Working Group on Mild Cognitive Impairment: Mild cognitive impairment: Beyond controversies, towards a consensus. J Intern Med 256:240-246, 2004.

CHAPTER 9

Spells

Spells are transient disorders that indicate reversible alterations in neuronal excitability. Transient disorders can affect the central or peripheral nervous system and can be focal or generalized. Examples of generalized transient disorders are generalized seizures, syncope, concussion, and cataplexy. Examples of focal transient disorders are focal seizures, transient ischemic attacks, migraine, transient mononeuropathies, paresthesias, muscle cramps, and tonic spasms.

The results of a neurologic examination of a patient who has a transient disorder are frequently normal because the disorder is caused by a physiologic rather than an anatomical mechanism. The nervous system transmits, stores, and processes information through electrical activity and the action of neurotransmitters. Alterations in neuronal excitability, either excess activity or loss of activity, can cause a transient disorder. Transient disorders can be caused by many mechanisms, including hypoxia, ischemia, seizures, electrolyte imbalances, drugs, and toxins. The absence of physical findings emphasizes the importance of taking a careful history. Accurate diagnosis may depend on additional information from the patient's family, friends, and coworkers.

Syncope, a nonepileptic loss of consciousness, indicates global diminution in brain metabolism. It has many causes; common ones include brain hypoperfusion from volume loss, inadequate postural reflexes, increased vagal tone, and cardiac dysfunction. Situational causes of syncope, such as micturition and cough, are due to a combination of mechanisms. Syncope can result from metabolic impairment despite adequate perfusion, as in hypoxia, carbon monoxide poisoning, anemia, and hypoglycemia. Syncope caused by acute intracranial hypertension, which may be due to a mass, hemorrhage, or cerebrospinal fluid obstruction, is less frequent.

The differential diagnosis of spells is extensive. Determining whether the spell has focal signs or symptoms is essential for making an accurate diagnosis. The common causes of focal spells are transient ischemic attacks, migraine, and focal seizures. Spells without focal signs or symptoms can include confusional states in which the patient's reactions to environmental stimuli are inappropriate. Confusional states occur in complex partial and absence seizures, toxic encephalopathies, confusional migraine, and psychiatric illness. Transient episodes of memory loss, as in transient global amnesia, are spells without focal symptoms. Patients with transient global amnesia have anterograde amnesia that can last for several hours. Drop attacks, which are episodes of sudden loss of postural tone without impairment of consciousness, also can cause spells without focal symptoms. Other spells without focal features include dizziness, psychiatric illness, sleep disorders, and pseudoseizures (Table 9.1).

Accurate diagnosis of spells depends on a careful medical history. As noted above, it is important to obtain additional history from others who have witnessed the spell or transient event. The patient's medical history, family history, and social history are necessary for differentiating the features of various spells. Laboratory studies, neuroimaging studies, electroencephalography (EEG), and prolonged EEG monitoring may be needed to establish the diagnosis. Important differentiating features of various spells are summarized in Table 9.2.

This chapter discusses common neurologic transient disorders, including seizures and sleep disorders. Other causes of spells, such as syncope, migraine, paroxysmal vertigo, and transient ischemic attacks, are discussed in other chapters.

SEIZURES

Diagnostic Approach to a First Seizure

In the case of a patient with a spell, the first diagnostic step is to determine whether the episode was an epileptic seizure or a nonepileptic event. The differential diagnosis for seizures is the same as for spells (Table 9.1). A convulsive epileptic seizure, or ictus, is the result of abnormal and excessive discharge of nerve cells and can be caused by many factors. When patients have a seizure, it is important to remind them that it is a symptom, not a condition. The features

consistent with an epileptic seizure include the loss of consciousness, tonic (continuous muscle contraction) and clonic (alternating contraction and relaxation of muscle) motor activity, injury, bladder incontinence, and postictal confusion. Syncope can be distinguished from seizure activity clinically by its relation to posture, usual occurrence during the day, and associated cardiovascular features. Convulsive activity, injury (eg, a bitten tongue), postictal confusion, amnesia, and incontinence rarely occur in syncope. Convulsive syncope, a seizure that occurs as a result of anoxia, can be a diagnostic challenge.

The second step in the evaluation is to determine whether the seizure was provoked or unprovoked. Provoked seizures are caused by factors that can disrupt cerebral function. Possible precipitating factors are drug ingestion or withdrawal, structural lesions of the brain, physical injuries, vascular insults, infections, and metabolic or toxic abnormalities. Some frequent causes of provoked seizures and investigative factors that may help elicit the cause are listed in Table 9.3. If the seizure occurs within 1 week after a precipitating factor, it is classified as an *acute symptomatic seizure*. The term *remote symptomatic seizure* is used if the known provoking factor occurred more than 1 week before the seizure, for example, a seizure that occurs several years after a skull fracture. A seizure that occurs in the absence of any identifiable factor is an *unprovoked seizure*. The term *idiopathic*, or *cryptogenic*, is used to describe seizures with no identifiable cause. If the seizure is caused by a specific provoking factor and that factor can be corrected, no further treatment is required. For example, if a patient has a seizure after an episode of excessive alcohol consumption, the avoidance of alcohol is preferred to treatment with anticonvulsants. Management of unprovoked seizures is more complicated, and the risks of recurrent seizure need to be assessed and discussed with the patient and family.

Table 9.1. Differential Diagnosis of Spells

Spells without focal symptoms	Spells with focal symptoms
Syncope	Transient ischemic attack
Confusional states	Partial seizures
Absence seizures	Migraine
Migraine	Multiple sclerosis
Dialysis dysequilibrium	Movement disorders
Porphyria	
Psychiatric disease	
Fluctuating encephalopathies (medication, metabolic, toxic)	
Memory loss	
Transient global amnesia	
Drug effect (benzodiazepines, anticholinergic drugs)	
Fugue states	
Alcoholic blackouts	
Drop attacks	
Vertebrobasilar ischemia	
Anterior cerebral artery ischemia	
Foramen magnum and upper spinal cord lesions	
Cataplexy	
Acute vestibulopathies	
Sleep disorders	
Narcolepsy	
Parasomnias	
Dizziness	
Vertigo	
Temporal lobe seizures	
Psychiatric	
Panic attacks, anxiety disorders	
Episodic dyscontrol	
Pseudoseizures	

Modified from Drislane, FW: Transient events. In Samuels, MA, and Feske, SK (eds): Office Practice of Neurology, ed 2. Churchill Livingstone, Philadelphia, 2003, pp 126-137. Used with permission.

The third step is to determine whether the seizure was generalized or focal. Focal seizures can become generalized seizures. For appropriate classification, prognosis, and treatment, it is important to distinguish between secondary generalized focal seizures and primary generalized seizures. Focal seizures are associated with a focal brain lesion and require a thorough investigation with imaging studies. Focal seizures are also a risk factor for recurrent seizure activity. The

Table 9.2. Differentiating Features of Spells Without Focal Symptoms

Confusional spells

Complex partial seizures: stereotyped spells, with automatisms (eg, lip smacking), EEG is helpful

Absence seizures: may have previous history of seizures, EEG confirms diagnosis

Migraine: headache associated, family history of headache

Toxic encephalopathies: history of chronic illness, medications, infections

Spells associated with memory loss

Transient global amnesia: sudden anterograde amnesia lasting hours, patient repeats same question during spell

Drug effect: use of benzodiazepines or anticholinergic drugs

Fugue state: prolonged episode of purposeful behavior, history of psychiatric illness

Drop attacks

Vertebrobasilar ischemia: older patients, other symptoms of brainstem ischemia

Anterior cerebral artery ischemia: cerebrovascular risk factors, rare

Foramen magnum and upper spinal cord lesions: brainstem or myelopathic features

Cataplexy: precipitated by emotion, associated with narcolepsy

Sleep disorders

Narcolepsy: excessive daytime somnolence, cataplexy, hypnagogic hallucinations

Parasomnias: sleepwalking, night terrors

Dizziness

Vertigo: benign positional vertigo, Ménière disease

Psychiatric

Panic attacks: discrete episodes of apprehension and fear and autonomic symptoms

Episodic dyscontrol: associated with head injury, well-defined precipitant

Pseudoseizures: bizarre spells, high frequency in epilepsy patients

EEG, electroencephalography.

From Adams, AC: Neurology in Primary Care. FA Davis, Philadelphia, 2000, p 156. Used with permission of Mayo Foundation for Medical Education and Research.

history of a patient with a seizure should include information from anyone who witnessed the event.

Warning signs and symptoms that precede the convulsion and indicate focal seizure activity include automatisms (eg, lip smacking, chewing, and complex pattern movements such as repetitively buttoning and unbuttoning clothing) and an aura. Examples of a preceding aura are an epigastric or "abdominal rising" sensa-tion, a sense of fear or apprehension, and other sensory symptoms (taste, smell, visual, or auditory hallucinations). A period of unresponsiveness and focal or asymmetrical motor activity are also common in focal seizure activity. Persistent weakness lasting less than 24 hours after a seizure is called *Todd paralysis* and is evidence of a focal seizure disorder.

A common focal seizure disorder of childhood, called *benign childhood epilepsy with*

Table 9.3. Causes of Provoked Seizures and Investigative Evaluation

Cause	Evaluation
Genetic and birth factors	History about pregnancy, birth, and delivery
Genetic influence	Family history
Congenital abnormalities	
Antenatal factors: infections, drugs, anoxia	
Perinatal factors: birth trauma, infections	
Infectious disorders	History: infections, HIV risk factors
Meningitis, encephalitis	Examination: nuchal rigidity, increased
Brain, epidural, or subdural abscess	temperature
	Laboratory: increased leukocyte count and
	ESR, positive serologic tests, CSF
	pleocytosis
	CT or MRI: mass or abscess
Toxic and metabolic	
Hypoglycemia, nonketotic hyperglycemia	Glucose level
Hypoxia	Blood gas values
Hyponatremia, hypomagnesemia,	Sodium, magnesium, calcium levels
hypocalcemia	
Uremia	Creatinine, blood urea nitrogen
Liver failure	Liver function tests
Drugs and drug withdrawal, alcohol	Toxic screen: cocaine, amphetamines,
	phencyclidine, hypnotic agents
	Alcohol level
Neoplasms	MRI
Primary intracranial	
Metastatic	
Lymphoma and leukemia	
Trauma	CT or MRI
Acute craniocerebral injury	
Subdural or epidural hematoma	
Vascular insult	
Ischemic stroke	Cerebrovascular risk factors
Hemorrhagic stroke	CT or MRI
Heredofamilial	Characteristic clinical features on
Neurofibromatosis, tuberous sclerosis,	examination
Sturge-Weber syndrome	
Degenerative disease	History of dementia
Alzheimer disease	

CSF, cerebrospinal fluid; CT, computed tomography; ESR, erythrocyte sedimentation rate; HIV, human
  immunodeficiency virus; MRI, magnetic resonance imaging.
From Adams, AC: Neurology in Primary Care. FA Davis, Philadelphia, 2000, p 157. Used with permission of Mayo Foundation for Medical Education and Research.

centrotemporal spikes, or *benign rolandic epilepsy*, is not associated with an underlying focal brain lesion. The onset is between the ages of 3 and 13 years. The child often awakens from sleep with motor and sensory symptoms of the face and hand. Drooling and arrest of speech are common. This benign disorder has a characteristic EEG pattern (Fig. 9.1). Neurologic examination findings are normal, and the disorder usually remits in adolescence.

For determining prognosis, it is crucial to know whether the event was the patient's first seizure. Studies have suggested that the risk of a recurrent seizure after the first unprovoked seizure is 30% to 50%. After a second unprovoked seizure, this risk increases to 70% to 80%. The patient should be asked if he or she ever had a seizure, a fit, or a convulsion with a fever as a young child. The risk for recurrent seizure after a second seizure is high, and treatment with antiepileptic drugs is often initiated at this time. Information about the patient's gestation, birth, delivery, and childhood development is important with

regard to complications associated with seizures (Table 9.3). A history of head trauma or serious infection may also indicate the possibility of remote symptomatic seizure. Any information about drug use is important. Central nervous system stimulants such as amphetamines, cocaine, and phencyclidine can induce seizure activity. Phenothiazines, atypical neuroleptics, penicillin, theophylline, and some tricyclic antidepressants reduce seizure threshold in susceptible persons. The family history is extremely important because a positive family history of epilepsy is a risk factor for recurrent seizure.

Focus the physical examination on detecting any underlying medical illness that would suggest a symptomatic seizure. Focal neurologic signs indicate focal seizure activity and increase the risk of recurrent seizure activity. Skin abnormalities may provide clues to an underlying neuroectodermal disorder, for example, café-au-lait spots in neurofibromatosis or angiofibromas alongside the nose of patients with tuberous sclerosis (Fig. 9.2).

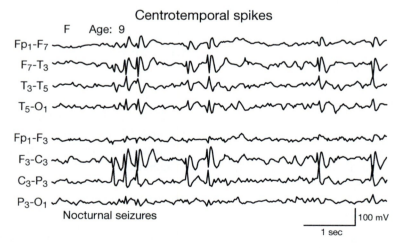

Fig. 9.1. Characteristic EEG in benign rolandic epilepsy. (From Westmoreland, BF: Clinical EEG Manual. Available from: http://mayoweb.mayo.edu/man-neuroeeg/images/3-04.jpg. Used with permission of Mayo Foundation for Medical Education and Research.)

EEG is indispensable in the evaluation of patients who have seizures. Its findings help determine the prognosis for recurrent seizure and help in classifying the seizure type as focal or generalized. EEG abnormalities, including focal and generalized epileptiform discharges and focal slowing, are associated with a higher risk of seizure recurrence. EEG should be performed as soon after the seizure as possible and should include a sleep recording to maximize the chance of detecting epileptiform abnormalities. Remember that normal EEG findings do not exclude the possibility of epilepsy, and repeat studies may be needed in certain clinical situations.

Magnetic resonance imaging (MRI) is the imaging study preferred for evaluating patients

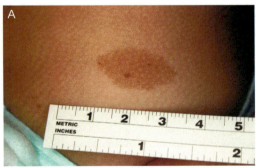

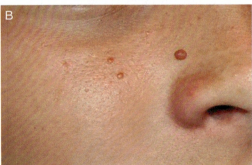

Fig. 9.2. *A*, Café-au-lait spot on the trunk of a patient with neurofibromatosis, and *B*, angiofibroma alongside the nose of a patient with tuberous sclerosis.

who have seizures. Compared with computed tomography (CT), MRI is more sensitive and accurate because of better soft tissue contrast, multiplanar imaging capability, and the absence of beam-hardening artifacts. The major structural causes of seizures, including tumors or any mass lesion, disorders of neuronal migration and cortical organization, vascular malformations, and mesial temporal sclerosis (Fig. 9.3), are visualized best with MRI. It also can detect evidence of previous brain injury from trauma, infection, inflammation, or infarction. Any structural abnormality seen on an imaging study increases the risk of recurrent seizure.

Functional neuroimaging in seizure disorders is becoming increasingly important, particularly for the presurgical evaluation of patients. Functional neuroimaging studies include magnetic resonance spectroscopy, magnetoencephalography, positron emission tomography, single-photon emission computed tomography, and subtraction ictal single-photon emission computed tomography coregistered to MRI, or SISCOM (Fig. 9.4). Functional neuroimaging

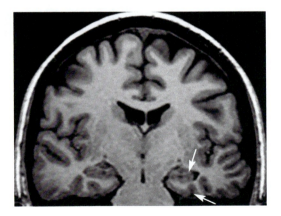

Fig. 9.3. Mesial temporal sclerosis. Oblique coronal T1-weighted MRI showing asymmetry of the hippocampal formation, with marked volume loss of the left hippocampus (*top arrow*), amygdala, and entorhinal cortex (*bottom arrow*).

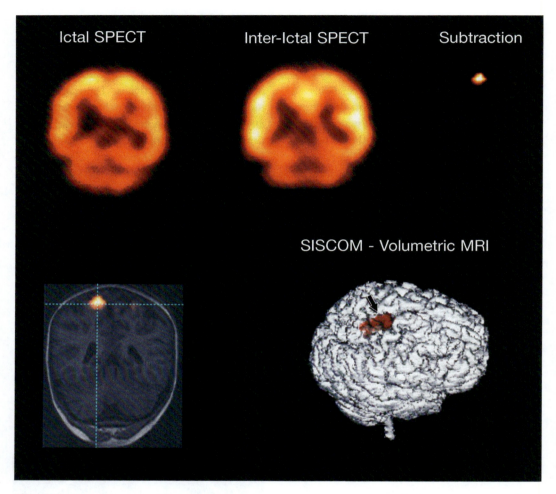

Fig. 9.4. Subtraction ictal single-photon emission computed tomography (SPECT) coregistered to MRI (SISCOM) showing probable location of seizure focus (*arrow*) on the surface of a 3-dimensional MRI. (From So, EL: Role of neuroimaging in the management of seizure disorders. Mayo Clin Proc 77:1251-1264, 2002. Used with permission of Mayo Foundation for Medical Education and Research.)

may be indicated for patients with negative MRI findings, indeterminate ictal EEG findings, multifocal EEG and MRI abnormalities, and EEG and MRI findings and seizure features that are not concordant.

After the diagnostic evaluation, decide about treatment. The purpose of treatment is to prevent recurrent seizures and the associated complications. Although antiepileptic drugs decrease the risk for recurrent seizures, there is no evidence that treatment affects long-term prognosis. Several complications are associated with antiepileptic drugs. Up to 10% of patients who take these drugs develop a skin rash, and almost 25% of newly treated patients have unacceptable side effects. The cost of the drugs, laboratory evaluations, and follow-up visits needs to be considered. Treatment also has implications for employment, insurance eligibility, and the social stigma of being labeled "epileptic."

The risk of recurrent seizures after a single unprovoked seizure is approximately 35% for the following 5 years. The range varies from less than 20% to 100%, depending on the presence or absence of risk factors. Risk factors for recurrent seizure include a previous provoked seizure, a focal seizure, abnormal results on neurologic examination, a family history of epilepsy, abnormal EEG findings, and structural abnormalities seen on MRI.

The decision about whether to treat an adult with an anticonvulsant medication depends on the estimate of recurrent risk. Also, an assessment should be made of the consequences of a recurrent seizure, including the potential effect on the patient's social, occupational, and psychologic status. The patient and family should participate in the decision-making process, and the patient's preferences should be considered. For a child or adolescent who has experienced a first seizure, the risk of another seizure versus the risk of cognitive, behavioral, physical, and psychosocial effects of antiepileptic drugs needs to be assessed. According to the recommendations of the American Academy of Neurology and Child Neurology Society, antiepileptic drugs are not indicated for preventing the development of epilepsy and treatment may be considered if the benefits of reducing the risk of a second seizure outweigh the risks of pharmacologic and psychosocial side effects.

Treatment with antiepileptic drugs is usually considered for provoked seizures when the provoking factor cannot be corrected. Treatment is recommended after a second unprovoked seizure because the risk of recurrent seizure increases to 70% to 80%. Some seizure types, such as absence and myoclonic seizures, are recurrent and usually treated. The decision-making steps for treating a patient who has a first-time seizure are shown in Figure 9.5.

After a patient has a seizure, several important safety issues need to be discussed. Patients should not engage in any situation in which they would injure themselves or others were a recurrent seizure to occur. Driving regulations must be discussed and the conversation documented in the medical record. Know the current driving regulations of the state in which you practice. Some states require that the physician report seizures or any episode of loss of consciousness. Most states require the patient to have a seizure-free period (30 days–1 year) before being allowed to drive. Exceptions vary by state. Periodic medical updates are required in many states. Consult the state's Department of Motor Vehicles for this information.

Epilepsy Classification

The International League Against Epilepsy has standardized the classification and terminology for epileptic seizures and syndromes. Seizures can be characterized by ictal signs and symptoms, seizure type, syndromes, etiology, and impairment. The classification scheme evolves as new information becomes available. This classification scheme is summarized in Table 9.4.

Treatment of Seizure Disorders

After the decision has been made to treat a seizure disorder, many factors determine which antiepileptic drug is prescribed. These factors include the effectiveness of the drug in controlling seizures, tolerability of side effects, pharmacokinetic properties, patient characteristics, drug interactions, and cost of therapy. The best antiepileptic drug is the one that controls seizures without causing unacceptable side effects. Therapy needs to be individualized. The dose of one antiepileptic drug should be increased gradually until seizure control is

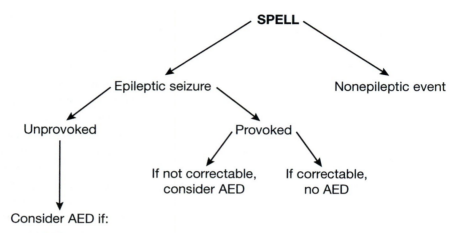

Fig. 9.5. Algorithm for evaluating spells. AED, antiepileptic drug; EEG, electroencephalogram. (From Adams, AC: Neurology in Primary Care. FA Davis, Philadelphia, 2000, p 159. Used with permission of Mayo Foundation for Medical Education and Research.)

achieved without provoking unacceptable adverse effects. Anticonvulsant levels are a guide to therapy, but it is the patient's clinical response that determines the effectiveness of the therapy. Antiepileptic drugs and their class and initial dose are listed in Table 9.5.

One of the first steps in selecting an antiepileptic drug is to determine whether the seizure is generalized or focal. Valproate (Depakote) is effective for controlling generalized seizures, including absence seizures, myoclonic seizures, and primary generalized tonic-clonic seizures. Ethosuximide (Zarontin)

is efficacious for absence seizures but is not effective for generalized tonic-clonic seizures. Lamotrigine (Lamictal) is a second-line drug for absence and myoclonic seizures, as is clonazepam (Klonopin) for myoclonic seizures. In addition to valproate, other first-line medications considered for generalized tonic-clonic seizures are carbamazepine (Tegretol), oxcarbazepine (Trileptal), and lamotrigine.

First-line therapy for focal seizures, including simple, complex, and secondary generalized seizures, are carbamazepine, gabapentin (Neurontin), lamotrigine, levetiracetam (Keppra), oxcarbazepine, topiramate (Topamax), valproate, and zonisamide (Zonegran). Although felbamate (Felbatol) is effective in treating focal seizures, it is reserved for treating catastrophic seizures because of the risk of aplastic anemia and liver failure. The selection of antiepileptic drug by seizure type and epilepsy syndrome is summarized in Table 9.6.

All antiepileptic drugs are associated with side effects. Many of the side effects a patient experiences at the initiation of therapy can be avoided by starting treatment at a low dose and gradually increasing it. Unless the clinical situation dictates prompt protection against seizure occurrence, avoid full or loading doses to minimize the chance of adverse effects. Common side effects associated with antiepileptic drugs are nausea and other gastrointestinal symptoms, sedation, dizziness, and incoordination. Before a patient drives a motor vehicle or operates dangerous equipment, he or she should determine whether the drug causes adverse effects that impair mental or motor performance. Within 6 weeks after starting treatment, approximately 10% of patients develop a rash. Rash is less likely with valproate or gabapentin (2% of patients) than with phenytoin (Dilantin), carbamazepine, or lamotrigine (10% of patients).

The risk of bone marrow suppression with antiepileptic drug treatment is low; however, this side effect is associated with carbamazepine. Avoid treatment with carbamazepine if the patient has a hematologic illness. Inform the patient or the patient's caregiver about the symptoms of early bone marrow suppression. Symptoms of fatigue, postural dizziness, bruises, fever, and sore throat may indicate anemia, coagulopathy, or infection before changes are detected with laboratory tests. Also avoid treatment with carbamazepine if the patient has demonstrated hypersensitivity to tricyclic antidepressants or is also taking a monoamine oxidase inhibitor. Felbamate is associated with a marked increase in the incidence of aplastic anemia and should be reserved for only those patients with intractable epilepsy for whom the risk is deemed acceptable in relation to the benefit of the medication. Hematologic consultation should be considered.

Many antiepileptic agents are associated with behavioral and cognitive disturbances. Barbiturates, including phenobarbital and primidone, are associated most often with these adverse effects. These agents should be prescribed with extreme caution for patients who are mentally depressed, have suicidal tendencies, have a history of drug abuse, or are receiving other central nervous system depressants. Because of the undesirable side effects of barbiturates, treatment with these drugs should be avoided. The side effects of antiepileptic drugs are summarized in Table 9.7.

It is important to know the pharmacokinetics of antiepileptic drugs when selecting the most appropriate medication (Table 9.8). For example, reduced renal function can lead to the accumulation of renally excreted drugs such as gabapentin, levetiracetam, and topiramate. Low protein-bound medications such as levetiracetam and gabapentin are removed by hemodialysis, and supplemental doses may be needed for patients receiving dialysis. Highly protein-bound drugs such as phenytoin and valproate are affected more by hypoalbuminemia, renal dysfunction, and interactions with other highly protein-bound drugs than are drugs not highly protein bound. In patients with liver dysfunction, drugs that have no enzymatic activity may be preferred, for example, gabapentin, levetiracetam, and topiramate. Drugs such as valproate and felbamate should be avoided if patients have liver disease.

Drug interactions, which depend on metabolism, enzyme induction, and protein binding, are also important when selecting an antiepileptic

Table 9.4.   Summary of the Classification Scheme of the International League Against Epilepsy

Descriptors	Groups and examples
Ictal semiology	
Motor	Elementary motor (tonic, myoclonic, tonic-clonic, atonic)
	Automatisms (lip smacking)
Nonmotor	Aura
	Sensory—elementary (somatosensory, visual); experiential (affective, mnemonic)
	Dyscognitive (perception, emotion, memory)
Autonomic	Aura (cardiovascular, gastrointestinal, sudomotor, vasomotor)
Somatotopic modifiers	Laterality
	Body part
	Centricity (axial, proximal/distal limb)
Modifiers/descriptors of seizure timing	Incidence
	State dependent (drowsiness, sleep, wakefulness)
	Catamenial
Duration	Status epilepticus
	Brief seizure
Severity	Benign (benign neonatal seizure)
	Severe (severe myoclonic epilepsy)
Prodrome	Vague sensation
Postictal phenomenon	Lateralizing (Todd paralysis)
	Nonlateralizing (amnesia)
Seizure type	
Self-limited	Generalized (absence, tonic-clonic)
	Focal (focal motor or sensory seizure)
Continuous	Generalized (generalized tonic-clonic status epilepticus)
	Focal (epilepsia partialis continua)
Precipitating stimuli (reflex)	Visual, reading
Syndromes	
Epilepsy syndromes and related conditions	West syndrome, Lennox-Gastaut syndrome, juvenile myoclonic epilepsy
Epilepsy seizures without a diagnosis of epilepsy	Alcohol withdrawal seizures, febrile seizures

Table 9.4 **(continued)**

Etiology

Idiopathic	Familial
Symptomatic	Genetic (chromosomal abnormalities, Rett syndrome, mitochondrial disorders)
	Neurodevelopmental disorders (neurocutaneous disorders)
	Progressive myoclonic epilepsies (Lafora disease)
	Tumors
	Pre-/perinatal ischemia
	Postnatal infections or other insults
	Miscellaneous (Alzheimer disease)
Provoked	Febrile seizures

Modified from Galanopoulou, AS, and Lado, FA: Classification, pathophysiology, causes, differential diagnosis of paroxysmal events. Continuum: Lifelong Learning in Neurology 10 no. 4:11-41, August 2004. Used with permission.

drug. Drugs that induce liver enzymes, including carbamazepine, oxcarbazepine, and phenytoin, can decrease the concentration and effectiveness of other drugs metabolized by these enzymes, for example, oral contraceptives, theophylline, corticosteroids, and warfarin. Drugs that do not have enzymatic activity include ethosuximide, gabapentin, levetiracetam, tiagabine, and zonisamide. Before any medical therapy is initiated, it is prudent to investigate the potential for drug interactions. Common interactions with antiepileptic drugs are summarized in Table 9.9.

The longer serum half-life of a drug may be important for dosage schedule and patient compliance. For example, phenytoin and zonisamide may be preferred to other drugs because they can be taken once a day.

Weight gain or weight loss can occur with many of the antiepileptic drugs and may be an important issue in selecting which therapeutic agent to prescribe. Medications associated with weight gain include valproate, carbamazepine, gabapentin, and pregabalin (Lyrica). Antiepileptic drugs liable to cause weight loss include topiramate and zonisamide. Lamotrigine, levetiracetam, and phenytoin are weight-neutral.

After a patient starts receiving maintenance therapy with an antiepileptic drug, he or she should have follow-up clinical evaluation and laboratory testing. Clinical evaluation is more useful than laboratory testing. Drug levels should be used only as a guide to therapy. The dosage of an antiepileptic drug should not be changed on the basis of a drug level. The drug level can guide the decision about dosage, based on whether the patient is having seizures or toxic side effects. The level of an antiepileptic drug is not meaningful until the drug has reached steady state. Circumstances that may change drug dosage include growth (in children), weight change, medical illness, or drug interactions. The free fraction of an antiepileptic drug that has high protein binding (carbamazepine, phenytoin, valproate) needs to be monitored in conditions that affect protein binding, for example, liver and kidney disease, pregnancy, and hypoalbuminemia.

Liver function tests and complete blood counts are often performed to determine whether

Table 9.5. Antiepileptic Drugs

Drug	Class, mode of action	Adult dose
Carbamazepine (Tegretol, Carbatrol)	Dibenzazepine carboxamide Blocks sodium channel conductance; reduces neuronal calcium uptake	Oral suspension and tablets: initial, 100 mg (suspension) *orally* 4 times daily on the 1st day *or* 200 mg (tablets) twice daily on the 1st day; may increase dosage by 200 mg/day (suspension or tablets) at weekly intervals. Extended-release capsules: initial, 200 mg *orally* twice daily; may increase dosage by 200 mg/day at weekly intervals until optimal response
Clonazepam (Klonopin)	Benzodiazepine GABA	0.5 mg *orally* 3 times daily
Ethosuximide (Zarontin)	Succinimide Blocks calcium channel conductance	500 mg/day *orally* adjusted by 250-mg increments every 4-7 days to desired therapeutic effect
Felbamate (Felbatol)	Carbamate Possible block of NMDA receptors and modulation of sodium channels	*Warning*: increased incidence of aplastic anemia; 1,200 mg/day *orally* (in 3-4 divided doses); may increase dosage in 600-mg/day increments every 2 weeks to 2,400 mg/day as needed and thereafter to 3,600 mg/day if clinically indicated
Gabapentin (Neurontin)	GABA Modulates N-type calcium channels	300 mg *orally* 3 times daily; may increase up to 1,800 mg/day (in 3 divided doses)
Lamotrigine (Lamictal)	Phenyltriazine Blocks voltage-dependent sodium conductance	50 mg/day *orally* for 2 weeks, then 100 mg/day (in 2 divided doses) for 2 weeks; may increase dosage by 100 mg/day *orally* every 1-2 weeks to the usual maintenance dose of 300-500 mg/day (in 2 divided doses)
Levetiracetam (Keppra)	Anticonvulsant Affects calcium channel and GABA	500 mg twice daily *orally* or *IV*; may increase dosage by 1,000 mg/day every 2 weeks (in 2 divided doses) to maximal recommended daily dose of 3,000 mg

Table 9.5 (continued)

Drug	Class, mode of action	Adult dose
Oxcarbazepine (Trileptal)	Dibenzazepine carboxamide Blocks sodium channels; increases potassium conductance	300 mg *orally* twice daily, then increase the dosage by 300 mg/day every 3rd day to 1,200 mg/day
Phenobarbital (Luminal)	Barbiturate Enhances activity of $GABA_A$ receptors; depresses glutamate excitability; reduces sodium, potassium, and calcium conductance	60-250 mg/day *orally* (single or divided doses)
Phenytoin (Dilantin)	Hydantoin Blocks sodium channels; reduces neuronal calcium uptake	100 mg *orally* 3 times daily, then 300 mg as a single dose
Pregabalin (Lyrica)	GABA Modulates N-type calcium channels	75 mg *orally* twice daily *or* 50 mg *orally* 3 times daily (150 mg/day) and increased to maximal dose of 600 mg/day in divided doses (either 2 or 3 times daily) based on response and tolerability
Primidone (Mysoline)	Barbiturate Enhances activity of $GABA_A$ receptors; depresses glutamate excitability; reduces sodium, potassium, and calcium conductance	100-125 mg *orally* at bedtime for 3 days; increase dose by 100-125 mg/day (divided doses) every 3 days to reach dose of 250 mg 3 times daily
Tiagabine (Gabitril)	GABA Uptake inhibitor Inhibits GABA reuptake	Adjunct: (adjunctive therapy for patients taking enzyme-inducing antiepileptic drugs) 4 mg *orally* once daily; may increase dosage by 4-8 mg/day at weekly intervals to maximal dose of 56 mg/day (in 2-4 divided doses)
Topiramate (Topamax)	Fructopyranose sulfamate Blocks sodium channels, enhances GABA-mediated chloride influx and modulatory effects of $GABA_A$	Initial monotherapy: 1st week, 25 mg *orally* twice daily (morning and evening); 2nd week, 50 mg *orally* twice daily; 3rd week, 75 mg *orally* twice daily; 4th week, 100 mg *orally* twice daily; 5th

Table 9.5   (continued)

Drug	Class, mode of action	Adult dose
	receptors and actions of the AMPA receptor	week, 150 mg *orally* twice daily; 6th week (maximal dose) 200 mg *orally* twice daily
Valproate (Depakote)	Valproic acid Affects GABA glutaminergic activity, reduces threshold of calcium and potassium conductance	10-15 mg/kg daily *orally*; may increase dosage 5-10 mg/kg per week to achieve optimal clinical response
Zonisamide (Zonegran)	Sulfonamide Blocks sodium, potassium, and calcium channels; inhibits glutamate excitation	100 mg/day *orally*; may increase dosage by 100 mg/day every 2 weeks to usual effective dosage range of 100-600 mg/day (in 1-2 divided doses)

AMPA, α-Amino-3-hydroxy-5-methyl-4-isoxazole propionic acid; GABA, γ-aminobutyric acid; IV, intravenously; NMDA, N-methyl-D-aspartate.

serious complications of hepatitis or hematologic suppression have developed. However, it is more important that the patient recognize the early symptoms of these serious complications. Often, minor laboratory abnormalities are not clinically significant. Laboratory values that are significant include a leukocyte count less than 3,000 cells/mm³ (3×10^9/L), a neutrophil count less than 1,500/mm³ (1.5×10^9/L), platelets less than 100,000/mm³ (100×10^9/L), and liver enzyme values more than 2.5 times normal. Asymptomatic patients with any of these values should be followed closely, and the dose of the antiepileptic drug should be decreased.

Epilepsy in Women

When treating women for seizures or epilepsy, several special issues need to be considered. Seizure disorders and antiepileptic drugs affect oral contraceptives, the menstrual cycle, and pregnancy. Tell women who have seizures that the failure rate of oral contraceptives is four times higher than normal when they are being treated with an enzyme-inducing antiepileptic drug. Enzyme-inducing antiepileptic drugs include carbamazepine, phenytoin, topiramate, phenobarbital, felbamate, and oxcarbazepine. Women who take these antiepileptic drugs should take oral contraceptives with at least 50 µg of ethinyl estradiol and avoid low-dose formulations of oral contraceptives. Gabapentin, levetiracetam, pregabalin, tiagabine, valproate, and zonisamide do not have this effect. Oral contraceptives can affect lamotrigine levels; thus, when they are added to or removed from the regimen of women taking lamotrigine, the women should be monitored for seizures and lamotrigine toxicity.

Menstrual dysfunction—anovulatory cycles, amenorrhea, oligomenorrhea, and abnormal cycle intervals—is more common in women with epilepsy than in those without epilepsy. Seizures affect the hypothalamic-pituitary-gonadal axis. Also, antiepileptic drugs affect hormone-binding globulin, which in turn can disrupt estrogen and progesterone binding. Up

Table 9.6. Antiepileptic Drug Selection by Seizure Type and Epilepsy Syndrome

Drug	Seizure type and epilepsy syndrome
Carbamazepine (Tegretol, Carbatrol)	**Focal:** simple, complex, secondary generalized tonic-clonic, benign rolandic (first-line) *Contraindicated for absence, myoclonic*
Clonazepam (Klonopin)	**Generalized:** myoclonic, juvenile myoclonic, infantile spasms (second-line), Lennox-Gastaut syndrome (third-line)
Ethosuximide (Zarontin)	**Generalized:** absence (first-line), adolescent-onset absence (second-line)
Felbamate (Felbatol)	**Generalized and focal:** *See drug warning*, juvenile myoclonic, Lennox-Gastaut syndrome, focal (third-line)
Gabapentin (Neurontin)	**Focal:** simple, complex, secondary generalized tonic-clonic, benign rolandic (first-line)
Lamotrigine (Lamictal)	**Generalized and focal:** generalized tonic-clonic, Lennox-Gastaut syndrome, focal simple, complex, secondary generalized tonic-clonic (first-line); absence, myoclonic, benign rolandic, juvenile myoclonic (second-line); infantile spasm (third-line)
Levetiracetam (Keppra)	**Generalized and focal:** focal simple, complex, secondary generalized tonic-clonic (first-line); benign rolandic, juvenile myoclonic (second-line); myoclonic, generalized tonic-clonic (third-line)
Oxcarbazepine (Trileptal)	**Focal:** simple, complex, secondary generalized tonic-clonic (first-line)
Phenobarbital (Luminal)	**Generalized and focal:** generalized tonic-clonic, focal simple, complex, secondary generalization (second-line)
Phenytoin (Dilantin)	**Generalized and focal:** generalized tonic-clonic, focal simple, complex, secondary generalization (second-line) *Contraindicated for absence, myoclonic*
Primidone (Mysoline)	**Generalized and focal:** generalized tonic-clonic, myoclonic, focal simple, complex, secondary generalization (second-line)
Topiramate (Topamax)	**Generalized and focal:** simple, complex, secondary generalized tonic-clonic (first-line); generalized tonic-clonic, benign rolandic, juvenile myoclonic, Lennox-Gastaut syndrome (second-line); myoclonic, infantile spasms (third-line)
Valproate (Depakote)	**Generalized and focal:** generalized tonic-clonic, absence, myoclonic, juvenile myoclonic, focal simple, complex, secondary generalized tonic-clonic (first-line)
Zonisamide (Zonegran)	**Generalized and focal:** focal simple, complex, secondary, generalized tonic-clonic (first-line); myoclonic, infantile spasms (third-line)

Table 9.7. Side Effects of Antiepileptic Drugs

Drug	Warnings and precautions	Common side effects	Other side effects to consider	Idiosyncratic effects
Carbamazepine (Tegretol, Carbatrol)	Use with care in patients with mixed seizure disorder that includes atypical absence	Dizziness, diplopia, light-headed-ness	Hyponatremia, cardiac dysrhythmias	Aplastic anemia, agranulocytosis
Clonazepam (Klonopin)	CNS depression Can cause generalized seizures in patients with mixed seizure disorder Contraindicated in acute narrow-angle glaucoma	Sedation, ataxia	Tolerance to anticonvul-sant activity may develop	Confusion, depression
Ethosuximide (Zarontin)	Caution in kidney and liver dysfunction Abrupt with-drawal can precipitate absence status May increase generalized tonic-clonic convulsions when used in mixed seizure disorders	Nausea, vomiting	Aggressive-ness, psychosis	Agranulocytosis, Stevens-Johnson syndrome
Felbamate (Felbatol)	Need informed consent Aplastic anemia Liver failure	Anorexia, vomiting, nausea	Headache, insomnia, weight loss	Aplastic anemia, liver failure
Gabapentin (Neurontin)	CNS depression Abrupt discontin-uation may pre-cipitate status epilepticus	Peripheral edema, fatigue, somnolence, dizziness, ataxia		Not established

Table 9.7   (continued)

Drug	Warnings and precautions	Common side effects	Other side effects to consider	Idiosyncratic effects
Lamotrigine (Lamictal)	CNS depression Liver dysfunction Platelet and coagulation tests should be performed periodically	Abnormal thinking, dizziness, ataxia, diplopia, nausea, weight gain	Rash	Stevens-Johnson syndrome
Levetiracetam (Keppra)	Reduced levels with hemodialysis Potential toxicity with renal impairment Suicides have occurred	Loss of appetite, vomiting, somnolence, hostile behavior	Suicide attempts	
Oxcarbazepine (Trileptal)	Alcohol may cause additive sedative effect Reduces effectiveness of oral contraceptive	Nausea, vomiting, diplopia, fatigue	Hyponatremia	Stevens-Johnson syndrome, multiorgan hypersensitivity reaction
Phenobarbital (Luminal)	CNS depression May be habit-forming	Sedation	Behavioral and cogntive disturbance	May cause paradoxical hyperactivity
Phenytoin (Dilantin)	Abrupt withdrawal may cause status epilepticus Lymphadenopathy Hyperglycemia	Nystagmus, ataxia, rash	Gingival hyperplasia, hirsutism, coarsening of facial features, atrioventricular defect and ventricular automaticity	Stevens-Johnson syndrome
Pregabalin (Lyrica)	Congestive heart failure with increased risk of peripheral edema Alcohol may cause additive sedative effect Ocular conditions	Edema, weight gain, vision changes, dizziness		Potential for tumorigenicity

Table 9.7 continued on next page

Table 9.7   (continued)

Drug	Warnings and precautions	Common side effects	Other side effects to consider	Idiosyncratic effects
Primidone (Mysoline)	CNS depression May be habit-forming Use with care in patients with depression	Sedation, dizziness, ataxia	Behavioral and cognitive disturbance, diminished libido, impotence	May cause paradoxical hyperactivity
Tiagabine (Gabitril)	May cause seizures Liver dysfunction Care with driving until effects are known	Dizziness, nervousness, tremor	Seizures in patients without history of seizures	Unexplained sudden death
Topiramate (Topamax)	CNS depression Proper hydration to avoid urinary tract calculi	Somnolence, fatigue	Memory dysfunction, weight loss	Urinary tract calculi
Valproate (Depakote)	CNS depression Liver dysfunction Platelet and coagulation tests should be performed periodically	Nausea, vomiting, tremor, thrombocytopenia	Weight gain, hair loss, neural tube defects in pregnancy, association with hyperandrogenism	Agranulocytosis, Stevens-Johnson syndrome, liver dysfunction
Zonisamide (Zonegran)	Older patients require cautious dosage titration	Somnolence, dizziness, agitation	Memory impairment	Agranulocytosis, Stevens-Johnson syndrome

CNS, central nervous system.

Modified from Adams, AC: Neurology in Primary Care. FA Davis, Philadelphia, 2000, pp 162-163. Used with permission of Mayo Foundation for Medical Education and Research.

to 50% of women with epilepsy report that their seizures vary with the menstrual cycle.

Many important issues are related to seizures, antiepileptic drugs, and pregnancy. At the beginning of the therapeutic relation with a woman of childbearing age, discuss seizures, antiepileptic drugs, and pregnancy. Although more than 90% of women with epilepsy have uneventful pregnancies, they need to know about the teratogenic potential of antiepileptic drugs and the potential harm to the fetus from a seizure. Seizure frequency can

Table 9.8. Pharmacokinetics of Antiepileptic Drugs

Drug	Protein binding, %	Enzymatic activity	Elimination half-life, hours	Elimination route (%)
Carbamazepine (Tegretol, Carbatrol)	75	Broad-spectrum inducer	9-15	Liver (99)
Clonazepam (Klonopin)	85	Induces cytochrome CYP2B	20-60	Liver (>90) Renal (<5)
Ethosuximide (Zarontin)	0	None	30-60	Liver (>80) Renal (<20)
Felbamate (Felbatol)	25	Induces cytochrome CYP3A4, inhibits CYP2C19	13-22	Liver (50) Renal (50)
Gabapentin (Neurontin)	0	None	5-7	Renal (100)
Lamotrigine (Lamictal)	55	Induces UDP-glucurono-syltransferase	12-62	Liver (90) Renal (10)
Levetiracetam (Keppra)	<10	None	6-8	Renal (100)
Oxcarbazepine (Trileptal)	40	Induces cytochrome CYP3A4 and UDP-glucuronosyltransferase, inhibits CYP2C19	9	Liver (99) Renal (1)
Phenobarbital (Luminal)	45	Broad-spectrum inducer	75-110	Liver (75) Renal (25)
Phenytoin (Dilantin)	90	Broad-spectrum inducer	9-36	Liver (95) Renal (5)
Tiagabine (Gabitril)	96	None	7-9	Liver (98) Renal (2)
Topiramate (Topamax)	15	Induces cytochrome CYP3A4, inhibits CYP2C19	12-24	Liver (35) Renal (65)
Valproate (Depakote)	90	Broad-spectrum inhibitor	6-18	Liver (98) Renal (2)
Zonisamide (Zonegran)	40	None	63	Liver (65) Renal (35)

CYP, cytochrome P-450; UDP, uridine diphosphate.

Modified from Lacerda, G, et al: Optimizing therapy of seizures in patients with renal or hepatic dysfunction. Neurology 67 Suppl 4:S28-S33, 2006. Used wth permission.

Table 9.9. Antiepileptic Drug Interactions

Carbamazepine
- Decreases: doxycycline, folic acid, haloperidol, oral contraceptives, theophylline, warfarin
- Drugs increasing carbamazepine levels: calcium channel blockers, cimetidine, danazol, diltiazem, erythromycin, fluoxetine, imipramine, isoniazid, propoxyphene
- Drugs decreasing carbamazepine levels: alcohol (long-term use), folic acid, phenobarbital, phenytoin

Phenytoin
- Decreases: chloramphenicol, cyclosporine, dexamethasone, doxycycline, folic acid, furosemide, haloperidol, meperidine, methadone, oral contraceptives, quinidine, theophylline, vitamin D
- Increases: warfarin
- Drugs decreasing phenytoin levels: alcohol (long-term use), antacids, carbamazepine, folic acid, rifampin, valproate
- Drugs increasing phenytoin levels: alcohol (short-term use), amiodarone, chloramphenicol, chlordiazepoxide, cimetidine, disulfiram, fluconazole, fluoxetine, imipramine, isoniazid, metronidazole, omeprazole, propoxyphene, sulfonamides, trazodone

Valproate
- Decreases: carbamazepine, oral contraceptives, phenobarbital, phenytoin
- Increases: alcohol, aspirin, benzodiazepines, cimetidine

From Adams, AC: Neurology in Primary Care. FA Davis, Philadelphia, 2000, p 164. Used with permission of Mayo Foundation for Medical Education and Research.

increase during pregnancy, and the importance of compliance with medication and close medical follow-up should be emphasized. Recommend a multivitamin with folate (4 mg) for all women of childbearing age. Folate must be present within the first 25 days after conception to protect against neural tube defects.

Discontinuing or switching to another antiepileptic drug should be done before the patient becomes pregnant. If the patient has been seizure-free for more than a year, consider withdrawal of drug treatment. Withdrawal of drug treatment is most likely to be successful in patients who have been seizure-free for 2 to 5 years while taking an antiepileptic drug, have a single type of partial or generalized seizure, have normal findings on neurologic examination, have a normal IQ, and whose EEG results normalize with treatment. Most seizures recur in the first 6 months after withdrawal of antiepileptic drug therapy; thus, advise the patient that during this period she should not become pregnant or drive a motor vehicle.

If withdrawal of the antiepileptic drug is not a possibility, the patient should receive maintenance therapy with one drug that, at the lowest dose possible, best controls her seizures. It is best for the patient to receive maintenance therapy with the antiepileptic drug that she already takes. The risk of fetal injury is twice normal and is increased with higher doses and with multiple medications. Antiepileptic drug monotherapy with divided doses is recommended. The free fraction of the drug should be determined before conception and checked every 3 months throughout pregnancy. Major malformations can be detected with ultrasonography, alpha fetoprotein testing, amniocentesis, and chorionic villus sampling. Enzyme-inducing antiepileptic drugs (carbamazepine, phenytoin, and phenobarbital) have been associated with an increased risk of neonatal bleeding because of low levels of vitamin K. Thus, vitamin K, 10 mg/day, should be taken during the final month of pregnancy if the patient is taking one of these medications.

Breastfeeding by women who take antiepileptic drugs is usually successful despite the concentration of these drugs in breast milk. The amount of drug in breast milk is inversely related to the degree of protein binding. Breastfeeding should be discontinued if sedation, poor feeding, or irritability occurs in the infant.

Epilepsy Surgery

Patients who have medically intractable seizures should be evaluated for possible surgical treatment. Focal cortical resection of an epileptogenic zone or lesion pathology has been successful in selected patients with focal seizures.

Vagal nerve stimulation has shown some efficacy as adjunctive therapy for medically refractory epilepsy. This treatment consists of a device that provides a programmable stimulus from a chest-implanted generator to electrodes on the left cervical vagus nerve. Deep brain stimulation is also being investigated as a surgical option for patients with epilepsy and seizures. Subspecialty evaluation with an epileptologist is recommended for patients who have medically refractory epilepsy.

Status Epilepticus

Status epilepticus is a condition of continuous seizure activity of 30 minutes or two or more seizures without recovery (returning consciousness) between seizures. The management of this medical emergency is summarized in Figure 9.6.

SLEEP DISORDERS

The International Classification of Sleep Disorders divides sleep disorders into 1) insomnias, 2) sleep-related breathing disorders, 3) hypersomnias of central origin, 4) circadian rhythm sleep disorders, 5) parasomnias, 6) sleep-related movement disorders, 7) isolated symptoms, and 8) other sleep disorders. Table 9.10 lists examples in each of these categories.

The term *dyssomnia* can include both insomnia and excessive sleepiness. Intrinsic dyssomnias are the primary sleep disorders that develop in the body or arise from causes in the body. Intrinsic dyssomnias that cause insomnia include psychophysiologic insomnia and restless legs syndrome. Narcolepsy is an example of a dyssomnia that causes excessive sleepiness. Obstructive sleep apnea is a dyssomnia that can produce either excessive sleepiness or insomnia.

Parasomnias are disorders of arousal, partial arousal, and sleep-wake transition. Changes in the autonomic nervous system and muscle tone are predominant features of parasomnias. Sleep walking, sleep terrors, sleep talking, and nightmares are examples of parasomnias.

The neurologic disorders often associated with sleep disturbance are cerebral degenerative disorders such as dementia and Parkinson disease. Sleep-related epilepsy refers to epilepsy that occurs during sleep and epilepsy exacerbated by sleep. Some forms of headache, for example, cluster headache, can occur predominantly in sleep and are included under the category of sleep-related headaches.

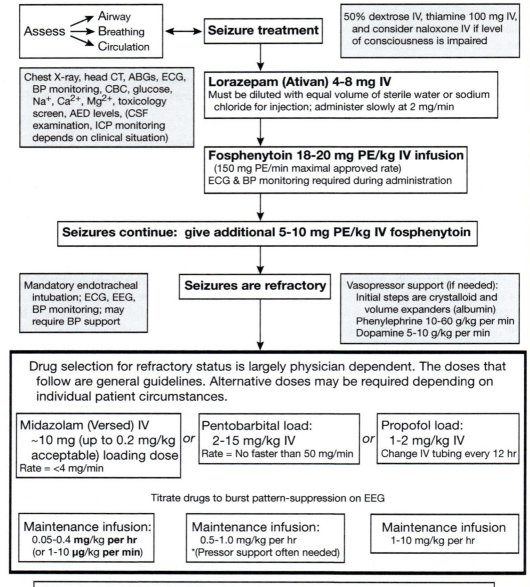

Fig. 9.6. Guideline for the management of status epilepticus in adults. ABG, arterial blood gas; AED, antiepileptic drug; BP, blood pressure; CBC, complete blood count; CSF, cerebrospinal fluid; CT, computed tomography; ECG, electrocardiography; EEG, electroencephalography; ICP, intracranial pressure; IV, intravenous; PE, phenytoin equivalent.

For a patient who has a sleep disorder, begin the evaluation with a thorough history and physical examination. Obtain information about the patient's sleep pattern: what time the patient goes to bed, length of time before falling asleep, time in bed, hours of sleep at night, time awake, time needed to feel restored and rested, and the number of daytime naps. Often, information needs to be obtained from bed partners, other family members, coworkers, or caregivers. Sleep dairies covering a 2- to 3-week period may be needed to provide an accurate accounting of the patient's sleep pattern.

A formal sleep evaluation can include polysomnography, multiple sleep latency test, maintenance of wakefulness test, pupillography, and actigraphy. Basic polysomnography involves monitoring eye movement, respiratory variables, electrocardiography, electromyography, and the EEG. The multiple sleep latency test is a standardized measure of the physiologic tendency to fall asleep during normal waking hours; it measures the same variables that are monitored in polysomnography. The maintenance of wakefulness test is similar to the multiple sleep latency test but measures the ability to remain awake. Pupillography measures pupil size; the interpretation of results is based on the observation that pupils constrict during drowsiness and sleep. Actigraphy records movement and nonmovement over time to supplement the sleep diary.

Excessive Daytime Somnolence

Most often, excessive daytime somnolence is the result of sleep deprivation. The amount of sleep needed by a person is the amount required for the person to feel rested and restored after awakening. For adults, the range is from 4 to 10 hours (mean, 8 hours). Make-up sleep is the only way to diminish sleepiness due to sleep deprivation. If excessive daytime sleepiness is not associated with sleep deprivation,

evaluate for narcolepsy, idiopathic central nervous system hypersomnia, or sleep apnea.

Narcolepsy is a hypersomnia of central origin with features of excessive daytime somnolence, cataplexy, sleep paralysis, and hypnagogic hallucinations. It is a sleep disorder in which sleep/wake phenomena are dissociated. The components of rapid eye movement (REM) sleep and non-rapid eye movement (NREM) sleep appear in the wakeful state. The control of the onset and offset of both REM and NREM sleep is impaired, causing nighttime sleep fragmentation and intrusion of REM and NREM sleep components into daytime wakefulness.

The *sleepiness of narcolepsy* is defined as the tendency to fall asleep easily in a relaxed or sedentary situation. Patients without sleepiness but with complaints of fatigue and tiredness tend not to fall asleep in these situations. The patient's sleep pattern may help distinguish between narcolepsy and sleep deficiency. A person with sleep deprivation tends to have different patterns on weekdays and weekends, whereas the person with narcolepsy tends to have the same sleep pattern (time in bed, hours of sleep, and number of daytime naps) throughout the week.

The sudden loss of muscle tone induced by emotion is called *cataplexy*, which occurs in about two-thirds of patients with narcolepsy. It is the inappropriate activation of descending neural pathways that promote atonia. The duration of cataplexy is short and neither consciousness nor memory is impaired. *Hypnagogic* (occurring at sleep onset) and *hypnopompic* (occurring at sleep offset) *hallucinations* are hallucinations that occur during the transition between sleep and waking. They may have vivid features, similar to dreams, but the person can be aware of his or her surroundings. *Sleep paralysis* is the inability to move during the onset and offset of sleep; it can last from seconds to minutes.

Table 9.10. The International Classification of Sleep Disorders

I. Insomnias

Adjustment insomnia, psychophysiologic insomnia, paradoxical insomnia, idiopathic insomnia, insomnia due to mental disorder, inadequate sleep hygiene, behavioral insomnia of childhood, insomnia due to drug or substance, insomnia due to medical condition, insomnia not due to substance or known physiologic condition (unspecified), physiologic insomnia (unspecified)

II. Sleep-related breathing disorders

Central sleep apnea syndrome, obstructive sleep apnea syndromes, sleep-related hypoventilation/hypoxemic syndromes, other sleep-related breathing disorder

III. Hypersomnias of central origin not due to a circadian rhythm sleep disorder, sleep-related breathing disorder, or other cause of disturbed nocturnal sleep

Narcolepsy with cataplexy, narcolepsy without cataplexy, narcolepsy due to a medical condition, narcolepsy (unspecified), recurrent hypersomnia, idiopathic hypersomnia with long sleep time, idiopathic hypersomnia without long sleep time, behaviorally induced insufficient sleep syndrome, hypersomnia due to a medical condition, hypersomnia due to drug or substance, hypersomnia not due to substance or known physiologic condition, physiologic hypersomnia (unspecified)

IV. Circadian rhythm sleep disorders

Delayed sleep phase type, advanced sleep phase type, irregular sleep-wake type, free-running type, jet lag type, shift work type, circadian rhythm sleep disorder due to a medical condition, other circadian rhythm sleep disorder, other circadian rhythm sleep disorder due to drug or substance

V. Parasomnias

Disorders of arousal (from NREM sleep)

Confusional arousals, sleepwalking, sleep terrors

Parasomnias usually associated with REM sleep

REM sleep behavior disorder, recurrent isolated sleep paralysis, nightmare disorder

Other parasomnias

Sleep-related dissociative disorders, sleep enuresis, sleep-related groaning, exploding head syndrome, sleep-related hallucinations, sleep-related eating disorder, parasomnia (unspecified), parasomnia due to drug or substance, parasomnia due to medical condition

VI. Sleep-related movement disorders

Restless legs syndrome, periodic limb movement disorder, sleep-related leg cramps, sleep-related bruxism, sleep-related rhythmic movement disorder, sleep-related movement disorder (unspecified), sleep-related movement disorder due to drug or substance, sleep-related movement disorder due to medical condition

Table 9.10   (continued)

VII. Isolated symptoms, apparently normal variants and unresolved issues

Long sleeper, short sleeper, snoring, sleep talking, sleep starts, benign sleep myoclonus of infancy, hypnagogic foot tremor and alternating leg muscle activation during sleep, propriospinal myoclonus at sleep onset, excessive fragmentary myoclonus

VIII. Other sleep disorders

Other physiologic sleep disorder, other sleep disorder not due to substance or known physiologic condition, environmental sleep disorder

NREM, non-rapid eye movement; REM, rapid eye movement.
Data from American Academy of Sleep Medicine: International Classification of Sleep Disorders, ed. 2: Diagnostic and Coding Manual. American Academy of Sleep Medicine, Westchester, IL, 2005.

Fewer than half the patients with narcolepsy have all four symptoms characteristic of the disorder. Furthermore, sleep paralysis and hypnagogic hallucinations can occur in persons without narcolepsy. Cataplexy may be part of somatization disorder or atonic seizures. Myoclonus may be mistaken for cataplexy. The diagnosis of narcolepsy can be confirmed with a formal sleep evaluation. The investigation includes all-night polysomnography, followed by a multiple sleep latency test, to determine the quality and quantity of the preceding night's sleep. The hypothalamic neuropeptide hypocretin (orexin) is not produced in patients with narcolepsy. For cases in which diagnosis is difficult, the absence of hypocretin may have diagnostic value.

The hypersomnolence of narcolepsy is treated with central nervous system stimulants. Modafinil, an α_1-adrenergic stimulant, has been approved for this use. Cataplexy, sleep paralysis, and hypnagogic hallucinations have been treated with tricyclic antidepressants, monoamine oxidase inhibitors, selective serotonin reuptake inhibitors, and anticholinergic medications. The mechanism of tricyclic antidepressants and monoamine oxidase inhibitors is likely suppression of REM sleep.

The term *idiopathic hypersomnia* describes a heterogeneous disorder of the central nervous system characterized by excessive daytime somnolence. Excessive daytime somnolence in the absence of symptoms suggestive of sleep deprivation, narcolepsy, or sleep apnea suggests idiopathic hypersomnia. If this rare disorder is suspected, consult a sleep disorder specialist.

After sleep deprivation, the most common cause of excessive daytime somnolence is sleep apnea, which is defined as repeated episodes of obstructive apnea and hypopnea during sleep. Its clinical features include complaints of fatigue and loud snoring. It is common among adults, especially males, postmenopausal women, and overweight persons. Remember that 25% to 30% of patients with sleep apnea are *not* overweight. A formal sleep study can confirm the diagnosis.

Behavioral interventions for sleep apnea include weight loss, avoidance of alcohol and sedatives, avoidance of sleep deprivation, and nocturnal positioning. First-line medical therapy includes positive pressure through a mask (continuous positive airway pressure, or CPAP). Other medical treatments include the use of an oral appliance, fluoxetine, protriptyline, and nocturnal oxygen. Upper airway bypass with tracheostomy and upper airway reconstruction are surgical options.

Insomnia

Insomnia is defined as trouble with the initiation, maintenance, duration, or quality of sleep that impairs daytime functioning. It is the most common sleep-related complaint and can be caused by medical, psychiatric, and drug-induced disorders. Neurologists often manage insomnia because of its frequent association with movement disorders. Insomnia is also a major complication of restless legs syndrome.

Insomnia that persists for more than 1 month, *chronic insomnia*, can be managed with cognitive behavioral and pharmacologic therapies. Some of the nonpharmacologic techniques used to treat chronic insomnia are summarized in Table 9.11. Medications for insomnia (Table 9.12) include benzodiazepines, benzodiazepine-receptor agonists, and melatonin-receptor agonist. Also, sedating antidepressants are often prescribed to treat insomnia. The long-term use of medications for the treatment of insomnia usually is not recommended because of dependency and tolerance.

Restless legs syndrome is characterized by a distressing need or urge to move the legs, usually accompanied by an uncomfortable deep-seated sensation in the legs that is brought on by rest and relieved with moving or walking. These leg paresthesias are prominent during periods of inactivity, particularly during the transition from wakefulness to sleep. Movement of the legs provides transient relief. The discomfort is difficult to describe, and patients describe it as "creeping," "crawling," "itching," "pulling," and "drawing." The symptoms usually involve the legs but can occur in the arms.

Most patients with restless legs syndrome have periodic movements of sleep. These are brief (1-2 seconds) jerks of one or both legs. Movement may involve only dorsiflexion of the big toe or flexion of the entire leg(s). The movements occur periodically, every 20 to 40 seconds. The patient is often aroused during sleep but is not aware of the arousal. Periodic movements of sleep can be extremely disruptive for the bed partner. Although up to 80% of patients with restless legs syndrome have periodic movements of sleep, not all people with periodic movements of sleep have restless legs syndrome. Periodic movements of sleep may have no clinical significance.

Restless legs syndrome is common; it has been estimated that it occurs in up to 15% of the population. This syndrome is classified as primary (or idiopathic) and secondary. The majority of patients who have primary restless legs syndrome report a positive family history. Secondary restless legs syndrome is related most often to iron deficiency. The syndrome is associated with several medical conditions, including iron deficiency anemia, pregnancy, peripheral neuropathy, thyroid disease, rheumatoid arthritis, and uremia.

Peripheral neuropathies may mimic restless legs syndrome, but movement does not relieve the paresthesias. Patients with fibromyalgia may have lower extremity pain that resembles the syndrome, but the pain does not increase with rest and inactivity. Akathisia, the motor restlessness often caused by dopamine receptor blocking drugs, is included in the differential diagnosis of restless legs syndrome. The restless movements or inner restlessness of akathisia is not worse at night or with lying down.

The first step in the management of a patient who has restless legs syndrome is to assess if there is evidence of iron deficiency or if the patient is taking medications that can worsen or cause the syndrome. Tricyclic antidepressants, antihistamines, and dopamine receptor blocking drugs can aggravate restless legs syndrome. Switching to a different medication in the same or different class may solve

Table 9.11. Cognitive Behavioral Therapy for Insomnia

Sleep hygiene

Correct extrinsic factors affecting sleep (eg, pets, snoring bed partner)

Exercise regularly during daytime

Avoid large meals at night

Avoid caffeine, tobacco, and alcohol

Avoid bright light (including television), noise, and temperature extremes

Reduce evening fluid intake

Reduce attention to bedtime clock

Stimulus-control therapy

Go to bed only when sleepy

Use the bedroom only for sleep and sex

Go to another room when unable to sleep in 15-20 minutes, engage in quiet activity and
return to bed when sleepy; repeat if necessary

Maintain consistent wake time regardless of duration of sleep

Avoid daytime napping

Cognitive therapy

Education to alter faulty attitude and beliefs about sleep, eg, 8 hours is necessary

Sleep-restriction therapy

Reduce time in bed to estimated total sleep time (minimum, 5 hours)

Increase time in bed by 15 minutes every week when estimated sleep efficiency (ratio of
time asleep to time in bed) is at least 90%

Relaxation therapy

Physical: progressive muscle relaxation, biofeedback

Mental: imagery training, meditation, hypnosis

Modified from Silber, MH: Chronic insomnia. N Engl J Med 353:803-810, 2005. Used with permission.

the problem. If the serum level of ferritin is less than 50 μg/L or if iron saturation is less than 16%, the patient should be treated for iron deficiency: 325 mg ferrous sulfate and 100 mg vitamin C can be given daily until the serum ferritin level is more than 50 μg/L or iron saturation is more than 20%. Common side effects of iron supplementation are constipation and gastric upset.

The patient should be educated about good sleep habits, decreasing caffeine and alcohol consumption, and performing moderate exercise daily. Dopaminergic medications are considered the first-line medication therapy for restless legs syndrome. This is based on the presumed dopaminergic dysfunction and abnormal brain iron metabolism in patients with the syndrome. Carbidopa-levodopa is effective but more associated with "augmentation" (increasing symptoms earlier in the day) than dopa agonists. Gabapentin, benzodiazepines, and opioids have also been effective medications (Table 9.13). If the patient does not have a response to one medication, try a

Table 9.12. Medications for Insomnia

Medication	Type	Duration of action	Half-life, hours	Dose, mg
Estazolam (ProSom)	Benzodiazepine	Intermediate	10-24	0.5-2
Eszopiclone (Lunesta)	Benzodiazepine receptor agonist	Intermediate	5-7	1-3
Ramelteon (Rozerem)	Melatonin receptor agonist	Short	2-5	8
Temazepam (Restoril)	Benzodiazepine	Intermediate	8-15	7.5-30
Triazolam (Halcion)	Benzodiazepine	Short	2-5	0.125-0.25
Zaleplon (Sonata)	Benzodiazepine receptor agonist	Ultrashort	1	5-20
Zolpidem (Ambien)	Benzodiazepine receptor agonist	Short	3	5-10

different agent, even in the same class. A combination of these drugs may be necessary to control the symptoms.

Parasomnias

Undesirable behavioral or experiential events that occur during sleep or are exacerbated by sleep are called *parasomnias*. Common examples include nightmares and sleepwalking. The differential diagnosis of paroxysmal nocturnal events or nighttime spells includes seizures and parasomnias.

Parasomnias are categorized by the stage of sleep in which they occur (Table 9.10). The disorders of arousal include confusional arousals, sleep walking, and sleep terror. These disorders occur during stages 3 and 4 of NREM sleep. Patients often have a positive family history for these events, suggesting a genetic component. These disorders are common in childhood and decrease in frequency with increasing age. Arousal disorders are characterized by confusion and automatic behavior following sudden arousal. Sleep terror is the most dramatic type, with the aroused person having a piercing scream or cry and autonomic and behavioral manifestations of intense fear. The person cannot be consoled but is usually amnestic for the event.

These disorders may not need to be evaluated, but polysomnography is recommended if there is violent behavior, excessive daytime somnolence, or atypical clinical features. Treatment should include removing anything that may precipitate arousal and avoiding caffeine and alcohol. Clonazepam can be effective by decreasing the arousal threshold.

REM sleep behavior disorder, a parasomnia that occurs during REM sleep, is frequently associated with neurologic disease. This sleep disorder is characterized by the loss of atonia characteristic of REM sleep; thus, the person is able to act out a dream. The result may be an elaborate motor behavior that is potentially injurious to the person or bed partner. Unlike the arousal disorders during NREM sleep, the person may recall the dream associated with the motor behavior. REM sleep behavior disorder is often mistaken for hallucinations or posttraumatic stress disorder.

Table 9.13. **Medications for Restless Legs Syndrome**

Medication	Dose	Clinical comment
Ferrous sulfate	325 mg orally daily	Prescribe if serum ferritin is <50 μg/L Can cause constipation and gastric upset
Carbidopa-levodopa (Sinemet)	50/200 mg sustained release, one or two tablets 1 hour before bedtime	Augmentation of symptoms Can cause nausea, orthostatic hypotension
Pramipexole (Mirapex)	Dose titration 0.125 mg 1-2 hours before symptoms, up to 1.5 mg divided in 2-3 doses	Can cause sudden sleepiness Can cause nausea, orthostatic hypotension
Ropinirole (Requip)	Dose titration 0.25 mg 1-3 hours before symptoms, up to 4 mg divided in 2-3 doses	Can cause sudden sleepiness Can cause nausea, orthostatic hypotension
Gabapentin (Neurontin)	Dose titration 300 mg, up to 2,400 mg in 3 doses, 1,500 mg in single dose	Can cause sedation, dizziness, somnolence
Clonazepam (Klonopin)	0.25 mg, one to two tablets at bedtime	Can cause tolerance, sedation
Propoxyphene + acetaminophen (Darvocet)	100 mg, can increase to 600 mg in 2-3 doses	Can cause dependence, sedation, constipation

Most patients with REM sleep behavior disorder are men. The disorder occurs in many neurodegenerative conditions, including Parkinson disease, multiple system atrophy, dementia with Lewy bodies, and progressive supranuclear palsy. It has been described in patients with Machado-Joseph disease, Guillain-Barré syndrome, narcolepsy, amyotrophic lateral sclerosis, limbic encephalitis, autism, Tourette syndrome, corticobasal degeneration, and Alzheimer disease. REM sleep behavior disorder can be the presenting symptom in Parkinson disease. Drug withdrawal, selective serotonin reuptake inhibitors, noradrenergic antagonists, and tricyclic antidepressants can induce the syndrome. Clonazepam is effective treatment, starting at a dose of 0.5 mg that can be increased up to 2 mg as needed. Melatonin (3-9 mg at bedtime has been prescribed) may be an option if clonazepam cannot be used.

SUGGESTED READING

Aldrich, MS: Diagnostic aspects of narcolepsy. Neurology 50 Suppl 1:S2-S7, 1998.

Allet, JL, and Allet, RE: Somatoform disorders in neurological practice. Curr Opin Psychiatry 19:413-420, 2006.

American Academy of Sleep Medicine: International Classification of Sleep Disorders, Revised: Diagnostic and Coding Manual. American Academy of Sleep Medicine, Chicago, 2001. Available from http://www.absm.org/PDF/ICSD.pdf.

Benbadis, SR: The EEG in nonepileptic seizures. J Clin Neurophysiol 23:340-352, 2006.

Biton, V: Weight change and antiepileptic drugs: Health issues and criteria for appropriate selection of an antiepileptic agent. Neurologist 12:163-167, 2006.

Britton, JW, and So, EL: Selection of antiepileptic drugs: A practical approach. Mayo Clin Proc 71:778-786, 1996.

Cascino, GD: Generalized convulsive status epilepticus. Mayo Clin Proc 71:787-792, 1996.

Cascino, GD: Clinical indications and diagnostic yield of video-electroencephalographic monitoring in patients with seizures and spells. Mayo Clin Proc 77:1111-1120, 2002.

Chabolla, DR, et al: Psychogenic nonepileptic seizures. Mayo Clin Proc 71:493-500, 1996.

Chen, DK, So, YT, and Fisher, RS, Therapeutics and Technology Assessment Subcommittee of the American Academy of Neurology: Use of serum prolactin in diagnosing epileptic seizures: Report of the Therapeutics and Technology Assessment Subcommittee of the American Academy of Neurology. Neurology 65:668-675, 2005.

Drislane, FW: Transient events. In Samuels, MA, and Feske, SK (eds): Office Practice of Neurology, ed 2. Churchill Livingstone, Philadelphia, 2003, pp 126-137.

Engel, J, Jr, and International League Against Epilepsy (ILAE): A proposed diagnostic scheme for people with epileptic seizures and with epilepsy: Report of the ILAE Task Force on Classification and Terminology. Epilepsia 42:796-803, 2001.

EURAP Study Group: Seizure control and treatment in pregnancy: Observations from the EURAP epilepsy pregnancy registry. Neurology 66:354-360, 2006. Epub 2005 Dec 28.

Gagnon, JF, Postuma, RB, and Montplaisir, J: Update on the pharmacology of REM sleep behavior disorder. Neurology 67:742-747, 2006.

Graves, TD: Ion channels and epilepsy. QJM 99:201-217, 2006. Epub 2006 Feb 22.

Harden, CL, and Leppik, I: Optimizing therapy of seizures in women who use oral contraceptives. Neurology 67 Suppl 4:S56-S58, 2006.

Hauser, WA, et al: Seizure recurrence after a 1st unprovoked seizure: An extended follow-up. Neurology 40:1163-1170, 1990.

Hauser, WA, et al: Risk of recurrent seizures after two unprovoked seizures. N Engl J Med 338:429-434, 1998.

Hirtz, D, et al, Quality Standards Sub-committee of the American Academy of Neurology; Practice Committee of the Child Neurology Society: Practice parameter: Treatment of the child with a first unprovoked seizure: Report of the Quality Standards Subcommittee of the American Academy of Neurology and the Practice Committee of the Child Neurology Society. Neurology 60:166-175, 2003.

Hitiris, N, and Brodie, MJ: Modern antiepileptic drugs: Guidelines and beyond. Curr Opin Neurol 19:175-180, 2006.

Hrachovy, RA, and Frost, JD, Jr: The EEG in selected generalized seizures. J Clin Neurophysiol 23:312-332, 2006.

Jack, CR, Jr: Magnetic resonance imaging in epilepsy. Mayo Clin Proc 71:695-711, 1996.

Kaplan, PW: The clinical features, diagnosis, and prognosis of nonconvulsive status epilepticus. Neurologist 11:348-361, 2005.

Lacerda, G, et al: Optimizing therapy of seizures in patients with renal or hepatic dysfunction. Neurology 67 Suppl 4:S28-S33, 2006.

LaRoche, SM, and Helmers, SL: The new antiepileptic drugs: Scientific review. JAMA 291:605-614, 2004.

Mahowald, MW, et al: Sleep disorders. Continuum: Lifelong Learning in Neurology 3:9-158, 1997.

Mahowald, MW, and Schenck, CH: Insights from studying human sleep disorders. Nature 437:1279-1285, 2005.

Mendez, OE, and Brenner, RP: Increasing the yield of EEG. J Clin Neurophysiol 23:282-293, 2006.

Morrell, MJ: Guidelines for the care of women with epilepsy. Neurology 51 Suppl 4:S21-S27, 1998.

Mosewich, RK, and So, EL: A clinical approach to the classification of seizures and epileptic syndromes. Mayo Clin Proc 71:405-414, 1996.

Nadkarni, S, LaJoie, J, and Devinsky, O: Current treatments of epilepsy. Neurology 64 Suppl 3:S2-S11, 2005.

O'Brien, TJ, et al: Subtraction peri-ictal SPECT is predictive of extratemporal epilepsy surgery outcome. Neurology 55:1668-1677, 2000.

Pohlmann-Eden, B, et al: The first seizure and its management in adults and children. BMJ 332:339-342, 2006.

Quality Standards Subcommittee of the American Academy of Neurology: Practice parameter: A guideline for discontinuing antiepileptic drugs in seizure-free patients: Summary statement. Neurology 47:600-602, 1996.

Quality Standards Subcommittee of the American Academy of Neurology in cooperation with American College of Emergency Physicians, Amerian Association of Neurological Surgeons, and American Society of Neuroradiology: Practice parameter: Neuroimaging in the emergency patient presenting with seizure: Summary statement. Neurology 47:288-291, 1996.

Riviello, JJ, Jr, et al, American Academy of Neurology Subcommittee; Practice Committee of the Child Neurology Society: Practice parameter: Diagnostic assessment of the child with status epilepticus (an evidence-based review): Report of the Quality Standards Subcommittee of the American Academy of Neurology and the Practice Committee of the Child Neurology Society. Neurology 67:1542-1550, 2006.

Roberts, R: Differential diagnosis of sleep disorders, non-epileptic attacks and epileptic seizures. Curr Opin Neurol 11:135-139, 1998.

Ryvlin, P: When to start antiepileptic drug treatment: Seize twice might not harm. Curr Opin Neurol 19:154-156, 2006.

Shuster, EA: Epilepsy in women. Mayo Clin Proc 71:991-999, 1996.

Silber, MH: Clinical practice: Chronic insomnia. N Engl J Med 353:803-810, 2005. Erratum in: N Engl J Med 353:2827, 2005.

Strollo, PJ, Jr, and Rogers, RM: Obstructive sleep apnea. N Engl J Med 334:99-104, 1996.

Thorpy, MJ: New paradigms in the treatment of restless legs syndrome. Neurology 64 Suppl 3:S28-S33, 2005.

Trenkwalder, C, Walters, AS, and Hening, W: Periodic limb movements and restless legs syndrome. Neurol Clin 14:629-650, 1996.

Varelas, PN, and Spanaki, M: Management of seizures in the critically ill. Neurologist 12:127-139, 2006.

Walters, AS, and The International Restless Legs Syndrome Study Group: Toward a better definition of the restless legs syndrome. Mov Disord 10:634-642, 1995.

Westmoreland, BF: Epileptiform electroencephalographic patterns. Mayo Clin Proc 71:501-511, 1996.

Zupanc, ML: Antiepileptic drugs and hormonal contraceptives in adolescent women with epilepsy. Neurology 66 Suppl 3:S37-S45, 2006.

CHAPTER 10

Pain

The word *pain* is derived from the Latin word *poena*, meaning fine or penalty. The International Association for the Study of Pain has described pain as an unpleasant sensory and emotional experience associated primarily with tissue damage and/or described in terms of such damage. Pain can be categorized as *neuropathic*, *nociceptive*, or *idiopathic* (Table 10.1). This chapter discusses neuropathic pain, which is pain caused by dysfunction of the nervous system. Nociceptive pain is the result of tissue damage that may or may not include damage to the nervous system. A well-known type of nociceptive pain is arthritis pain. Idiopathic pain encompasses several poorly understood pain disorders that are not associated with tissue damage and includes many pain disorders that have been considered psychogenic in origin. The sensation of *acute pain* is familiar to everyone and is one of the earliest and most common symptoms of disease. Pain is the number one reason that patients seek medical attention. It is an alarm mechanism warning of tissue damage and potential danger. However, *chronic pain* is a unique sensory experience. The management of patients who complain of chronic pain is extremely challenging, and

frustration is common on the part of the patient and the clinician.

The evaluation of chronic pain has many diagnostic problems. A major problem is the inability to establish a cause for the pain. It is not possible to test for several conditions because of limitations of available technology; for example, electromyography does not demonstrate small-fiber neuropathies, and a bone scan is of no use in detecting structural or functional change in early reflex sympathetic dystrophy. Examples of conditions not amenable to diagnostic tests are myofascial pain syndromes and postconcussive headache. Other conditions such as atypical facial pain and fibromyalgia have no etiologic specificity. Also, psychiatric issues, including depression, personality disorders, and posttraumatic stress disorder, can complicate the diagnosis. Other factors that complicate the evaluation of chronic pain are medical-legal issues, drug abuse, and physical and sexual abuse. Many chronic pain disorders, including fibromyalgia, somatization disorder, factitious disorder, and malingering, need to be understood from a historical perspective. Previous medical records are essential in the evaluation of a patient who has chronic pain, and they often constitute the most important diagnostic test.

Table 10.1. Categories of Pain and Examples

Neuropathic	Nociceptive	Idiopathic
Polyneuropathies	Arthritic	Myofascial pain syndrome
Complex regional pain syndrome	Acute postoperative	Somatoform pain disorder
Central pain syndromes	Posttraumatic	
Postherpetic neuralgia		

From Adams, AC: Neurology in Primary Care. FA Davis, Philadelphia, 2000, p 172. Used with permission of Mayo Foundation for Medical Education and Research.

A question that further complicates the evaluation of pain is why some patients have a chronic pain syndrome after injury to the nervous system and others with the same type of injury do not. The information available about the anatomy and physiology of pain provides only partial answers. Two aspects of pain need to be considered: the sensory-discriminative aspect involves identifying a nociceptive (pain) stimulus (mechanical, thermal, or chemical) and determining its location, intensity, and timing (onset and duration of stimulus). The motivational-affective aspect involves recognizing the unpleasantness and aversive quality of the stimulus and reacting to it. This is the "suffering" aspect of pain and is unique to the person. In addition to neural pathways involved in the transmission of pain, there is an antinociceptive pathway that modulates the transmision of pain.

Pain can produce a functional change in the nervous system. For example, sensitization is a feature of nociceptors (pain receptors) in which noxious stimuli lower the threshold of the receptors to subsequent stimulation, even to the point that innocuous stimuli can activate the receptors. It is important to understand that pain is an alarm system which changes the psychologic state of the person and causes a behavioral response. This emphasizes the importance of addressing the psychologic issues of patients who experience chronic pain.

GENERAL MANAGEMENT PRINCIPLES

Pain, like any other presenting complaint, warrants an appropriate investigation. However, several management principles in the treatment of chronic pain apply in general. First, the pain is real. You must convey to the patient your belief that the symptom is genuine. Believing the patient, caring about the patient's welfare, and showing a willingness to work with the patient to improve the functional aspects of his or her life are keys to successful management of chronic pain. Doubting the authenticity of the complaint has no therapeutic benefit. Instances in which the patient cannot be believed (eg, malingering and factitious disorder) are rare.

Treat any pain aggressively and as early as possible. Treating pain early may avoid the structural-functional changes in the nervous system that lead to chronic pain. The psychologic issues associated with the patient's pain must be incorporated into the management plan. Some of the issues are depression, fear, interpersonal relationships, financial compensation, and disability. The patient needs to understand that these psychologic factors can influence the intensity and tolerance of pain. Ask the patient to imagine how the pain would be if he or she won a million-dollar lottery and to compare this with how the pain would be if his or her spouse died or fire destroyed the house.

It is essential to establish appropriate goals before initiating treatment. A complete "cure" is not a realistic goal, but a reduction in the patient's level of pain with improvement in functional status is a realistic goal. Factors that influence pain, such as depression, physical inactivity or regression, drug addiction, and emotional regression, can be treated.

DIAGNOSTIC APPROACH

Begin the evaluation of a patient who complains of chronic pain by obtaining previous medical records. Because these patients tend to have had extensive diagnostic testing, obtaining previous medical records is an important and cost-effective diagnostic tool.

The pain history should include the temporal course of the symptoms, the location and intensity of the pain, and associated symptoms. The patient's description of the pain may provide diagnostic information as well as help in making decisions about treatment. Neuropathic pain is often described as "sharp," "burning," and "shooting" and is associated with skin sensitivity. Patients with peripheral nerve or nerve root pain report an aching sensation "like a toothache." Neuropathic pain is often described as "icky" or as an abnormal noxious sensation (*dysesthesia*). Features of neuropathic pain include *allodynia* (a nonnoxious stimulus perceived as painful) and *hyperalgesia* (increased pain response to a noxious stimulus).

Also, the pain history should include an evaluation of the patient's mood, functional status, and sleep pattern and how the patient copes with pain. It is important to know how the pain has affected the patient's employment, recreational activities, and relationships with family and friends. It is also important to know

about the patient's use of alcohol or illicit drugs for the pain or the use of these substances before the onset of pain. Although the medical records provide information about previous treatments, get the patient's perspective by asking what treatments have been tried and what the response was. It is important to know the medication dose and length of use. If this information is not known, a repeat trial of medication can be attempted.

The patient's behavior while the medical history is being taken may be important in determining the reasons for previous treatment failure and may influence your interpretation of the examination findings. Excessive pain behavior, a description of severe disabling pain with little objective evidence of pain, anger, a sense of entitlement, depression, and information that previous treatment was negligent are all meaningful. The history should identify psychosocial stressors and the patient's expectations. It may be useful to ask the patient what his or her plans are if the pain lessens or worsens. The absence of future plans or goals may indicate that the patient does not plan to get better. Before treatment is begun, it is important to know if the illness is being used to avoid responsibilities or problems. Identify financial and disability issues. If the pain lessens, does it change the patient's legal or financial status?

The physical examination should include systemic, musculoskeletal, dermatologic, and neurologic evaluations. Testing the range of motion of the spine and joints and palpating soft tissues for tightness and tenderness are important in the evaluation of myofascial pain disorders. Complex regional pain disorders or reflex sympathetic dystrophy can be associated with abnormalities in skin color, swelling, and temperature. The neurologic examination should focus on the sensory examination. Pain due to damage of the central nervous system, called *central pain*, is associated with a deficit in thermal sensation. In addition to evidence of sensory loss, the presence of allodynia or hyperalgesia suggests a neuropathic pain condition.

TREATMENT

The treatment of chronic pain may involve several types of therapy, including medications, physical and occupational therapy, injections of anesthetic agents, behavioral therapy, invasive analgesic therapies (spinal administration of medications), and surgical options (eg, deep brain stimulation and motor cortex stimulation). Also, treatment may require the participation of many healthcare professionals. Referral to a pain specialist should be considered—not necessarily as a last resort.

Many pharmacologic agents are available for treating pain (Table 10.2). Sequential drug trials may be needed to determine which drug provides the best pain relief. The response of a patient to one drug may vary, even with drugs of the same class. It is important to titrate one drug at a time, beginning with the lowest dosage and increasing it until pain relief is obtained or intolerable side effects develop. Slow increments in dosage can reduce the chance of side effects. Only a few medications (tricyclic antidepressants and mexiletine) have toxic serum levels. The addition of a second drug should be avoided unless the first drug produces only partial pain relief or higher doses cause intolerable side effects.

Opioids

Whether narcotics should be used to treat chronic pain is a difficult question. Narcotic analgesia is well accepted as a treatment for pain due to malignancy or for palliative care but not for pain due to a nonmalignant cause. Some clinicians advocate early and aggressive treatment with these agents, whereas others think they should be prescribed only after all reasonable attempts at analgesia have failed. The problem with narcotics is the rapid development of tolerance, with the patient taking the agent for withdrawal symptoms instead of pain relief. In addition to losing efficacy over time, narcotics can induce hyperalgesia. However, the risk of opioid narcotic abuse is considered small if the patient has been evaluated for psychologic comorbid conditions, disability, and a history of substance abuse. If the patient is being cared for by several clinicians, only one should be designated to prescribe opioid narcotics. Close follow-up is needed, with attention to pain relief, adverse effects, and aberrant drug-related behavior.

When treating chronic pain with opioids, it is important to remember that these agents are at least two times more potent when administered intravenously than orally. When changing opioid drug or route, doses must be changed. Several opioids and the analgesic equivalent of 10 mg of intramuscular (potency considered the same as intravenous) morphine are summarized in Table 10.3.

It is also important to keep in mind the potential problems that can result when treating chronic pain with opioids that are combined with acetaminophen or aspirin. Patients who take these medications may be at risk for exposure to unsafe doses of aspirin and acetaminophen. Generally, it is best to use a long-acting medication with a minimal dose of short-lasting medication for initial titration of dose and breakthrough pain. The use of different types of opioid narcotics may be ineffective because of competition at the receptor site. For example, the combination of tramadol and oxycodone may be less effective than oxycodone alone (immediate release and controlled release). Other guidelines for treatment with opioid narcotics are summarized in Table 10.4.

Table 10.2. Pain Medications

Drug	Type of drug or mechanism	Initial dose (oral unless specified)	Adverse effects
Acetaminophen (APAP, Tylenol)	Nonopioid analgesia	650 mg every 4-6 hours	Hepatotoxicity
NSAIDs	Nonsteroidal antiinflammatory		Gastropathy
Aspirin (ASA)		650 mg every 4-6 hours	Platelet inhibition
Ibuprofen (Motrin)		400 mg every 4-6 hours	
Naproxen (Naprosyn)		250 mg every 6-8 hours	
Opioids	Opioid		Constipation, sedation, impaired ventilation
Codeine		15-60 mg, titrate	Toxicity >1.5 mg/kg
Fentanyl (Duragesic)		25 µg/hour, titrate (transdermal)	
Hydrocodone, with APAP or ASA (Vicodin)		10 mg every 3-4 hours, titrate	Hepatotoxicity with APAP
Hydromorphone (Dilaudid)		4-8 mg, titrate	
Methadone (Dolophine)		5-10 mg every 6-8 hours, titrate	
Morphine		15-30 mg, titrate	
Oxycodone (Oxycontin, Percocet, Percodan)		7.5-10 mg, titrate	Gastropathy with ASA
Tramadol (Ultram)	Mu-opiate receptor agonist, serotonin and norepinephrine reuptake inhibitor	50 mg every 4-6 hours, titrate	Dizziness, nausea, sweating
Tricyclic antidepressants	Block reuptake of serotonin and norepinephrine, sodium channel blockade		Drowsiness, xerostomia, constipation, weight gain
Amitriptyline (Elavil)		10-25 mg at bedtime	

Table 10.2   (continued)

Drug	Type of drug or mechanism	Initial dose (oral unless specified)	Adverse effects
Nortriptyline (Pamelor)		10-25 mg at bedtime	
SSRI antidepressants	Selective serotonin reuptake inhibitors		Insomnia, nausea
Fluoxetine (Prozac)		20 mg every AM	
Paroxetine (Paxil)		10 mg every AM	
Mixed reuptake inhibitor antidepressants	Block reuptake of serotonin and norepinephrine, sodium channel blockade		
Duloxetine (Cymbalta)		60 mg daily	Nausea, constipation, xerostomia
Nefazodone (Serzone)		100 mg twice daily	Headache, insomnia
Venlafaxine (Effexor)		25 mg 2 or 3 times daily	Hypertension
Anticonvulsants			
Carbamazepine (Tegretol)	Blocks sodium channel conductance; reduces neuronal calcium uptake	100-200 mg daily	Dizziness, diplopia, light-headedness
Clonazepam (Klonopin)	Benzodiazepine, GABAergic	0.5 mg daily	Sedation, ataxia, physical and psychologic dependence
Gabapentin (Neurontin)	GABA modulation of N-type calcium channels	100-300 mg daily	Peripheral edema, fatigue, somnolence, dizziness, ataxia
Lamotrigine (Lamictal)	Blocks voltage-dependent sodium conductance	25 mg daily	Rash, abnormal thinking, dizziness, ataxia, diplopia, nausea, weight gain

Table 10.2   (continued)

Drug	Type of drug or mechanism	Initial dose (oral unless specified)	Adverse effects
Levetiracetam (Keppra)	Calcium channel and GABA activity	250-500 mg twice daily	Loss of appetite, vomiting, somnolence, hostile behavior
Oxcarbazepine (Trileptal)	Sodium channel blockade; increases potassium conductance	75-150 mg twice daily	Nausea, vomiting, diplopia, fatigue
Phenytoin (Dilantin)	Sodium channel blockade; reduces neuronal calcium uptake	300 mg daily	Nystagmus, ataxia, rash
Pregabalin (Lyrica)	GABA modulation of N-type calcium channels	150 mg daily	Edema, weight gain, vision changes, dizziness
Tiagabine (Gabitril)	Inhibits GABA reuptake	4 mg daily	Dizziness, nervousness, tremor
Topiramate (Topamax)	Blocks sodium channels; enhances GABA-mediated chloride influx and modulatory effects of $GABA_A$ receptors and actions of AMPA receptors	25 mg daily	Somnolence, fatigue, urinary tract calculi
Valproate (Depakote)	Affects GABA glutaminergic activity; reduces threshold of calcium and potassium conductance	250 mg 3 times daily	Nausea, vomiting, tremor, thrombocytopenia, weight gain
Zonisamide (Zonegran)	Blocks sodium, potassium, and calcium channels; inhibits glutamate excitation	100 mg daily	Somnolence, dizziness, agitation

Table 10.2   (continued)

Drug	Type of drug or mechanism	Initial dose (oral unless specified)	Adverse effects
Antiarrhythmic			
Mexiletine (Mexitil)	Blocks sodium channels	150 mg daily, titrate	Cardiac (consider cardiology consultation), nausea, anxiety
Sympatholytic			
Clonidine (Catapres)	α_2-Adrenergic agonist	0.1 mg (transdermal)	Hypotension
Topical agents			
Capsaicin (Zostrix)	Depletion of substance P		Burning sensation
Lidocaine (Lidoderm)	Blocks sodium channels	1-3 patches for up to 12 hours in a 24-hour period	Hypotension, skin irritation
Lidocaine and prilocaine (EMLA)	Blocks sodium channels	See package insert	Caution in liver disease
NMDA antagonists			
Dextromethorphan (several over-the-counter cough preparations)	Blocks NMDA receptors	15 mg daily, titrate	Dizziness, somnolence
Ketamine (Ketalar)	Blocks NMDA receptors	10 mg/mL (intravenous), titrate	Vivid dreams, hypertension
Antispasmodic			
Baclofen (Lioresal)	? GABAergic	5 mg 3 times daily	Drowsiness, hypotension, seizures with abrupt withdrawal

AMPA, α-Amino-3-hydroxy-5-methyl-4-isoxazole propionic acid; GABA, γ-aminobutyric acid; NMDA, N-methyl-D-aspartate; NSAID, nonsteroidal antiinflammatory drug; SSRI, selective serotonin reuptake inhibitor.

Antidepressant Medications

Many antidepressant medications are effective in treating neuropathic pain. The analgesic effect of antidepressant medications is independent of an antidepressant response. Tricyclic antidepressants, such as amitriptyline and nortriptyline, block the reuptake of serotonin and norepinephrine, and the change in

Table 10.3. Opioid Dose Equivalent

	Oral or intramuscular	Intravenous
Morphine	30 mg oral 10 mg intramuscular	4 mg/hour intravenous
Fentanyl (Duragesic)		100 µg/hour
Hydromorphone (Dilaudid)	7.5 mg oral 1.5 mg intramuscular	
Levorphanol (Levo-Dromoran)	4 mg oral 2 mg intramuscular	
Methadone (Dolophine)	20 mg oral 10 mg intramuscular	
Oxycodone (Oxycontin, Percocet, Percodan)	20 mg oral	

Modified from Portenoy, RK: Contemporary Diagnosis and Management of Pain in Oncologic and AIDS Patients. ed 3. Handbooks in Health Care, Newton, PA, 2000, pp 82-87. Used with permission.

serotonin and norepinephrine activity is thought to be the mechanism of the analgesic properties of these antidepressants. There is increasing evidence that tricyclic antidepressants may act like local anesthetics and block sodium channels, decreasing the generation of ectopic discharges. Tricyclic antidepressants also act at cholinergic, histaminergic, and adrenergic receptor sites. The common side effects of the drugs include the anticholinergic symptoms of blurred vision, dry mouth, and constipation and the antihistaminergic symptoms of sedation and weight gain. The side effects can be minimized if the dose is titrated very slowly. Amitriptyline can be started at 10 to 25 mg at bedtime and increased every week by the same amount. It rarely is necessary to exceed 100 mg, and serum levels can be determined if necessary. Nortriptyline has fewer side effects than amitriptyline. The patient needs to know that it may take up to 6 weeks before a therapeutic effect occurs and that adverse symptoms tend to diminish as the patient adapts to the medication.

Selective serotonin reuptake inhibitors (SSRIs) have not been as effective as tricyclic antidepressants for treating neuropathic pain. However, SSRIs are effective antidepressants and should be considered when depression is a prominent symptom. Antidepressants categorized as "mixed reuptake inhibitors" inhibit the reuptake of serotonin and norepinephrine and have some local anesthetic properties. They may have fewer adverse effects than tricyclic antidepressants do. Duloxetine is a selective serotonin and norepinephrine reuptake inhibitor and is the first drug approved by the US Food and Drug Administration for the treatment of diabetic peripheral neuropathy.

When prescribing any antidepressant, it is important to be aware of the potential of these medications to increase the risk of suicide in patients with depression. This is especially important with regard to children and adolescents. The patient should be asked about suicidal ideation before treatment and then be observed for increasing depression or agitation that would warrant psychiatric referral.

Table 10.4. Recommendations for Use of Long-term Opioid Therapy

- Patient and physician need to recognize that long-term use of narcotics is a serious commitment and requires close monitoring and follow-up
- Consider a written contract setting out terms of goal-directed therapy, terms for discontinuing treatment, and risks and benefits
- Use long-acting opioids and minimize use of short-acting opioids for initial titration of dose and breakthrough pain
- Use one type of long-acting medication and short-acting medication for breakthrough pain to avoid receptor competition
- Do not exceed recommended doses of acetaminophen or aspirin in combination medications
- There should be only one prescribing provider
- The patient should use only one pharmacy
- Refills should be anticipated and not provided by after-hour coverage
- Document carefully

Data from Ballantyne, JC: Opioids for chronic nonterminal pain. South Med J 99:1245-1255, 2006.

Anticonvulsants

Many anticonvulsants can be effective in treating neuropathic pain. Paroxysmal pain or neuralgia-like pain (sharp, lancinating pain) is often responsive to treatment with anticonvulsants. The modulation of N-type calcium channels by γ-aminobutyric acid (GABA) appears to be the mechanism of action of gabapentin and pregabalin. Carbamazepine, oxcarbazepine, phenytoin, and lamotrigine act by blocking sodium channels. These medications have variable effects at different doses and serum levels. Slow titration can reduce the problem of adverse effects.

Gabapentin has been prescribed extensively for neuropathic pain. It has no drug interactions and a low incidence of adverse effects. The initial dose is 300 mg per day, and this can be increased by 300 mg every 3 to 7 days until a therapeutic effect is achieved or intolerable side effects develop. The effective dose varies (usual range, 2,100-3,600 mg daily in divided doses); 6,000 mg is considered the maximal dose.

Other Agents

Sodium channel antagonists inhibit the spontaneous discharge from nerve sprouts and cell bodies of injured primary afferent neurons. This inhibition is the presumed mechanism of action of mexiletine and lidocaine, two local anesthetic antiarrhythmic agents effective in treating certain neuropathic pain problems. Before initiating treatment with mexiletine, be sure the patient has no evidence of cardiac disease. Cardiology consultation should be considered if the patient has a history of cardiac abnormality, abnormal electrocardiographic findings, or cardiac symptoms. In pain clinics, an intravenous infusion of lidocaine is often used to predict the response to oral mexiletine.

Several chronic neuropathic pain syndromes, including complex regional pain syndrome and small-fiber neuropathies, may be due partly to abnormal activity in the sympathetic nervous system. Sympatholytic agents used to treat pain include adrenergic receptor blockers such as phentolamine mesylate and prazosin and the α2-agonist clonidine. Phentolamine mesylate has been administered intravenously to identify which patients with sympathetically mediated pain may have a response to sympathetic blocks or surgical sympathectomy. Transdermal clonidine is effective in treating painful peripheral neuropathies. Hypotension, impotence, and other autonomic side effects limit the use of sympatholytic agents.

Several topical agents have been useful in treating peripheral neuropathic pain. Capsaicin cream, an extract of chili peppers, has been used to treat peripheral neuropathies and postherpetic neuralgia. The efficacy of this treatment has been mixed. The mechanism of action is thought to involve the depletion of substance P from small nociceptive fibers, which in turn reduces spontaneous activity and evoked input from damaged afferent nerves. The cream is applied three times daily. Burning pain is noted after each application and usually resolves after 1 week of treatment. Some patients have reported that this treatment exacerbated their pain. Care must be taken to avoid contact with the mouth or eyes, but capsaicin has no systemic side effects. Local anesthetics such as lidocaine and a combination of lidocaine and prilocaine are available as topical agents. These preparations have little systemic effect but are often limited by poor absorption.

Antagonists of the *N*-methyl-D-aspartate (NMDA) receptor for glutamate are being investigated for the treatment of neuropathic pain. Ketamine has shown some usefulness as a third-line agent in the treatment of neuropathic pain. Dextromethorphan, the active ingredient in many over-the-counter cough preparations, has a modest effect on painful neuropathies. The doses that have been used are high (380 mg/day), and sedation and ataxia have been common side effects. NMDA antagonists also may have a role in opioid therapy. They potentiate the analgesic effect of opioids and may block or reduce tolerance to opioids.

Baclofen, considered a nonopioid analgesic and skeletal muscle relaxant, has been used to treat spasticity in multiple sclerosis and spinal cord injury. It has limited efficacy in treating painful paroxysms that occur in both peripheral and central neuropathic pain conditions.

Transcutaneous electrical nerve stimulation (TENS) is a physical method that can provide pain relief in a few neuropathic pain disorders. The mechanism of action of the TENS unit is to evoke sensation proximal to a nerve injury to inhibit the pain sensation. For this method to be effective, paresthesias need to be induced in the painful area. Local skin irritation is the only adverse effect. The few data available about the effectiveness of TENS in chronic pain are contradictory.

The data about the efficacy of acupuncture for the treatment of chronic pain are also contradictory. There are several methods of acupuncture, and all of them require inserting needles into various points on the body. Evidence suggests that acupuncture needling causes the release of enkephalin and dynorphin in the spinal cord, activation of opioid receptors in the periaqueductal gray matter and release of norepinephrine and serotonin, and the release of adrenocorticotropic hormone and β-endorphin from the pituitary gland. Little information is available about the use of acupuncture in the treatment of neuropathic pain.

Neurosurgical Treatment of Pain

The neurosurgical options available for the treatment of pain include the delivery of intraspinal medication, ablative surgery, and stimulation, including spinal cord stimulation, motor cortex stimulation, and deep brain stimulation.

The delivery of intraspinal medications involves the insertion of a catheter (mid-lumbar subdural space) attached to a programmable implanted pump. A trial with an outside reservoir can be performed before the pump is implanted. Intrathecal medication avoids the large systemic doses of medications and their adverse effects. Obstruction and leakage are the equipment-related complications.

Ablative surgery for pain includes cordotomy, dorsal root entry zone lesions (rhizotomy), sympathectomy, myelotomy, mesencephalotomy, and cingulotomy. Many of these procedures have been replaced by stimulation therapies.

Spinal cord stimulation involves the insertion of electrodes, attached to a programmable generator, into the epidural space. As with intraspinal delivery of medication, the electrodes can be attached to an external stimulator for a trial period before the generator is implanted in a subcutaneous pocket. Spinal cord stimulation is effective in selected cases of back pain, complex regional pain syndromes I and II, peripheral nerve injuries, and peripheral neuropathies.

The use of motor cortex stimulation is increasing for several intractable pain syndromes, particularly facial pain. An electrode is placed in the epidural space overlying the motor cortex. The mechanism of this neuromodulation is not known. The use of deep brain stimulation in the management of pain is under intensive investigation. The sites for implantation include the sensory thalamus and periaqueductal gray matter.

POLYNEUROPATHIES

Polyneuropathies are discussed in Chapter 6. Painful polyneuropathies include neuropathies due to diabetes mellitus, vasculitis, amyloid deposition, human immunodeficiency virus (HIV) infection, chronic alcoholism, toxic effects of arsenic or thallium, paraneoplastic disease, and Fabry disease. Hereditary sensory neuropathy is also associated with pain.

The most common of these is diabetic neuropathy. Pain can be associated with distal neuropathy as well as with the proximal asymmetric form, diabetic radiculoplexus neuropathy. The pain is thought to reflect axonal injury caused by metabolic disturbance from diabetes and by diffuse microvascular infarcts of the nerve. Diabetic radiculoplexus neuropathy may involve immune-mediated occlusion of arterioles that supply the nerves. A reasonable treatment for diabetic radiculoplexus neuropathy is narcotic opioids, because remission usually occurs within 3 to 6 months from onset. Immunosuppressant medication is being investigated for treating diabetic neuropathy.

Tricyclic antidepressants and mixed reuptake inhibitors are effective in treating painful polyneuropathies. The effectiveness of SSRIs has been disappointing, and they are not recommended. Gabapentin and pregabalin are efficacious and have few side effects. Treatment with mexiletine is beneficial; however, this drug can be administered only if the patient has normal heart function. Transdermal clonidine has been beneficial in some cases of diabetic neuropathy, which reflects the heterogeneity of this painful disorder and the role of the sympathetic nervous system.

COMPLEX REGIONAL PAIN SYNDROMES

Complex regional pain syndrome type 1 (CRPS 1), previously known as "reflex sympathetic dystrophy," is usually caused by minor trauma to an extremity (eg, sprain or fracture) or a medical event (eg, myocardial infarction). After the trauma or event, sensory and inflammatory symptoms develop and spread. The symptoms are disproportionate to the injury. CRPS 1 is characterized by burning pain. Autonomic abnormalities associated with CRPS include swelling, hyperhidrosis or hypohidrosis, vasodilatation or vasoconstriction, and changes in skin temperature. Common trophic changes associated with the syndrome include abnormal nail growth, increased or decreased hair growth, thin skin, and osteoporosis. Weakness, tremor, dystonia, and neglect-like symptoms of the affected extremity are the motor abnormalities associated with CRPS.

CRPS 2 is used to describe causalgia. CRPS 2 is caused by partial injury of a peripheral nerve. Its clinical features are comparable to those of CRPS 1 and include burning pain, allodynia, edema, and skin changes. The distinction between type 1 and type 2 is partial injury of a peripheral nerve in CRPS 2.

The pathophysiology of CRPS is not understood completely. An inflammatory reaction has been proposed in the acute phase of CRPS. In CRPS 2, abnormal characteristics of primary afferents have been described, including spontaneous discharge, sensitization, ectopic mechanosensitivity, and responsiveness to norepinephrine. Spontaneous discharges from the accumulation of sodium channels in the terminal membrane may be part of the mechanism of CRPS. In the central nervous system, both NMDA receptor–mediated hyperexcitability in the spinal cord dorsal horn and spinal cord neuronal hyperexcitability may be involved in the pathophysiologic mechanism. Reorganization of the primary somatosensory cortex has been demonstrated in CRPS, and reversal has been shown coincident with clinical improvement.

CRPS is a clinical diagnosis. In addition to spontaneous pain, the patient can experience hyperalgesia to mechanical and thermal stimulation. The autonomic, vascular, and motor changes listed above support the diagnosis. Three-phase bone scanning, quantitative sensory testing, and autonomic testing may aid in the diagnosis.

The management of patients with CRPS is difficult, and a multidisciplinary approach with a pain specialist, physiatrist, and psychiatrist is recommended. The medications that have been shown in controlled trials to be efficacious include gabapentin, corticosteroids, and calcium-modulating drugs (calcitonin, clodronate, pamidronate, and alendronate). The medications listed in Table 10.2 have also been used to treat CRPS. Interventional techniques that have been used include intravenous regional sympathetic blockade, local anesthetic sympathetic blockade, spinal cord stimulation, and sympathetic denervation.

POSTHERPETIC NEURALGIA

The varicella-zoster virus is omnipresent; the primary infection with this virus is varicella (chickenpox). The virus becomes latent in dorsal root ganglia, and its reactivation causes herpes zoster (shingles). This virus can cause several painful conditions. Preherpetic neuralgia is the radicular pain that precedes the skin eruption, usually by 2 to 4 days. The pain of acute herpes zoster occurs from the time the rash appears to the time of vesicular crusting. Postherpetic neuralgia is the pain that persists for more than 3 months in the region of the cutaneous lesions.

Postherpetic neuralgia occurs in 10% of patients with herpes zoster. Those at increased risk for postherpetic neuralgia include the elderly and persons with depressed immune function from malignancy, chemotherapy, surgery, or HIV infection. Also at increased risk are patients who had involvement of the face (especially the ophthalmic branch of the trigeminal nerve), intense acute herpetic pain, severe skin lesions, or permanent sensory loss in the affected area. Increased psychosocial stress and postherpetic neuralgia appear to be correlated.

The pain of postherpetic neuralgia is described as "constant deep aching" or "burning pain." Intermittent paroxysms of lancinating or jabbing pain with allodynia are also common. Movement and any tactile stimulation of the area, including stimulation produced by clothing, are avoided. Neurologic examination shows a loss of pin prick and thermal sensations in the affected area.

It is expected that with the widespread use of the virus vaccine, postherpetic neuralgia will be prevented. Antiviral treatment at the time of the herpes zoster infection decreases herpetic pain in the short term and has a modest effect in decreasing the likelihood that postherpetic neuralgia will develop. Treatment with intravenous acyclovir followed by oral valacyclovir has been shown to lessen the pain of postherpetic neuralgia, suggesting that a viral ganglionitis may contribute to the pain of this syndrome. Corticosteroids may reduce the pain of an acute infection, but they have not been shown to reduce the incidence or severity of postherpetic neuralgia. Nerve blocks early in the course of the disease have not been shown to prevent postherpetic neuralgia.

Tricyclic antidepressants are effective for treating postherpetic neuralgia. As with other painful conditions, these agents are started at a low dose and increased until a therapeutic response is achieved or intolerable side effects develop. Many anticonvulsants have been used to treat postherpetic neuralgia; efficacy has been shown with gabapentin and pregabalin. Topical analgesics are useful because the area involved is well defined and these agents have no systemic side effects. Spinal cord stimulation and other neuromodulation techniques may need to be pursued if these measures are not effective.

CENTRAL PAIN

Central pain is caused by a lesion within the central nervous system, for example, stroke, spinal cord trauma, or multiple sclerosis. Central pain may be overlooked because of the delay in the onset of painful symptoms. The delay can be for days, months, and (rarely) years after the central nervous system lesion. Frequently complicating the diagnosis of central pain is the paucity of physical findings. A consistent finding is loss of temperature sensation.

Some of the adjectives patients use to describe central pain are "superficial pain," "deep pain," "burning," "aching," "pricking," and "lancinating." Temperature changes, emotional stimuli, and movement can trigger the pain. Features of central pain include poor localization, impaired sensory discrimination, prolonged aftersensations, and delayed sensory latency.

Treating central pain can be difficult. Reassure patients by educating them about the cause of the pain, and provide psychosocial support throughout treatment. For short-term treatment of central pain, benefit has been demonstrated with intravenous lidocaine, propofol, and ketamine. Tricyclic antidepressants, anticonvulsants such as gabapentin and lamotrigine, and opioid analgesics are first-line drug therapy. For intractable central pain, neuromodulation with spinal cord stimulation and deep brain stimulation is an option.

NEUROPATHIC CANCER PAIN

Neuropathic cancer pain can be due to direct involvement of neural structures by tumor or it can be related to cancer therapy. Toxic neuropathies result from treatment with chemotherapeutic agents, including cisplatin, vincristine, and paclitaxel. Postsurgical pain due to thoracotomy, mastectomy, or amputation is another example of a clinical pain syndrome related to cancer. Other examples of neuropathic cancer pain are postradiation pain (myelotomy and plexopathy) and postherpetic neuralgia. Many of these pain syndromes are heterogeneous and involve neural, myofascial, bone, and visceral pain symptoms.

The most important aspect in the evaluation of the pain of a patient with cancer is to determine whether the cancer causes the symptom. Postthoracotomy pain and postmastectomy pain are distinct clinical syndromes. In the cancer population, postthoracotomy pain should be considered to have a neoplastic origin until repeat evaluations over several months are negative. Recurrent neoplasm has been discovered in more than 90% of patients who had increasing pain after the incisional pain resolved. In contrast, the pain following mastectomy is often caused by surgical injury to the intercostobrachial nerve. This pain occurs in the distribution of the T2 dermatome and can begin several months to years after the operation. In the case of this characteristic clinical syndrome, the patient can be reassured and extensive evaluation avoided.

Treatment of the underlying cancer is the best treatment of pain in patients with cancer. When pain is caused by tumor compressing a nerve, consider surgical decompression, chemotherapy, or radiation (or a combination). Because most cancer pain syndromes are heterogeneous, pharmacologic treatment often requires multiple medications. A combination of opioids, tricyclic antidepressants, and anticonvulsants is frequently prescribed for neuropathic cancer pain.

The World Health Organization lists three categories of pain to guide analgesic drug therapy. Nonopioid drugs with or without adjuvant therapy are used first for mild pain (eg, aspirin and other nonsteroidal antiinflammatory drugs and acetaminophen). For mild to moderate pain, the addition of opioids such as codeine and oxycodone is considered. Morphine or fentanyl is considered for moderate to severe pain. The dose of the drug that is chosen should be increased aggressively to prevent persistent pain without causing intolerable side effects. Around-the-clock dosing with long-acting medications should be used to prevent pain. Rescue medications (medications used to provide relief for breakthrough pain) should be available. The approximate dose of the rescue medication should be equal to the dose of the regular medication given for the interval. For example, 30 mg of immediate-release morphine every 4 hours is the rescue dose for a patient taking 90 mg of sustained-release morphine every 12 hours.

The route of administration of analgesic drugs is important. If the patient cannot take medication orally, consider a rectal, transdermal, spinal, intrathecal, or intraventricular route. Anticipate the common side effects of the medications so they can be managed or prevented. Constipation is a common side effect of opioid analgesics. If one opioid analgesic is not tolerated, switch to another. The initial dose of a sequential analgesic should be 25% to 50% less than the estimated equivalent dose (Table 10.3) to allow for incomplete cross-tolerance. All adjuvant analgesics listed in Table 10.2 are reasonable to try for treating the heterogeneous pain disorders associated with cancer.

PALLIATIVE CARE

As shown in a large study, more than 50% of patients experienced moderate to severe pain in the last 3 days of life. It is important for the neurologist to understand palliative care not only in the context of treating pain but also for other chronic and progressive neurologic diseases such as amyotrophic lateral sclerosis, severe stroke, high cervical spinal cord injuries, advanced dementia, and advanced multiple sclerosis. Palliative care is defined by the World Health Organization as "the active total care of patients whose disease is not responsive to curative treatment." The control of pain, other symptoms, and psychologic, social, and spiritual problems is paramount. The goal of palliative care is to achieve the best quality of life for patients and their families. The goals of palliative care according to the World Health Organization are listed in Table 10.5.

MENTAL DISORDERS AND PAIN

Chronic pain is frequently a symptom of mental disorders, including somatization disorder, hypochondriasis, and factitious physical disorders. Pain is also associated with psychologic factors and malingering. Other psychiatric disorders (eg, depression, anxiety, panic, and posttraumatic stress disorders) exert a strong influence on chronic pain. Psychiatric treatment concurrent with medical treatment is recommended for these disorders.

The concept of abnormal illness behavior is useful in understanding mental disorders and pain. How a person behaves when ill is called *illness behavior*. Normal illness behavior is behavior appropriate to the level of the disease present. Exaggerated or amplified behavior, that is, out of proportion to the level of the disease present, is abnormal and called *illness-affirming behavior*. Illness-affirming behavior is seen in conversion disorder, somatization disorder, hypochondriasis, and pain associated with psychologic factors. All four of these conditions have unconscious motivation and production of signs and symptoms (ie, the patient is unaware of the production of symptoms or the motivation behind the behavior). However, in malingering and factitious disorder, illness-affirming behavior is associated with the conscious production of signs and symptoms. Patients with malingering are aware of the motive behind the behavior, whereas those with factitious disorder are not.

The diagnostic criteria for somatization disorder include multiple physical complaints before the age of 30 years. The physical complaints occur over several years and cause notable impairment or the seeking of medical attention. The presence of four pain complaints,

Table 10.5. Palliative Care

- Provides relief from pain and other distressing symptoms
- Affirms life and regards dying as a normal process
- Intends neither to hasten nor to postpone death
- Integrates the psychologic and spiritual aspects of patient care
- Offers a support system to help patients live as actively as possible until death
- Offers a support system to help the family cope during the patient's illness and in their own bereavement
- Uses a team approach to address the needs of patients and their families, including bereavement counseling, if indicated
- Will enhance quality of life and may also positively influence the course of illness
- Is applicable early in the course of illness, in conjunction with other therapies that are intended to prolong life, such as chemotherapy or radiation therapy, and includes those investigations needed to better understand and manage distressing clinical complications

From Palliative care. World Health Organization, Geneva, Switzerland [cited 2007 Aug 22]. Available from: http://www.who.int/cancer/palliative/en. Used with permission.

two gastrointestinal symptoms, one sexual symptom, and one pseudoneurologic symptom complete the criteria. Management of somatization disorder requires that one clinician coordinate medical treatment and schedule regular visits. This prevents the unnecessary use of invasive procedures. Also, with this coordinated treatment, the patient does not need to develop new symptoms to maintain the relationship with the clinician.

Patients with hypochondriasis are preoccupied by the belief or fear that they have serious disease. Normal aches and pains may be misinterpreted as signs of severe disease. The preferred method of management is reassurance and follow-up appointments for reassessment.

Pain associated with psychologic factors was previously called "somatoform" or "psychogenic" pain. Pain is the predominant focus of the clinical presentation and causes distress or functional impairment. Psychologic factors have an important role in the onset, severity, exacerbation, and maintenance of pain. A previous history of physical complaints without organic findings, prominent guilt, or a history of physical or sexual abuse confirms the diagnosis. Individual, group, and marital therapy; psychiatric treatment; physical therapy; biofeedback; and antidepressant medications are all reasonable treatments.

Factitious disorder should be considered if illness-affirming behavior is present and the symptoms appear to be produced on a voluntary or conscious basis. If there is no apparent motivation for the behavior, factitious disorder should be suspected. A patient with factitious disorder has periods of improvement followed by relapses. Other clues to this disorder include a willingness of the patient to undergo invasive procedures, difficulty obtaining previous medical records, and the patient's resistance to psychiatric consultation. Malingering differs from factitious disorder by the identification of a motive for the behavior, for example, avoiding jail, seeking narcotics, and obtaining disability payments. Psychiatric consultation is recommended.

SUGGESTED READING

Allen, RR: Neuropathic pain in the cancer patient. Neurol Clin 16:869-888, 1998.

Aronoff, GM: Approach to the patient with chronic pain. In: Strategies. Neurology 45 Suppl 9:S11-S16, 1995.

Backonja, MM, and Galer, BS: Pain assessment and evaluation of patients who have neuropathic pain. Neurol Clin 16:775-790, 1998.

Bajwa ZH, Lehmann, LJ, and Fishman, SM: Anatomy and physiology of pain. In: Samuels, MA, and Feske, S (eds): Office Practice of Neurology. Churchill Livingstone, New York, 1996, pp 1157-1162.

Ballantyne, JC: Opioids for chronic nonterminal pain. South Med J 99:1245-1255, 2006.

Benarroch, EE: Sodium channels and pain. Neurology 68:233-236, 2007.

Beric, A: Central pain and dysesthesia syndrome. Neurol Clin 16:899-918, 1998.

Casey, KL, et al: Pain. Continuum 2:7-74, 1996.

Cluff, RS, and Rowbotham, MC: Pain caused by herpes zoster infection. Neurol Clin 16:813-832, 1998.

Dawson, DM, and Sabin, TD: Pain. In: Samuels MA, and Feske, S (eds): Office Practice of Neurology. Churchill Livingstone, New York, 1996, pp 36-40.

Eisenberg, E, McNicol, ED, and Carr, DB: Efficacy and safety of opioid agonists in the treatment of neuropathic pain of nonmalignant origin: Systematic review and meta-analysis of randomized controlled trials. JAMA 293:3043-3052, 2005.

Eisendrath, SJ: Psychiatric aspects of chronic pain. Neurology 45 Suppl 9:S26-S34, 1995.

Fargas-Babjak, A: Acupuncture, transcutaneous electrical nerve stimulation, and laser therapy in chronic pain. Clin J Pain 17 Suppl:S105-S113, 2001.

Galer, BS: Painful polyneuropathy. Neurol Clin 16:791-812, 1998.

Giller, CA: The neurosurgical treatment of pain. Arch Neurol 60:1537-1540, 2003.

Gonzales, GR: Central pain: Diagnosis and treatment strategies. Neurology 45 Suppl 9:S11-S16, 1995,

Hocking, G, and Cousins, MJ: Ketamine in chronic pain management: An evidence-based review. Anesth Analg 97:1730-1739, 2003.

Irving, GA: Contemporary assessment and management of neuropathic pain. Neurology 64 Suppl 3:S21-S27, 2005.

Kanner, RM: Pharmacological approaches to pain management. Continuum: Lifelong Learning in Neurology 11(6) Pain and Palliative Care:137-154, 2005.

Levy, MH: Pharmacologic treatment of cancer pain. N Engl J Med 335:1124-1132, 1996.

Maihofner, C, et al: Cortical reorganization during recovery from complex regional pain syndrome. Neurology 63:693-701, 2004.

Nicholson, BD: Evaluation and treatment of central pain syndromes. Neurology 62 Suppl 2:S30-S36, 2004.

Payne, R: Principles of palliative medicine and pain management in neurologic illness. Continuum: Lifelong Learning in Neurology 11(6) Pain and Palliative Care:13-32, 2005.

Quan, D, et al: Improvement of postherpetic neuralgia after treatment with intravenous acyclovir followed by oral valacyclovir. Arch Neurol 63:940-942, 2006. Epub 2006 May 8.

Rowbotham, MC: Chronic pain: From theory to practical management. Neurology 45 Suppl 9:S5-S10, 1995.

Rowbotham, MC: Pharmacologic managment of complex regional pain syndrome. Clin J Pain 22:425-429, 2006.

Sharma, A, Williams, K, and Raja, SN: Advances in treatment of complex regional pain syndrome: Recent insights on a perplexing disease. Curr Opin Anaesthesiol 19:566-572, 2006.

Wernicke, JF, et al: A randomized controlled trial of duloxetine in diabetic peripheral neuropathic pain. Neurology 67:1411-1420, 2006.

CHAPTER 11

Cerebrovascular Disease

Transient ischemic attack (TIA) is an episode of focal neurologic dysfunction caused by ischemia. The clinical symptoms usually last less than 1 hour, and there is no evidence of acute infarction. A *minor stroke* is defined as persistent neurologic deficit that is not disabling. The characteristic temporal profile of a TIA or stroke is sudden onset of neurologic signs or symptoms, with maximal deficit occurring within seconds or a few minutes after onset. Vascular injury to the nervous system presents suddenly, and patients can report the exact time of onset unless they awaken with the symptoms or if language or consciousness is involved. TIAs are focal events, and the symptoms and signs of neurologic deficit should correspond to a known vascular distribution (Fig. 11.1 and 11.2). Patients with TIAs are at risk for developing a disabling stroke; it has been estimated that between 10% and 20% will have such a stroke within 90 days after a TIA. The specific risk can vary depending on the mechanism of the ischemic event. Evaluation and intervention need to be initiated immediately.

DIAGNOSTIC APPROACH

Five questions need to be answered in the diagnostic evaluation of a patient who has a cerebrovascular event:

1. Is it a vascular event?
2. Is hospitalization required?
3. Is the event hemorrhagic or ischemic?
4. Does the event localize to the anterior or posterior circulation?
5. What is the mechanism?

Is It a Vascular Event?

The first diagnostic consideration is to determine whether the event represents a TIA. TIAs are focal events with focal symptoms, in contrast to the generalized symptoms that occur with syncope, presyncope, and hypoglycemia. Migraine with neurologic symptoms can often be confused with TIAs because of the abrupt onset of focal symptoms. However, migraine symptoms tend to be positive phenomena, for example, scintillating scotomas, fortification spectrum, and tingling paresthesias. Visual or sensory loss is considered a negative phenomenon, and negative phenomena more likely

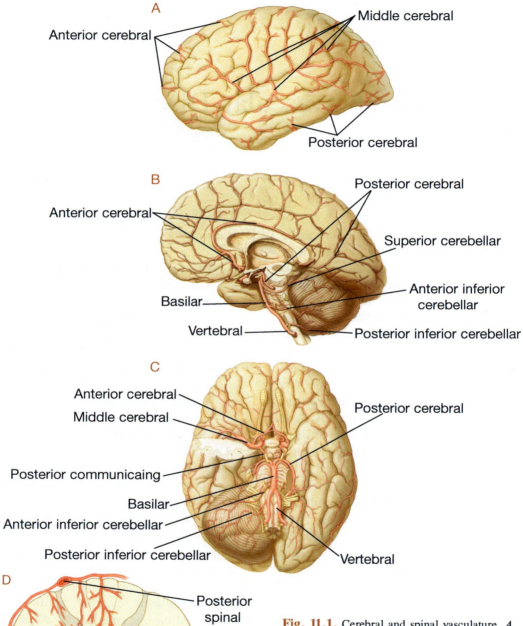

A

Anterior cerebral

Middle cerebral

Posterior cerebral

B

Anterior cerebral

Posterior cerebral

Superior cerebellar

Anterior inferior cerebellar

Basilar

Vertebral

Posterior inferior cerebellar

C

Anterior cerebral

Middle cerebral

Posterior cerebral

Posterior communicaing

Basilar

Anterior inferior cerebellar

Posterior inferior cerebellar

Vertebral

D

Posterior spinal artery

Anterior spinal artery

Fig. 11.1. Cerebral and spinal vasculature. *A*, Lateral surface of brain; *B*, medial surface of brain; and *C*, ventral surface of brain. *D*, Cross section of spinal cord vascular pattern. (From Adams, AC: Neurology in Primary Care. FA Davis, Philadelphia, 2000, p 186. Used with permission of Mayo Foundation for Medical Education and Research.)

Artery	Anatomical distribution	Clinical findings
Anterior cerebral	Medial surface	Weakness, clumsiness, and sensory loss affecting contra-lateral leg
Middle cerebral	Lateral surface	Hemiparesis, hemisensory loss, hemianopia, and aphasia (left hemisphere)
Posterior cerebral	Medial surface	Hemianopia or quadrantanopia with macular sparing
Vertebrobasilar	Base of brain	Diplopia, cranial nerve signs, bilateral motor and sensory signs, ataxia, vertigo, and facial weakness
	Anterior spinal artery	Anterior spinal artery syndrome: weakness and loss of pain and temperature sense below the level of the lesion, with sparing of vibration and joint position sense

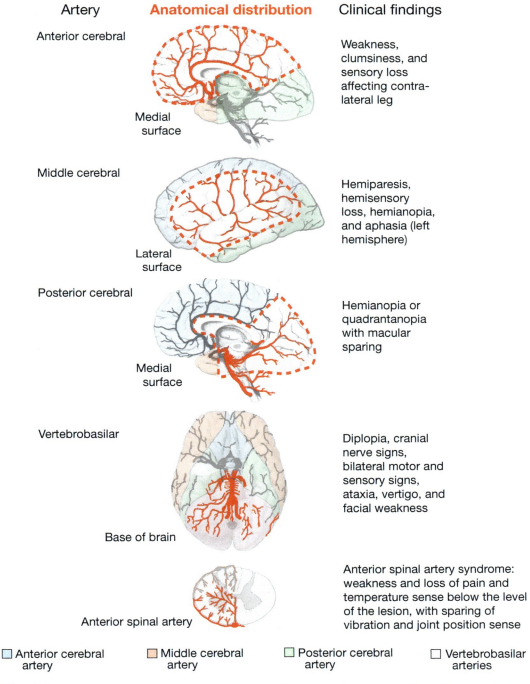

☐ Anterior cerebral artery   ☐ Middle cerebral artery   ☐ Posterior cerebral artery   ☐ Vertebrobasilar arteries

Fig. 11.2. Anatomical distribution of the major cerebral arteries, with common clinical features. (From Adams, AC: Neurology in Primary Care. FA Davis, Philadelphia, 2000, p 187. Used with permission of Mayo Foundation for Medical Education and Research.)

occur with ischemic attacks. Without the characteristic headache, a patient with migraine may have a previous history of headaches, a positive family history for headaches, and fewer cardiovascular risk factors than a patient with a TIA.

Partial seizure activity can mimic TIAs. However, symptoms of partial seizures, like those of migraine, tend to be positive phenomena. For example, in a partial seizure, focal tonic and clonic movement of an extremity is more likely than motor weakness. The time to maximal deficit is longer in partial seizures, and there is a tendency for the symptoms to "march"; that is, motor or sensory symptoms may begin in the hand and, over minutes, spread to the face and then to the leg. Stereotyped spells are characteristic of seizure activity, although stereotyped episodes occurring in a single vascular distribution can occur in focal arterial stenosis.

An inner ear problem such as labyrinthitis or vestibulopathy may present acutely and is included in the differential diagnosis of TIA. Vertigo without other brainstem or cerebellar symptoms or vertigo associated with auditory symptoms is due most often to an inner ear lesion. For example, a patient with vertigo due to lateral medullary ischemia can have vertigo, ataxia, dysarthria, dysphagia, and sensory symptoms (Fig. 11.3).

Multiple sclerosis can present with sudden focal neurologic symptoms, but the rapid resolution of symptoms in minutes is uncommon. Neurologic signs and symptoms due to multiple sclerosis are not restricted to a single vascular area. Patients with multiple sclerosis are often younger and have fewer cerebrovascular risk factors than patients with TIAs.

Hemorrhage into a neoplasm can present suddenly, but the signs and symptoms usually

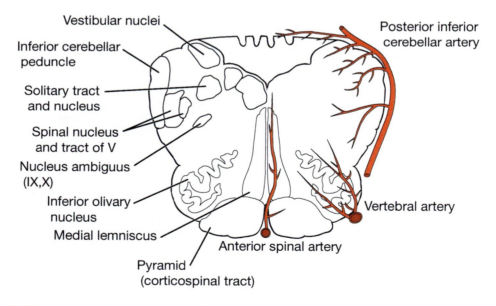

Fig. 11.3. Vascular supply of the medulla. Signs and symptoms of the lateral medullary syndrome include ataxia, vertigo, dysarthria, dysphagia, Horner syndrome, and loss of pain and temperature sense on ipsilateral face and contralateral body.

are not transient. Focal signs and symptoms from a neoplasm have a stuttering or progressive temporal profile. Neuroimaging will usually resolve any diagnostic questions.

Is Hospitalization Required?

After the event has been determined to be vascular, the next step is to determine whether hospitalization is necessary. This question is not always easy to answer and opinions differ. The most important point is whether the evaluation of the patient as an inpatient or outpatient is performed without delay. The patient should be hospitalized if he or she is at high risk for recurrent vascular events or is medically unstable. Clinical features that suggest high risk are patients older than age 60 years, symptom duration of more than 10 minutes, symptoms of motor weakness or language impairment, and patients with diabetes mellitus.

If a cardioembolic source is suspected, the patient, like those with atrial fibrillation or recent myocardial infarction, should be given anticoagulation, which may require hospitalization. Patients who have multiple events and events that are increasing in frequency and duration should be hospitalized.

Patients often delay in presenting for evaluation, and if the event occurred 2 weeks before the assessment, an expedited work-up in the following 1 or 2 days is reasonable. Immediately start treatment with aspirin, 81 to 325 mg daily, while the evaluation is in progress. If the patient has an aspirin allergy, it is important to remember that other antiplatelet agents do not have an immediate onset of action like aspirin. Clopidogrel has an initial antiplatelet response in 2 hours, but it takes 3 to 7 days for the peak antiplatelet effect to occur.

Is the Event Hemorrhagic or Ischemic?

The next step in the evaluation of a patient with cerebrovascular symptoms is to determine whether the vascular event is hemorrhagic or ischemic. The majority of vascular events are ischemic. Hemorrhagic stroke is more likely to present with severe headache, fluctuating levels of consciousness, and meningeal signs. Ischemic vascular events are more likely to involve a singular vascular territory, and the patient's status may improve early in the course of the event. Often, the distinction between ischemic and hemorrhagic events cannot be made solely on the basis of clinical information. Computed tomography (CT) without contrast is the test of choice for the immediate evaluation of a patient who has a cerebrovascular event. CT is able to identify intracerebral hemorrhages and most subarachnoid hemorrhages (Fig. 11.4). For a patient with a TIA, the CT findings should be normal and exclude hemorrhage, vascular tumor, and arteriovenous malformation. Eligibility guidelines for acute thrombolytic therapy are based on CT findings that exclude acute hemorrhagic stroke. Early in ischemic stroke, CT results may be negative or the scan may show only a poorly outlined area of decreased density with subtle gyral flattening. As the interval from the time of stroke to CT increases, the area of the ischemic stroke seen on CT increases, becomes better defined, and is hypointense to the surrounding tissue. The areas where hypodensity would appear on CT for each of the major cerebral arteries are illustrated in Figure 11.5.

Magnetic resonance imaging (MRI) is superior to CT for identifying small infarcts, especially those involving the posterior, or vertebrobasilar, circulation. Diffusion-weighted imaging is a sensitive method for detecting acute infarction. The abnormality may be seen as early as 30 minutes after the infarction and persist for 2 to 4 weeks (Fig. 11.6). Perfusion imaging can measure cerebral blood flow and can be used in conjuction with diffusion-weighted imaging to detect the ischemic penumbra

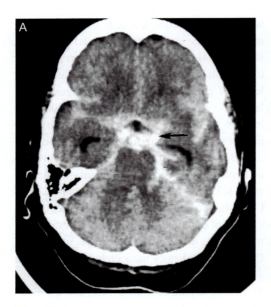
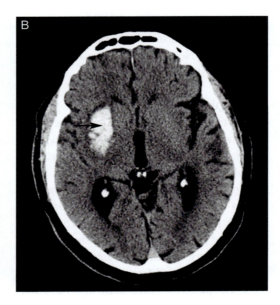

Fig. 11.4. Computed tomographic images of hemorrhagic stroke. *A*, Subarachnoid hemorrhage. Blood in subarachnoid space (*arrow*) is hyperdense. *B*, Intracerebral hemorrhage (*arrow*).

or brain tissue at risk for infarction (Fig. 11.7). The use of perfusion and diffusion-weighted imaging is being developed to improve intervention in acute stroke.

Does the Event Localize to the Anterior or Posterior Circulation?

The next diagnostic step is to localize the symptoms to either the anterior or the posterior circulation. The anterior circulation includes the territory supplied by the carotid artery system, which includes the internal carotid, anterior cerebral, and middle cerebral arteries. The posterior circulation includes the vertebral, basilar, and posterior cerebral arteries (Fig. 11.8). Localization is particularly important in patients who have multiple potential mechanisms for stroke. An example is a patient with vertigo and dysarthria (symptoms of posterior circulation involvement) who has carotid artery stenosis and atrial fibrillation. In this case, the

more relevant risk factor for the patient's ischemic symptoms would be atrial fibrillation. The common clinical features of anterior circulation (carotid system) and posterior circulation (vertebrobasilar system) dysfunction are summarized in Table 11.1.

What Is the Mechanism?

The major portion of the diagnostic evaluation of a patient who has a cerebrovascular event is determining the underlying mechanism of the event. Four major groups of diseases are associated with ischemic cerebrovascular disorders: 1) cardiac disorders; 2) large-vessel, or craniocervical, occlusive disease; 3) small-vessel, or intracranial, occlusive disease; and 4) hematologic disorders (Table 11.2). Embolus from a proximal artery or from the heart is the most common mechanism of ischemic strokes and TIAs. Atherosclerotic disease of the carotid artery in the region of the carotid bifurcation

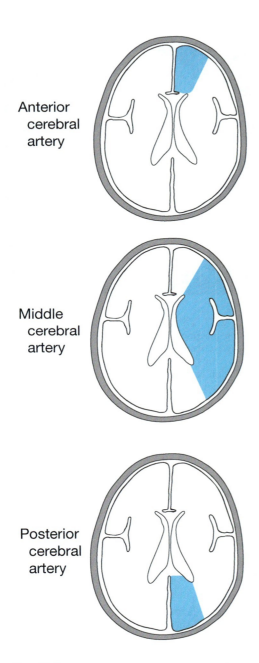

Anterior cerebral artery

Middle cerebral artery

Posterior cerebral artery

Fig. 11.5. Drawings of cranial CT scans showing the areas (blue) of hypodensity appearing with infarction of the major cerebral arteries. (From Adams, AC: Neurology in Primary Care. FA Davis, Philadelphia, 2000, p 189. Used with permission of Mayo Foundation for Medical Education and Research.)

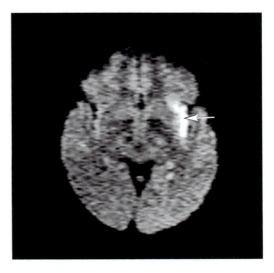

Fig. 11.6. Diffusion-weighted imaging showing acute ischemia in left insular cortex (*arrow*). Diffusion-weighted imaging provides a signal inversely proportional to the molecular diffusion of water molecules. In acute ischemia, with cytotoxic edema and the influx of water from the extracellular to intracellular space, the diffusion of water molecules is restricted, resulting in increased signal intensity.

is a common cause of carotid artery embolus. Cardiac emboli account for 20% of ischemic strokes and TIAs. Another 20% of ischemic strokes are related to decreased blood flow or occlusion of small penetrating brain arteries. Poorly controlled hypertension and diabetes mellitus often damage these small vessels. Despite extensive investigation, the mechanism of many ischemic events remains unknown or uncertain.

Identifying the underlying mechanism clinically can be difficult. Cardiac embolism should be suspected if the patient experienced a recent episode of chest pain, has a pulse irregularity suggestive of atrial fibrillation, has a history or examination findings suggestive of congestive heart failure, has prosthetic heart valves, has the onset of symptoms with a Valsalva maneuver, or has findings of deep

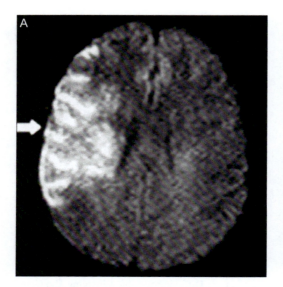

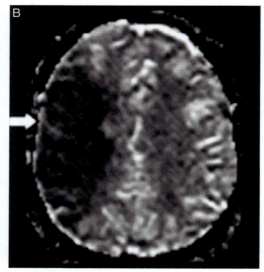

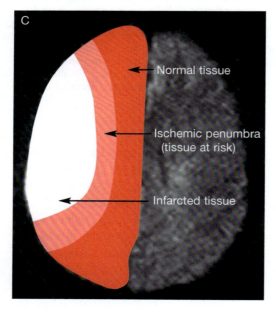

Fig. 11.7. Diffusion-weighted imaging and perfusion imaging in acute right middle cerebral artery ischemia (*white arrow*): *A*, diffusion abnormality; *B*, perfusion abnormality. *C*, If the perfusion abnormality is larger than the diffusion abnormality, it indicates the brain tissue at risk for infarction. This is called the ischemic penumbra.

venous thrombophlebitis in the lower extremities. Any history, examination, or neuroimaging findings that indicate the stroke involves more than one vascular territory are also suggestive of cardiac embolism.

Carotid artery stenosis is suggested by symptoms consistent with retinal artery ischemia.

Emboli to the first branch of the carotid artery, the ophthalmic artery, cause transient monocular blindness, or amaurosis fugax. Emboli from the carotid artery may lodge in the same branches of the intracranial circulation, causing stereotyped TIAs. The presence of a carotid bruit may indicate carotid artery stenosis.

The occlusion of small penetrating arterioles causes lacunar infarction, or small infarcts, in deep cortical sites and the brainstem (Fig. 11.9). Thus, aphasia, visual field deficits, seizures, or motor and sensory deficits in one limb are uncommon with these ischemic events. Common clinical syndromes associated with lacunar infarctions are pure motor hemiparesis, pure sensory hemianesthesia, and dysarthria–clumsy hand syndrome.

Posterior circulation　　**Anterior circulation**

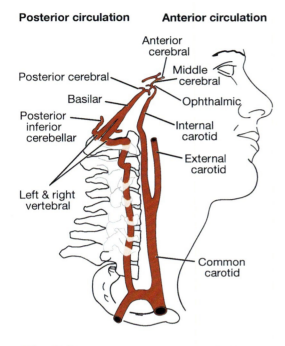

Fig. 11.8. Posterior and anterior circulations.

TIA or stroke in a patient younger than 55 years without obvious risk factors for cardiac disease or atherosclerosis should prompt an investigation for atypical causes of stroke. Arteriopathies, such as arteritis and dissection, or coagulation disorders are possible causes that should be investigated.

EVALUATION

The historical points that need to be ascertained for a patient presenting with cerebrovascular symptoms include cerebrovascular risk factors (Table 11.3), cardiac history, alcohol and drug use, use of hormone replacement or oral contraceptives, personal or family history of thrombotic disorders, history of miscarriages, history of migraine, recent trauma, hemorrhage, or surgery. The neurovascular examination should include blood pressure, pulse, auscultation for

Table 11.1.　Clinical Deficits Associated With the Anterior and Posterior Cerebral Circulations

Anterior (internal carotid) circulation	Posterior (vertebrobasilar) circulation
Hemiparesis	Hemiparesis
Contralateral body	Contralateral body
Contralateral face	Ipsilateral face
Hemisensory loss (cortical type)	Hemisensory loss
Contralateral body	Brainstem
Contralateral face	Contralateral body
Aphasia (left hemisphere)	Ipsilateral face
Monocular loss of vision	Thalamus—all modalities
	Contralateral body
	Contralateral face
	Homonymous hemianopia
	Diplopia
	Dysarthria
	Dysphagia
	Ataxia

Table 11.2. Mechanisms of Stroke

Cardiac disorders
  Valve-related emboli
    Calcific aortic stenosis, infective endocarditis, mitral valve prolapse, nonbacterial
      thrombotic endocarditis, prosthetic valves, rheumatic heart disease
  Intracardiac thrombus or tumor
    Atrial fibrillation, sick sinus syndrome, myocardial infarction, cardiac arrhythmias,
      congestive heart failure, cardiomyopathy, atrial myxoma, cardiac fibroelastoma
  Systemic venous thrombi and right-to-left cardiac shunt
    Atrial or ventricular septal defect, thrombophlebitis, pulmonary arteriovenous
      malformation
Large-vessel disease
  Atherosclerosis
    Cervical arteries, aortic arch, and major intracranial arteries
  Carotid artery dissection
    Traumatic, spontaneous, aortic dissection, fibromuscular dysplasia
  Other
    Fibromuscular dysplasia, Takayasu disease, vasospasm, moyamoya disease,
      homocystinuria, Fabry disease, pseudoxanthoma elasticum
Small-vessel disease
  Atherosclerosis or lipohyalinosis
  Infectious arteritis (from meningitis or any other infective process of the central nervous
    system)
  Noninfectious arteritis
  Systemic lupus erythematosus, polyarteritis nodosa, granulomatous angiitis, temporal
    arteritis, drug use, irradiation arteritis, Wegener granulomatosis, sarcoidosis, Behçet
    disease
Hematologic disorders
  Polycythemia, thrombocythemia, thrombotic thrombocytopenic purpura, sickle cell disease,
    dysproteinemia, increased homocysteine level, leukemia, disseminated intravascular
    coagulation, antiphospholipid antibody syndromes (lupus anticoagulant, anti-cardiolipin
    antibodies), protein C and protein S deficiencies, resistance to activated protein C,
    antithrombin III deficiency

Modified from Adams, AC: Neurology in Primary Care. FA Davis, Philadelphia, 2000, p 191. Used with permission of Mayo Foundation for Medical Education and Research.

bruits, assessment of peripheral pulses, and cardiac examination. The initial blood tests for evaluating patients who have cerebrovascular symptoms include a complete blood count, platelet count, electrolytes, glucose, creatinine, erythrocyte sedimentation rate, prothrombin time, activated partial thromboplastin time, and lipid analysis. Lipid analysis should include determining the levels of high-density lipoprotein and total cholesterol. The initial cardiac

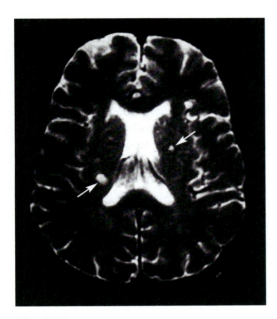

Fig. 11.9. MRI scan showing lacunar infarcts (*arrows*). (From Adams, AC: Neurology in Primary Care. FA Davis, Philadelphia, 2000, p 192. Used with permission of Mayo Foundation for Medical Education and Research.)

evaluation should include electrocardiography and chest radiography. The clinical presentation of the patient and the results of the initial tests will direct further evaluation. Many of the diagnostic tests used in the evaluation of cerebrovascular disorders and the indications for their use are summarized in Table 11.4.

TREATMENT

The treatment of TIA depends on the mechanism that causes the symptoms. For the majority of TIAs, antiplatelet agents are indicated. Other treatments could include anticoagulation, endovascular intervention, surgery, antibiotics, or immunosuppressant medication. All modifiable cerebrovascular risk factors should

be treated. If no evidence suggests a cardioembolic mechanism or high-grade vascular occlusive disease, antiplatelet therapy is recommended (Table 11.5). The effective dose of aspirin ranges from 50 mg once daily to 650 mg twice daily. The low-dose "baby aspirin" (81 mg) reduces the risk of adverse reactions that include gastrointestinal tract irritation, ulceration, and bleeding. The combination of aspirin and extended-release dipyridamole (Aggrenox) has been shown to be more effective than aspirin alone in the prevention of secondary stroke and TIA. This agent may be an option for patients who have recurrent TIAs while receiving aspirin therapy. Common side effects include headache, gastrointestinal irritation, and dizziness.

Other antiplatelet options include clopidogrel (Plavix) and ticlopidine (Ticlid). These agents are particularly important if the patient is allergic to or intolerant of aspirin. These agents, like the combination of aspirin and extended-release dipyridamole, may be an option for patients with recurrent TIAs who are receiving aspirin therapy. Ticlopidine has been associated with life-threatening hematologic effects and requires monitoring. Clopidogrel is an effective antiplatelet agent and does not require hematologic monitoring. The dose of clopidogrel is 75 mg once daily. The combination of clopidogrel and aspirin has been used to treat high-risk cardiovascular atherothrombotic disease, but it has not been shown to be effective for reducing the risk of ischemic stroke. The combination of aspirin and clopidogrel has been shown to increase the risk of bleeding complications.

Anticoagulation with warfarin is recommended if a cardiac source of emboli is identified as the mechanism of the TIA. Warfarin is also considered for patients with symptomatic intracranial stenosis for whom antiplatelet agents have failed. The therapeutic range of

Table 11.3. Cerebrovascular Risk Factors

Nonmodifiable
>   Heredity, male sex, older age, race and ethnicity

Modifiable
>   Hypertension, atrial fibrillation, tobacco smoking, hyperlipidemia, heavy alcohol use, asymptomatic carotid artery stenosis, transient ischemic attack, cardiac disease, diabetes mellitus, physical inactivity

Cardiac risk factors
>   Established
>>   Atrial fibrillation, valvular heart disease, dilated cardiomyopathy, recent myocardial infarction, intracardiac thrombus

>   Suspected
>>   Sick sinus syndrome, patent foramen ovale, aortic arch atheroma, myocardial infarction within the last 2 months, left ventricular dysfunction, atrial septal aneurysm, mitral anular calcification, mitral valve strands, spontaneous echocardiographic contrast (transesophageal echocardiographic finding)

Potential stroke risk factors
>   Antiphospholipid antibodies, increased homocysteine levels, infection (*Chlamydia pneumoniae*, *Helicobcter pylori*, peridontal infection), systemic inflammation, migraine, oral contraceptive use, sympathomimetic pharmaceuticals, illicit drug use, obesity, stress, snoring, sleep apnea, physical inactivity, impaired fasting glucose, poor diet or nutrition

From Adams, AC: Neurology in Primary Care. FA Davis, Philadelphia, 2000, p 194. Used with permission of Mayo Foundation for Medical Education and Research.

anticoagulation is an international normalized ratio (INR) between 2.0 and 3.0. A higher range, 2.5 to 4.5, is used for patients with mechanical heart valves, intracardiac thrombus, or recurrent cardiac embolus. If the patient is receiving anticoagulation with heparin, the treatment is usually continued until the patient reaches the therapeutic range with oral anticoagulation. Bleeding is the major complication of warfarin therapy, and hypertension and increasing age increase the risk of hemorrhagic complications. The usual starting dose is 5 mg daily but is adjusted according to the INR. The INR is monitored daily until the level of anticoagulation has stabilized, and it may be checked monthly after the maintenance dose of

warfarin has been established. Be aware of any potential drug interactions in a patient receiving warfarin therapy.

PREVENTION OF A FIRST STROKE

Stroke prevention strategies begin with identifying the patients who are at high risk for stroke and reducing or eliminating modifiable risk factors. Many of the identified cerebrovascular risk factors are listed in Table 11.3. Risk factors that cannot be modified include age, sex, heredity, and race or ethnicity. These nonmodifiable risk factors help identify patients who are at risk and may benefit from more aggressive

Table 11.4. Diagnostic Tests for Cerebrovascular Disorders

Test	Indication
Head CT without contrast medium*	Determine if hemorrhage or ischemia Eligibility for thrombolytic therapy
Complete blood count with platelet count*	Polycythemia, thrombocytosis, hematologic malignancy
Partial thromboplastin time, prothrombin time*	Coagulation disorder
Chemistry screen*	Liver and kidney function, glucose metabolism
Erythrocyte sedimentation rate*	Arteritis, systemic infection, or malignancy
Lipid analysis*	Hyperlipidemia with atheromatous plaques
Electrocardiography*	Cardiac arrhythmia, ischemia
Chest radiography*	Cardiopulmonary status
Additional cardiac evaluation: Holter monitoring, transthoracic echocardiography, transesophageal echocardiography, MRI of heart, cine-CT of heart	Emboli from heart valves, intracardiac thrombi from local stagnation and endocardial alterations, shunting of systemic venous thrombi into arterial circulation
Arterial evaluation: Carotid ultrasonography, transcranial Doppler, MRA, arteriography	Arterial occlusive disease, arteritis, arterial dissection, angiopathy
Homocysteine level, vitamin B_{12}, and folate	Increased homocysteine levels are associated with atherosclerotic vascular disease
Hematologic evaluation: Anticardiolipin antibodies, lupus anticoagulant, protein C, protein S, antithrombin III, serum fibrinogen, bleeding time, hemoglobin electrophoresis	Hematologic abnormalities, hypercoagulable state
Infectious: Treponemal antibody absorption test, blood cultures, CSF analysis	Syphilis, infective endocarditis, central nervous system infections
CSF analysis	Subarachnoid hemorrhage with negative imaging studies, meningitis, neurosyphilis
Electroencephalography	Coma, brain death
MRI	Small infarcts, posterior fossa infarcts, tumors, vascular malformations

CSF, cerebrospinal fluid; CT, computed tomography; MRA, magnetic resonance angiography; MRI, magnetic resonance imaging.
*Test for initial evaluation.
From Adams, AC: Neurology in Primary Care. FA Davis, Philadelphia, 2000, p 193. Used with permission of Mayo Foundation for Medical Education and Research.

Table 11.5. Antiplatelet Agents

Medication	Dose	Clinical comment
Aspirin	50 mg once daily to 650 mg twice daily	Lower dose reduces risk of side effects Onset of action is immediate Favorable cost
Aspirin/dipyridamole (Aggrenox)	25 mg/200 mg twice daily	Common side effects are headache, gastrointestinal symptoms, and dizziness
Clopidogrel (Plavix)	75 mg once daily	When combined with aspirin, may increase risk for bleeding Adverse effects include rash, diarrhea, and hematologic effects
Ticlopidine (Ticlid)	250 mg twice daily	Potential adverse hematologic effects limit use

preventative treatments. Increasing age is a risk factor for stroke, and the risk doubles each decade over the age of 55 years. Men have a greater risk than women. Both African Americans and Hispanic Americans have an increased incidence of stroke compared with that of whites. The stroke risk is also greater for persons whose parents had a stroke. The influence of heredity and environmental factors is an area of ongoing study.

Risk factors for which the value of modification has definitely been established include hypertension, atrial fibrillation, cigarette smoking, hyperlipidemia, heavy alcohol use, asymptomatic carotid artery stenosis, and TIA. Many other medical disorders and lifestyle issues can increase the risk for stroke.

The most prevalent and modifiable risk factor for stroke is hypertension. It is a risk factor for ischemic stroke and intracerebral and subarachnoid hemorrhage. Hypertension is defined as systolic pressure of 140 mm Hg or more and diastolic pressure of 90 mm Hg or more. The risk of stroke increases with an increase in both systolic and diastolic pressure as well as with isolated systolic hypertension. Treatment of hypertension decreases the risk of stroke. Blood pressure should be controlled in patients with hypertension who are most likely to develop stroke. Blood pressure should be measured as part of regular health care visits, and patients with hypertension should monitor their blood pressure at home.

The risk of ischemic stroke is increased after myocardial infarction, with the greatest risk during the first month after infarction. Anticoagulation with warfarin (INR, 2.0-3.0) is recommended after myocardial infarction in patients who have atrial fibrillation, decreased left ventricular function (ejection fraction, ≤28%), or left ventricular thrombi. Aspirin is recommended for the prevention of subsequent myocardial infarction. Lipid-lowering agents, particularly 3-hydroxy-3-methylglutaryl coenzyme A (HMG-CoA) reductase inhibitors (statin agents), reduce the risk of stroke after a myocardial infarction. The US Food and Drug Administration has approved pravastatin

(Pravachol) for patients who have had a myocardial infarction and have average cholesterol levels less than 240 mg/dL. Simvastatin (Zocor) has been approved for use in preventing stroke and TIA in patients with coronary heart disease and cholesterol levels of 240 mg/dL or more. In addition to the benefits of lipid-lowering therapy for patients with cardiovascular disease, it has been shown that this therapy can decrease the rate of stroke and other major vascular events.

Atrial fibrillation is an important risk factor for stroke. In comparison with patients without atrial fibrillation, the risk is 17 times higher for those with atrial fibrillation associated with valvular heart disease and 5 times higher for those with nonvalvular atrial fibrillation. The recommended guidelines for treating patients who have atrial fibrillation depend on age and the associated risk factors of previous stroke or TIA, hypertension, heart failure, and diabetes mellitus. Patients older than 75 years with or without risk factors should receive warfarin therapy. Patients 65 to 75 years old who have risk factors should also receive warfarin therapy, and those without risk factors should receive treatment with warfarin or aspirin. Patients younger than 65 years who have risk factors should receive warfarin and those without risk factors should receive aspirin.

Diabetes mellitus increases the risk of stroke in numerous ways. Large-artery atherosclerosis is accelerated by glycosylation-induced injury, adverse effects on cholesterol level, and promotion of plaque formation through hyperinsulinemia. Diabetes is associated with small-vessel ischemia, or lacunar infarction. Even patients with glucose intolerance (fasting blood glucose level, 110-125 mg/dL) have an increased risk of stroke. Patients with diabetes have an increased probability of hypertension, hyperlipidemia, and obesity. In addition to glycemic control to reduce microvascular complications and other complications of the disease, patients with diabetes should receive treatment directed at achieving good blood pressure control.

Carotid artery stenosis is another known risk factor for TIA and stroke. The course of action that should be taken for patients who have symptomatic carotid artery stenosis is better defined and less controversial than that for patients who have asymptomatic carotid artery stenosis. Published guidelines for asymptomatic carotid artery stenosis recommend endarterectomy for patients who have a stenosis of more than 60%, as defined with angiography, and a perioperative risk less than 3%. Despite this, many neurologists do not recommend endarterectomy because of the low rate of stroke in medically treated patients and several issues of controversy concerning asymptomatic carotid artery studies. The cardiac status and other medical illnesses of a patient need to be factored into the decision about endarterectomy. The status of the other carotid artery and the vertebral arteries is important in the decision about surgery. Patients with bilateral carotid artery occlusive disease or those with rapidly progressive stenosis may be at higher risk for stroke. Medical therapy for asymptomatic carotid arteries includes antiplatelet therapy plus modification of other cerebrovascular risk factors. Statin drugs may have a role in plaque stabilization.

Tobacco smoking is an independent risk factor for ischemic stroke and is dose related. The mechanisms for this increased risk include progression of atherosclerosis, enhanced platelet aggregation, increased blood pressure, and increased blood viscosity, coagulability, and fibrinogen levels. Smoking cessation leads to a reduction in stroke risk.

The risk of stroke from alcohol consumption is different for hemorrhagic and ischemic strokes. Alcohol has a direct dose-dependent effect on the risk of hemorrhagic stroke. Moderate alcohol consumption, defined as from one drink annually to two drinks daily, is independently associated with a decreased risk of ischemic stroke. Heavy alcohol consumption, defined as five or more drinks daily, is associated with an increased risk of ischemic stroke. The mechanisms for the increased risk include the induction of hypertension, hypercoagulable state, cardiac arrhythmias, and decreased cerebral blood flow. The mechanisms for the beneficial effect of light or moderate consumption include increasing high-density lipoprotein cholesterol levels and decreasing fibrinogen levels and platelet aggregation.

Several studies have demonstrated a benefit for stroke risk with physical activity. Regular exercise has well-established benefits for reducing cardiovascular disease and premature death. The protective effect of physical activity may be related to its role in reducing other risk factors such as hypertension and diabetes. The mechanisms include decreasing fibrinogen levels and platelet activity and increasing high-density lipoprotein concentrations. Moderate physical activity for 30 minutes each day, five days a week is recommended. The duration of physical activity recommended by various guidelines has consistently increased over the last several years.

An increased level of the amino acid homocysteine is associated with atherogenesis and thrombosis. Homocysteine levels can be lowered with folate (400 µg to 1 mg daily), vitamin B_{12} (500 µg daily), and vitamin B_6 (10-12.5 mg daily). Although no definitive benefit has been demonstrated with the use of vitamins, it is reasonable to consider recommending them to patients who have increased levels of homocysteine.

Other potential risk factors for stroke are being investigated (Table 11.3). Antiphospholipid antibodies (acquired autoantibodies directed against various phospholipids) are potential risk factors for stroke. These autoantibodies, which include lupus anticoagulant, anticardiolipin, and antiphosphatidylserine antibodies, are often found in patients who have autoimmune disease and are a risk factor for arterial and venous thrombosis. Inflammation and infection are also potential risk factors for stroke. Stroke prevention strategies will improve as cerebrovascular risk factors become better defined.

SYMPTOMATIC CAROTID ARTERY STENOSIS

The internal carotid artery supplies all the structures of the frontal and parietal lobes, including the part on the medial surface of the cerebral hemisphere, and the lateral portion and pole of the temporal lobe. Clinical findings of carotid artery disease include transient monocular blindness, contralateral hemiparesis, hemianesthesia, hemianopia, aphasia (left hemisphere), and hemineglect (right hemisphere).

A physical finding that indicates carotid artery disease is the presence of retinal emboli seen on ophthalmoscopic examination (Fig. 11.10). Retinal emboli are seen at the bifurcation of the retinal arterioles. Fibrin-platelet emboli are gray-white, and cholesterol emboli (Hollenhorst plaques) are shiny and orange-yellow. Both types are consistent with carotid embolization from ipsilateral atherosclerotic lesions.

A bruit (the sound of turbulent blood flow in the underlying artery) can be detected with auscultation by gently placing the bell of the stethoscope over the carotid artery. A localized or diffuse carotid bruit heard in a patient with cerebrovascular ischemic symptoms is 85% predictive of a moderate or high-grade stenosis. However, bruits are not detected in more than one-third of patients with high-grade stenosis. A carotid bruit is a poor predictor of stenosis.

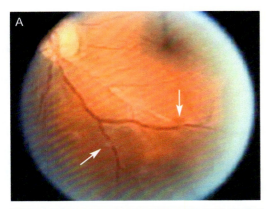

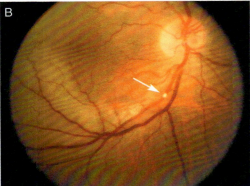

Fig. 11.10. Retinal emboli. *A*, Fibrin-platelet emboli (*arrows*); *B*, cholesterol embolus (Hollenhorst plaque) (*arrow*).

Clinical features alone are not sufficient for determining which patients would benefit from surgery. Carotid (Doppler) ultasonography can measure blood velocity and show arterial morphology with a high degree of accuracy. This is a useful method for investigating the cause of ischemic symptoms and for evaluating patients for possible surgical or endovascular treatment of carotid artery disease. Carotid ultrasonography cannot detect intracranial occlusive disease or provide information about collateral circulation (Fig. 11.11). Extracranial and intracranial magnetic resonance angiography (MRA) or CT angiography are recommended if carotid endarterectomy is to be pursued. Conventional angiography may be needed if ultasonography or MRA/CT angiography provide conflicting information or if these tests are not feasible (Fig. 11.12).

Carotid endarterectomy is a beneficial surgical procedure for preventing strokes in patients with symptomatic carotid stenosis. The surgical benefit depends on the risk of surgery. The combined morbidity and mortality for carotid endarterectomy is between 2% and 6% at experienced medical centers. Mortality rates are greater for surgeons (and hospitals) who perform few carotid endarterectomies.

Clinical trials have shown that carotid endarterectomy is better than medical therapy for patients with stenosis of 70% or more associated with recent (within 2-4 weeks) retinal or cerebral ischemia (TIA) or minor stroke. The benefit of endarterectomy is greatest within the first 2 to 3 years after the operation.

Endarterectomy provides a moderate reduction in the risk of stroke for patients with symptomatic carotid artery stenosis of 50% to 69%. The modest reduction emphasizes the importance of selecting a surgeon with established surgical skill and a patient with low surgical risk. If the risk of stroke or death from surgery exceeds 6%, the benefit of surgery is lost. Carotid endarterectomy should be performed only by surgeons with a low rate of complications, as determined by independent monitoring. A subgroup of patients with 50% to 69% stenosis that is more likely to benefit from surgery are older men and patients with irregular and ulcerated plaque. Medical management is recommended for patients with carotid artery stenosis less than 50%.

Many risk factors can influence perioperative risk and should be considered in the decision to pursue carotid endarterectomy. Medical risk factors include hypertension (blood pressure > 180/110 mm Hg), recent myocardial infarction, congestive heart failure, angina, chronic

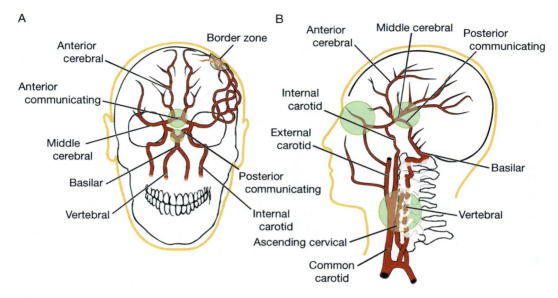

Fig. 11.11. Collateral circulation. *A*, Anteroposterior view. The anterior communicating artery connects the right and left carotid circulations. Leptomeningeal anastomoses form collateral pathways among the border zones of major arterial territories. *B*, Lateral view. Green circles indicate important collateral pathways. (From Pessin, MS, and Teal, PA: Cardinal clinical features of ischemic cerebrovascular disease in relation to vascular territories. In Samuels, MA, and Feske, S [eds]: Office Practice of Neurology. Churchill Livingstone, New York, 1996, pp 311-329. Used with permission.)

obstructive pulmonary disease, severe obesity, and age older than 70 years. Patients who have neurologic deficits from multiple cerebral infarctions, a progressive neurologic deficit, neurologic deficit less than 24 hours in duration, or daily TIAs are at increased risk for perioperative complications. Angiographic evidence of additional vascular disease is also associated with an increased risk.

The complications associated with carotid endarterectomy such as wound hematoma and infection can occur with any surgical procedure. Complications unique to carotid endarterectomy include postoperative carotid occlusion, TIA, and stroke. These complications usually result from technical errors. Increased cerebral blood flow after the procedure can cause headache, intracerebral hemorrhage, or brain edema. The nerves at risk for injury during the procedure

include the recurrent laryngeal, superior laryngeal, vagus, spinal accessory, and hypoglossal nerves. The potential complications of endarterectomy emphasizes the importance of the skill and experience of the surgical team.

Patients who have atherosclerotic carotid artery disease frequently have coronary artery disease. In fact, patients who survive an atherosclerotic stroke are more likely to die of a coronary event than recurrent stroke. Because carotid artery and cardiac diseases are coincident, questions arise about the possibility of simultaneous carotid endarterectomy and coronary artery surgery. The risk of perioperative ischemic stroke for any operation is 0.2%. For coronary bypass grafting, the risk is 1.4% to 2%. The risk increases to 8.5% for patients undergoing coronary bypass grafting who recently had a TIA or stroke. Carotid endarterectomy should be

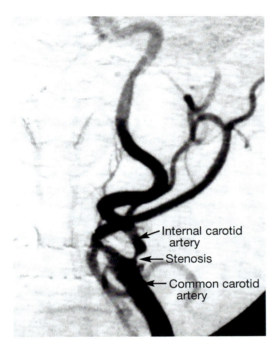

Internal carotid artery
Stenosis
Common carotid artery

Fig. 11.12. Angiogram showing internal carotid artery stenosis. (From Adams, AC: Neurology in Primary Care. FA Davis, Philadelphia, 2000, p 198. Used with permission of Mayo Foundation for Medical Education and Research.)

considered for patients with symptomatic disease before they have a general surgical procedure. For patients who have both symptomatic coronary and carotid stenoses, combined carotid and coronary surgery may be reasonable. Carotid artery stenting may be an option for these patients. The risk of perioperative stroke with asymptomatic carotid artery stenosis is low, and a preoperative or simultaneous prophylactic carotid endarterectomy is not necessary.

Carotid artery stenting and angioplasty are options to consider for patients who have carotid stenosis in a location not amenable to endarterectomy or for patients whose medical risk is too high for them to undergo endarterectomy. Neurosurgical consultation is recommended when considering these procedures.

STROKE IN YOUNG ADULTS

Stroke in persons younger than 45 years is uncommon. In addition to the usual mechanisms of cerebrovascular disease, the investigation of a young person with a stroke should include evaluation of the less common causes of stroke, such as angiopathies, unusual cardiac embolic disorders, inflammatory conditions, illicit drug use, and hematologic disorders.

Migrainous Stroke

The criteria for the diagnosis of migrainous stroke have been defined by the International Headache Society Classification of Head Pain. Migrainous stroke occurs in a patient who has a previous diagnosis of migraine with aura when that patient has one or more migrainous symptoms that persist longer than 60 minutes and neuroimaging confirms ischemic infarction in the relevant area. Migrainous stroke is diagnosed if other causes of infarction have been excluded by appropriate investigation. The four types of migraine-related stroke are the following:

1) A stroke that occurs remotely in time from a migraine attack
2) A stroke with migraine symptoms, sometimes called a migraine mimic (eg, arteriovenous malformation that causes symptoms of migraine)
3) A migraine-induced stroke (preceding symptoms resemble those of a previous migraine attack; other causes of stroke have been excluded)
4) Stroke of uncertain cause

The diagnosis of migraine-induced stroke is one of exclusion and a comprehensive cerebrovascular evaluation needs to be performed to determine whether there are other causes of stroke and to identify other risk factors. An increase in the risk of stroke has been reported for women with migraine who take oral contraceptives, especially high-dose estrogen preparations. This risk is even higher for patients who smoke. Advise patients to avoid these risk factors. Migraine prophylaxis should be optimized. Also, vasoconstrictive medications should be avoided or their use limited. Taking aspirin daily is reasonable for patients who have prolonged or frequent attacks of migraine with aura.

Arterial Dissection

If a young person has a stroke, consider nonatherosclerotic angiopathy. Arterial dissection is a potential cause of stroke by arterial narrowing or the formation of thrombus with secondary embolization. Common sites of dissection are the proximal internal carotid artery beyond the bifurcation and the distal extracranial vertebral artery. Arterial dissection is frequently associated with neck trauma, but it can occur spontaneously or in association with an angiopathy such as fibromuscular dysplasia. Patients with arterial dissection frequently complain of headache. If the carotid artery is involved, the pain may be referred to the eye, and involvement of the sympathetic fibers that course along the carotid artery may cause Horner syndrome (see Fig. 1.8). If the vertebral artery is involved, the patient may complain of pain in the neck or back of the head and have a lateral medullary syndrome (Fig. 11.3).

The diagnosis of arterial dissection can be made with angiography or MRA. If more than one vessel is involved, consider diseases of the arterial wall, such as fibromuscular dysplasia, Marfan syndrome, and Ehlers-Danlos syndrome. Treatment options are anticoagulant and antiplatelet therapies.

Illicit Drug Use

Illicit drug use is a potential cause of stroke in young adults. Drugs associated with both ischemic and hemorrhagic strokes include amphetamines, cocaine, heroin, phencyclidine, phenylpropanolamine, and lysergic acid diethylamide (LSD). The mechanisms of stroke include direct vascular effects, inflammatory and non-inflammatory arteritis, prothrombic state, cardiac arrhythmias, and endocarditis.

Hematologic and Systemic Disorders

Hematologic disorders also can cause both ischemic and hemorrhagic strokes. Sickle cell disease is one of the more common hematologic disorders associated with stroke in young people. Hypercoagulable states due to malignancies and other systemic disorders are potential causes of stroke. Other systemic disorders such as sarcoidosis and connective tissue disease can cause vasculitis, leading to stroke. Syphilis, Lyme disease, tuberculosis, and fungal and bacterial infections can all cause stroke.

Cardiac Causes

In addition to the cardiac causes in older adults, unusual causes of cardiac emboli may be found in young adults, including congenital heart disease, patent foramen ovale, postpartum cardiomyopathy, and cardiac tumors. Transesophageal echocardiography, MRI of the heart, and cardiology evaluation may be needed if a cardiac source of emboli is suspected.

TREATMENT OF ACUTE STROKE: THROMBOLYTIC THERAPY

The treatment of acute stroke has changed remarkably since the publication of the findings of the National Institute of Neurological Disorders and Stroke Study Group on tissue plasminogen activator (tPA) for acute ischemic stroke. The disability caused by stroke can be effectively reduced by acute early intervention. The effectiveness depends on many factors. Public education is essential so patients recognize a brain attack as a medical emergency. Potential candidates for treatment need to be identified correctly and transported immediately to an emergency department. Emergency departments, hospitals, and medical personnel need plans for correctly diagnosing and treating acute stroke within the limited therapeutic time. On admission to the emergency department, the following should be obtained: body weight, complete blood count, platelet count, electrolytes, glucose, aspartate aminotransferase, activated partial thromboplastin time, prothrombin time, electrocardiography, chest radiography, and CT (without contrast) of the head.

Patients with a severe or progressive ischemic stroke should be considered for thrombolytic therapy. *The onset of symptoms needs to be less than 3 hours before treatment is started.* For patients who awaken from sleep with a neurologic deficit, the time of symptom onset is the time they went to bed. CT should not show any evidence of intracranial hemorrhage, mass effect, or midline shift.

The pretreatment guidelines for administering tPA are summarized in Table 11.6. Exclusion criteria for thrombolytic therapy include patients with any of the following:

- A rapidly improving deficit
- Obtundation or coma
- Seizure
- Mild deficit
- Blood pressure greater than 185/110 mm Hg
- Gastrointestinal or urinary tract hemorrhage within the preceding 21 days
- Ischemic stroke or serious head trauma within the preceding 3 months
- A history of intracranial hemorrhage or bleeding diathesis
- Major surgical procedure within the preceding 2 weeks
- Arterial puncture at a noncompressible site or lumbar puncture within the preceding week

Laboratory abnormalities that exclude patients from thrombolytic therapy are 1) heparin treatment within the preceding 48 hours, with an increased activated partial thromboplastin time, 2) anticoagulant treatment, with a prothrombin time of more than 15 seconds, or 3) a glucose level less than 50 mg/dL or more than 400 mg/dL.

Thrombolytic therapy with tPA is effective in improving neurologic status if administered within 3 hours after the onset of symptoms. In the treatment trial, a greater proportion (12% greater absolute difference) of patients who received tPA had minimal or no deficit at 3 months compared with those who received placebo. More importantly, there was no increase in severe deficits or disability in the tPA group.

Intravenous tPA is given in a 0.9-mg/kg dose (maximum, 90 mg), with 10% given as a bolus and the rest given over 60 minutes. The patient's condition should be monitored in an intensive care unit, and blood pressure should be less than 185/105 mm Hg. Heparin and antiplatelet therapy should not be administered for 24 hours after tPA therapy.

The major complication of thrombolytic therapy is intracranial hemorrhage. This complication should be suspected if the neurologic status of the patient deteriorates. If CT confirms hemorrhage, consider replacement therapy with platelets and cryoprecipitate.

HEMORRHAGIC STROKE

Hemorrhagic stroke, including intracerebral and subarachnoid hemorrhage, accounts for 15% of all strokes. The diagnosis of hemorrhagic stroke can be made with CT (Fig. 11.4). The causes of spontaneous intracerebral hemorrhage include hypertension, aneurysm rupture, vascular malformations, bleeding diatheses, drug-related hemorrhage, tumors, and cerebral venous occlusive

Table 11.6. Pretreatment Guidelines for Tissue Plasminogen Activator (tPA)

	Consider tPA	No tPA
Clinical	≤3 hours* from focal anterior or posterior circulation ischemic symptom onset[†]	>3 hours from focal anterior or posterior circulation ischemic symptom onset[†]
	Fixed significant or progressive deficit	Rapidly resolving or minor deficit
	Alert or somnolent patient	Obtunded or comatose patient
	No seizure in association with stroke	Seizure at onset of stroke
	No history of intracranial hemorrhage or bleeding diathesis	History of intracranial hemorrhage or bleeding diathesis
	No history of ischemic stroke or serious head injury within 3 months	Ischemic stroke or serious head injury within 3 months[‡]
	BP elevations rapidly responsive to use of labetalol and similar agents and maintained at ≤185 mm Hg systolic, ≤110 mm Hg diastolic pretreatment	BP elevations persistently >185 mm Hg systolic, >110 mm Hg diastolic despite antihypertensive therapy; patients requiring aggressive therapy (eg, sodium nitroprusside) to maintain above levels are excluded
	Absence of GI, UT hemorrhage within 21 days	GI or UT hemorrhage within 21 days
	No major surgery within 14 days	Major surgery within 14 days
	No recent myocardial infarction	Recent myocardial infarction
	No recent arterial puncture at a noncompressible site	Recent arterial puncture at a noncompressible site[§]
	No recent lumbar puncture	Recent lumbar puncture[§]
	Female patient who is not pregnant	Pregnant female patient
	Normal aPTT (either on heparin in the last 48 hours or not on heparin); INR ≤1.7 (either on warfarin or not on warfarin)	On heparin in the last 48 hours with elevated aPTT or INR >1.7
	Platelet count ≥100,000/mm^3 (≥100×10^9 cells/L)	Platelet count <100,000/mm^3 (<100×10^9 cells/L)
	Glucose ≥50 mg/dL	Glucose <50 mg/dL
CT	No evidence for significant early infarction,[¶] hemispheric swelling, or hemorrhage	Evidence for significant early infarction[¶] with focal mass effect, hemispheric swelling, or hemorrhage
	Absence of intracranial tumor	Intracranial tumor

aPTT, activated partial thromboplastin time; BP, blood pressure; CT, computed tomography; GI, gastrointestinal; INR, international normalized ratio; UT, urinary tract.

Table 11.6   (continued)

There is no evidence that tPA administered 3-6 hours after the onset of symptoms is efficacious, and it typically is not given more than 3 hours after the onset of symptoms. Intra-arterial thrombolysis may still be considered for selected patients who have had symptoms for more than 3 hours.

†*For patients who wake up with stroke symptoms, the time they went to bed defines the time of symptom onset.*

‡*Selected patients with minor cerebral infarction within the last 3 months may be considered for tPA therapy depending on the clinical circumstances.*

§*The risk of hemorrhagic complication in the setting of a recent lumbar puncture or arterial puncture at a noncompressible site is uncertain. Treatment in these situations should be considered cautiously for selected patients after review of the findings of the lumbar puncture or arterial puncture and the clinical circumstances.*

¶*The safety and efficacy of tPA for patients with CT scan showing early infarct changes is controversial. However, tPA generally is not contraindicated for patients with early infarct changes. In most patients with early findings suggesting a significant cerebral infarction (ie, >1/3 of middle cerebral artery distribution), tPA typically is not administered because of hemorrhage risk and low likelihood of efficacy.*

disease (Fig. 11.13). Hypertensive hemorrhage, the most common cause of intracerebral hemorrhage, is most likely to occur in the putamen, thalamus, cerebellum, pons, and caudate nucleus (Fig. 11.14). Lobar hemorrhage, or bleeding into the cerebral cortex and subcortical white matter, can occur in any lobe of the brain and has many causes.

The clinical features of hemorrhagic stroke depend on the location of the hemorrhage. Unlike embolic stroke, which has a maximal deficit at the time of onset, hemorrhagic stroke can progress over several minutes to hours. Blood in the form of a hematoma can behave like a mass lesion. Headache, decreased level of consciousness, and seizure are more likely to occur in hemorrhagic stroke than in ischemic stroke.

The diagnostic evaluation of patients who have hemorrhagic stroke is the same as for those who have ischemic stroke (Table 11.4). MRA or cerebral angiography (or both) is essential to evaluate for aneurysms, vascular malformations, and arteriopathies. Repeat MRA or angiography in 2 to 3 months may be necessary if the initial study findings are negative. The hematoma may obscure a vascular abnormality or small tumor. Follow-up CT or MRI may be needed for the same reason.

In hemorrhagic stroke, the management concerns are to identify the cause of the hemorrhage and to control blood pressure. Surgical therapy may be necessary for progressively enlarging hematomas. Neurointensivist and neurosurgical consultation is recommended for the management of hemorrhagic strokes.

A

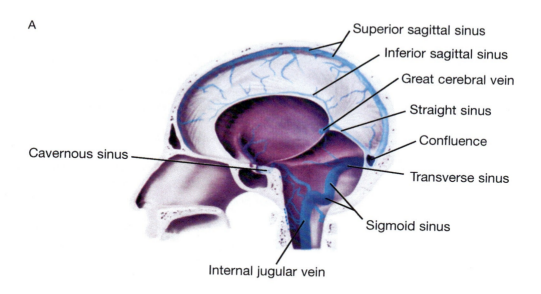

Superior sagittal sinus

Inferior sagittal sinus

Great cerebral vein

Straight sinus

Confluence

Transverse sinus

Cavernous sinus

Sigmoid sinus

Internal jugular vein

B

Superior sagittal sinus

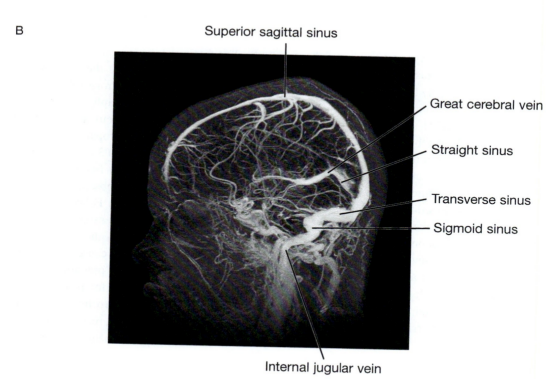

Great cerebral vein

Straight sinus

Transverse sinus

Sigmoid sinus

Internal jugular vein

Fig. 11.13. Venous sinuses. *A,* Cerebral veins and venous sinuses *B,* Magnetic resonance venography showing normal pattern (sagittal view). (*A* from Hanaway, J, et al: The Brain Atlas: A Visual Guide to the Human Central Nervous System. Fitzgerald Science Press, Bethesda, MD, 1998, p 28. Used with permission.)

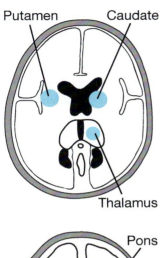

Putamen   Caudate

Thalamus   Hypertensive
              hemorrhage

Pons

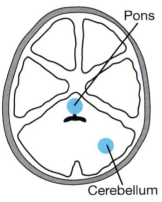

Cerebellum

Lobar
hemorrhage

Fig. 11.14. Locations of hypertensive and lobar hemorrhagic strokes. (From Adams, AC: Neurology in Primary Care. FA Davis, Philadelphia, 2000, p. 201. Used with permission of Mayo Foundation for Medical Education and Research.)

SUGGESTED READING

Albers, GW, et al, TIA Working Group: Transient ischemic attack: Proposal for a new definition. N Engl J Med 347:1713-1716, 2002.

Amarenco, P, et al, Stroke Prevention by Aggressive Reduction in Cholesterol Levels (SPARCL) Investigators: High-dose atorvastatin after stroke or transient ischemic attack. N Engl J Med 355:549-559, 2006.

Blacker, DJ, et al: The preoperative cerebrovascular consultation: Common cerebrovascular questions before general or cardiac surgery. Mayo Clin Proc 79:223-229, 2004.

Chaturvedi, S, et al, Therapeutics and Technology Assessment Subcommittee of the American Academy of Neurology: Carotid endarterectomy: An evidence-based review: Report of the Therapeutics and Technology Assessment Subcommittee of the American Academy of Neurology. Neurology 65:794-801, 2005.

Chimowitz, MI, et al, Warfarin-Aspirin Symptomatic Intracranial Disease Trial Investigators: Comparison of warfarin and aspirin for symptomatic intracranial arterial stenosis. N Engl J Med 352:1305-1316, 2005.

Donnan, GA, et al: Patients with transient ischemic attack or minor stroke should be admitted to hospital: for. Stroke 37:1137-1138, 2006. Epub 2006 Mar 16.

Elkind, MS: Inflammation, atherosclerosis, and stroke. Neurologist 12:140-148, 2006.

Eshaghian, S, et al: Role of clopidogrel in managing atherothrombotic cardiovascular disease. Ann Intern Med 146:434-441, 2007.

Flemming, KD, and Brown, RD, Jr: Secondary prevention strategies in ischemic stroke: Identification and optimal management of modifiable risk factors. Mayo Clin Proc 79:1330-1340, 2004.

Flemming, KD, et al: Evaluation and management of transient ischemic attack and minor cerebral infarction. Mayo Clin Proc 79:1071-1086, 2004.

Goldstein, LB, and Hankey, GJ: Advances in primary stroke prevention. Stroke 37:317-319, 2006. Epub 2006 Jan 12.

Goldstein, LB, and Simel, DL: Is this patient having a stroke? JAMA 293:2391-2402, 2005.

Hankey, GJ: Secondary prevention of recurrent stroke. Stroke 36:218-221, 2005. Epub 2005 Jan 6.

Hankey, GJ: Potential new risk factors for ischemic stroke: What is their potential? Stroke 37:2181-2188, 2006. Epub 2006 Jun 29.

Hankey, GJ, and Eikelboom, JW: Adding aspirin to clopidogrel after TIA and ischemic stroke: Benefits do not match risks. Neurology 64:1117-1121, 2005.

Howard, G, et al: Stroke and the statistics of the aspirin/clopidogrel secondary prevention trials. Curr Opin Neurol 20:71-77, 2007.

Johnston, SC, et al: National Stroke Association guidelines for the management of transient ischemic attacks. Ann Neurol 60:301-313, 2006.

Kittner, SJ, et al: Cerebral infarction in young adults: The Baltimore-Washington Cooperative Young Stroke Study. Neurology 50:890-894, 1998.

Lindley, RI: Patients with transient ischemic attack do not need to be admitted to hospital for urgent evaluation and treatment: against. Stroke 37:1139-1140, 2006. Epub 2006 Mar 16.

Mas, JL, et al, EVA-3S Investigators: Endarterectomy versus stenting in patients with symptomatic severe carotid stenosis. N Engl J Med 355:1660-1671, 2006.

National Institute of Neurological Disorders and Stroke rt-PA Stroke Study Group: Tissue plasminogen activator for acute ischemic stroke. N Engl J Med 333:1581-1587, 1995.

Prabhakaran, S: Reversible brain ischemia: Lessons from transient ischemic attack. Curr Opin Neurol 20:65-70, 2007.

Redgrave, JN, and Rothwell, PM: Asymptomatic carotid stenosis: What to do. Curr Opin Neurol 20:58-64, 2007.

Ringleb, PA: Thrombolytics, anticoagulants, and antiplatelet agents. Stroke 37:312-313, 2006. Epub 2006 Jan 12.

Rothwell, PM, and Johnston, SC: Transient ischemic attacks: Stratifying risk. Stroke 37:320-322, 2006. Epub 2006 Jan 12.

Touze E, et al: Risk of myocardial infarction and vascular death after transient ischemic attack and ischemic stroke: A systematic review and meta-analysis. Stroke 36:2748-2755, 2005. Epub 2005 Oct 27.

Wiebers, DO, Feigin, VL, and Brown, RD, Jr: Handbook of Stroke, ed 2. Lippincott Williams & Wilkins, Philadelphia, 2006.

CHAPTER 12

Movement Disorders

CLASSIFYING MOVEMENT DISORDERS

Movement disorders are neurologic syndromes in which movement is either excessive (*hyperkinesia*) or too little (*hypokinesia*). A general term used for both hyperkinesia and hypokinesia is *dyskinesia*, which is defined as difficulty with performing voluntary movements. The prototypic hypokinetic movement disorder is Parkinson disease. Other terms used to describe this movement disorder are *bradykinesia* (slowness of movement) and *akinesia* (loss of movement). Common hyperkinetic movement disorders include tremor, tics, and restless legs syndrome (see Chapter 9 for restless legs syndrome). The definition of many hypokinetic and hyperkinetic movement disorders and common clinical examples are listed in Table 12.1.

Movement is often classified as automatic, voluntary, semivoluntary, and involuntary. *Automatic movements* are motor behaviors that are performed without conscious effort, for example, the arm swing associated with walking. *Voluntary movements* are planned or intentional movements. They can also be induced by external stimuli, as in turning the head in response to a loud noise. *Semivoluntary movements* include the movements seen in tics, restless legs syndrome, and akathisia. They are induced by an inner sensory stimulus, not unlike the need to scratch an itch. They are also called "involuntary movements," because they are executed to negate an unwanted or unpleasant sensation. *Involuntary movements* include movements such as tremor and myoclonus. They are often nonsuppressible or only partially suppressible.

Movement disorders are associated frequently with disease or pathologic alterations of the basal ganglia or their connections: the caudate, putamen, globus pallidus, subthalamic nucleus, and substantia nigra (Fig. 12.1). Disorders of the cerebellum are associated with impaired coordination (asynergy and ataxia), impaired judgment of distance (dysmetria), and intention tremor. Myoclonus, or sudden shock-like involuntary movements caused by muscle contractions or inhibitions, can occur from disorders of any part of the central nervous system. Some rare movement disorders such as painful legs and moving toes syndrome are associated

Table 12.1. Definitions of Movement Disorders and Clinical Examples

Movement disorder	Definition	Clinical example
Hypokinetic		
Akinesia/bradykinesia	Absence or slowness of movement	Parkinson disease
Apraxia	Incapacity to execute purposeful movement not due to weakness, sensory loss, or incoordination	Parietal lobe lesion
Blocking tics	Motor phenomenon characterized by a brief interference of social discourse and contact	Tourette syndrome
Catatonia	Syndrome of psychomotor disturbances characterized by periods of physical rigidity, negativism, and bizarre mannerisms	Schizophrenia
Freezing phenomenon	Transient periods of several seconds in which motor act is halted	Parkinson disease
Hesitant gait	Slow cautious gait with wide base and short steps associated with fear of falling	Hydrocephalus
Rigidity	Increased muscle tone to passive motion	Parkinson disease
Stiff muscles	Continuous muscle contraction without muscle disease, rigidity, or spasticity	Stiff person syndrome
Hyperkinetic		
Akathisia	Inability to sit still, motor restlessness	Adverse effect of anti-dopaminergic drugs (eg, antipsychotic agents)
Asynergia or dyssynergia	Decomposition of movement from breakdown of normal coordinated execution of a voluntary movement	Cerebellar disease
Ataxia	Incoordination	Cerebellar disease
Athetosis	Slow, writhing, continuous involuntary movement	Perinatal injury
Ballism	Large jerking or shaking movements	Infarct of subthalamic nucleus (hemiballism)

Table 12.1   (continued)

Movement disorder	Definition	Clinical example
Chorea	Involuntary, irregular, purposeless, nonrhythmic, abrupt, rapid, unsustained movements that seem to flow from one body part to another	Huntington disease
Dysmetria	A form of dyssynergia	Cerebellar disease
Dystonia	A state of abnormal tone; twisting movements tend to be sustained at peak of movement and can be repetitive and progress to prolonged abnormal postures	Torticollis (cervical or focal dystonia)
Hemifacial spasm	Unilateral facial muscle contractions	Compression of facial nerve by aberrant blood vessels
Myoclonus	Sudden, brief, shocklike involuntary movements caused by muscle contractions or inhibitions	Asterixis (brief flapping of outstretched arms from metabolic encephalopathy)
Myokymia	Fine persistent quivering or rippling of muscles	Pontine lesion from multiple sclerosis
Stereotypy	Coordinated movements that are repeated continually and identically	Obsessive-compulsive disorder
Tics	Stereotyped, voluntary-appearing, purposeless movements	Tourette syndrome
Tremor	Oscillatory movements affecting one or more body parts	Essential tremor

From Adams, AC: Neurology in Primary Care. FA Davis, Philadelphia, 2000, pp 205-206. Used with permission of Mayo Foundation for Medical Education and Research.

with disorders of the peripheral nervous system. Many movement disorders are genetic, and the specific gene has been identified for several of them. Some of the more familiar inherited movement disorders are Huntington disease, Wilson disease, and familial essential tremor.

DIAGNOSTIC APPROACH TO MOVEMENT DISORDERS

If a patient has an abnormal movement, several questions need to be answered to distinguish among the different dyskinesias.

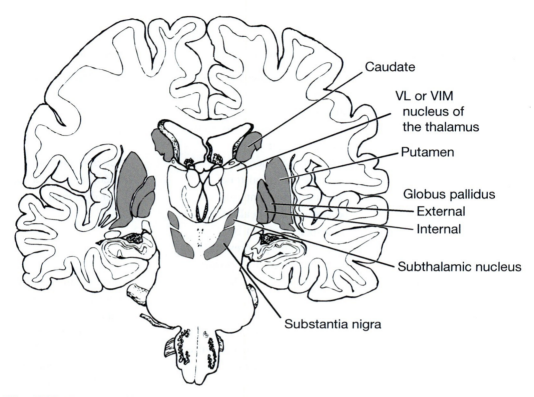

Fig. 12.1. The basal ganglia. VIM, ventral intermediate; VL, ventral lateral. (Modified from DeArmond, SJ, Fusco, MM, and Dewey, MM: Structure of the Human Brain: A Photographic Atlas. ed 3. Oxford University Press, New York, 1989, p 48. Used with permission.)

1) Is the movement rhythmical or arrhythmical? Tremor and myoclonus are rhythmical dyskinesias, and athetosis, ballism, chorea, and tic are arrhythmical movements.
2) What is the duration of movement? Most dyskinesias are brief, nonsustained movements. Focal dystonia such as torticollis or writer's cramp is a sustained abnormal movement.
3) What is the continuity of the contractions? Are the movements paroxysmal, as in tic? Are they continual, occurring over and over again, as in chorea? Are they continuous or unbroken, as in tremor?
4) Is there a relation to sleep? Most dyskinesias are diminished during sleep. However, periodic movements of sleep, hypnogenic dyskinesias, palatal myoclonus, myokymia, and moving toes are dyskinesias that appear or persist during sleep.

After initially observing the patient, determine whether the abnormal movement occurs at rest or with action. This is the major focus when evaluating a patient who has tremor. The tremor of Parkinson disease diminishes with action, whereas essential tremor occurs with action. Akathisic movement and restless legs are also associated with rest. The distribution of movement (focal or generalized), speed (fast or slow), and associated features help distinguish the various movement disorders.

PARKINSONISM

The diagnostic criteria for parkinsonism include bradykinesia, rest tremor, rigidity, and loss of postural reflexes. Other diagnostic features are flexed posture and freezing or motor blocks. The diagnosis is considered definitive if the patient has at least two of these features, with one of them being rest tremor or bradykinesia. The diagnosis of probable parkinsonism is made if rest tremor or bradykinesia is present alone. Without bradykinesia or rest tremor, at least two of the other features must be present for the diagnosis of possible parkinsonism (Table 12.2).

The four major categories of parkinsonism are primary, secondary, heredodegenerative, and multisystem degeneration. *Primary parkinsonism* is called *Parkinson disease*. *Secondary* (acquired or symptomatic) *parkinsonism* can result from anything that damages or interferes with the normal functioning of the motor control circuitry of the brain (eg, stroke, trauma, toxins, drugs, or infections), but the most common cause is exposure to dopamine receptor-blocking drugs (eg, antipsychotic or antiemetic agents). *Heredodegenerative parkinsonian disorders* are rare. The most familiar ones are Huntington disease and Wilson disease. *Multisystem degenerative*, or "parkinsonism plus," *disorders* include progressive supranuclear palsy, cortical-basal ganglionic degeneration, and multiple system atrophy disorders (eg, striatonigral degeneration, Shy-Drager syndrome, and sporadic olivopontocerebellar atrophy). The classification of parkinsonism is summarized in Table 12.3.

The diagnosis of parkinsonism can be difficult in the early stages of the disease. The primary focus of the evaluation of a patient with a hypokinetic movement disorder is to determine whether the diagnosis is "Parkinson disease" or "parkinsonism." This distinction is

Table 12.2. Diagnostic Criteria for Parkinsonism

1. **Rest tremor**
2. **Bradykinesia**
3. Rigidity
4. Loss of postural reflexes
5. Flexed posture
6. Motor blocks or freezing

Definite: At least two features must be present, with one being rest tremor or bradykinesia.
Probable: Either rest tremor or bradykinesia is present alone.
Possible: At least two of features 3 to 6 must be present.

important for prognosis and treatment. Patients with parkinsonism have a poorer prognosis and response to treatment than those with Parkinson disease.

The diagnosis of Parkinson disease is made clinically on the basis of the cardinal motor features of bradykinesia, rest tremor, rigidity, and postural instability. However, these clinical features are not specific and are of limited sensitivity for Parkinson disease. Autopsy studies have shown that the diagnosis of Parkinson disease is incorrect in approximately 25% of cases. The neuropathologic findings in the disease are Lewy bodies and loss of neurons in the substantia nigra.

Patients with early Parkinson disease rarely complain of slow movement. Instead, they usually complain of a feeling of weakness or fatigue. The term "weakness" is often used to describe difficulty with getting started or initiating movement. The most frequent complaints are trouble getting out of a car or bathtub, difficulty with turning in bed, difficulty buttoning clothing, stiffness, and tremor. Handwriting becomes slow and small (micrographia). Patients often describe the rigidity of Parkinson disease as

Table 12.3. Classification of Parkinsonism

Primary or idiopathic
   Parkinson disease
   Juvenile parkinsonism
Secondary
   Drugs: dopamine receptor blocking drugs (antipsychotic and antiemetic drugs)
   Infectious: postencephalitic, AIDS, SSPE, CJD, prion diseases
   Other: parathyroid abnormalities, hypothyroidism, hepatocerebral degeneration, brain
      tumors, paraneoplastic, normal-pressure hydrocephalus, psychogenic
   Toxins: MPTP, carbon monoxide, manganese, mercury, cyanide, methanol, ethanol
   Trauma
   Vascular: multi-infarct, Binswanger disease
Heredodegenerative
   Ceroid lipofuscinosis
   Disinhibition-dementia-parkinsonism
   Familial amyotrophy-dementia-parkinsonism
   Familial basal ganglia calcification
   Familial parkinsonism with peripheral neuropathy
   Familial progressive subcortical gliosis
   Gerstmann-Sträussler-Scheinker syndrome
   Hallervorden-Spatz disease
   Hereditary ceruloplasmin deficiency
   Hereditary hemochromatosis
   Hereditary juvenile dystonia-parkinsonism
   Huntington disease
   Lubag (X-linked dystonia-parkinsonism)
   Machado-Joseph disease
   Mitochondrial cytopathies with striatal necrosis
   Neuroacanthocytosis
   Olivopontocerebellar and spinocerebellar degeneration
   Parkinsonian-pyramidal syndrome
   Wilson disease
Multisystem degeneration
   Cortical-basal ganglionic degeneration
   Multiple system atrophy
   Olivopontocerebellar atrophy
   Pallidopyramidal disease
   Parkinsonism-dementia complex
   Parkinsonism-dementia-ALS complex of Guam
   Progressive pallidal atrophy
   Progressive supranuclear palsy or Steele-Richardson-Olszewski syndrome
   Shy-Drager syndrome
   Striatonigral degeneration

Table 12.3 (continued)

AIDS, acquired immunodeficiency syndrome; ALS, amyotrophic lateral sclerosis; CJD, Creuzfeldt-Jakob disease; MPTP, 1-methyl-4-phenyl-1,2,3,6-tetrahydropyridine; SSPE, subacute sclerosing panencephalitis.
Modified from Jankovic, J, and Lang, AE: Classification of movement disorders. In AANS Publications Committee/Germano, IM (eds): Neurosurgical Treatment of Movement Disorders. American Association of Neurological Surgeons, Park Ridge, IL, 1998, pp 3-18. Used with permission.

"stiffness" and think that it is related to arthritis. Family members and friends are likely to comment on the change in the patient's gait and voice. Patients are often told that they appear depressed because of reduced animation in their face, *masked facies*.

A large part of the physical examination of a patient who has a hypokinetic movement disorder can be conducted while the patient is walking to the examination room and during the history. Trouble getting up from a chair, flexed posture with reduced arm swing while walking, hand tremor, and masked facies are readily apparent physical findings. In patients with subtle disease, the reduced rate of eye blinking will become apparent if you blink only when the patient blinks.

Features of Parkinsonism

Tremor

The tremor of Parkinson disease is a distal rest tremor. It was this characteristic feature that led James Parkinson to refer to the disease as "shaking palsy." The tremor can occur in the hands, legs, or lips. It usually begins on one side. Asymmetrical onset of the tremor is more characteristic of Parkinson disease than of other parkinsonian disorders. The usual tremor is "pill-rolling" of the fingers or flexion-extension or pronation-supination of the hands. The tremor stops with active movement of the limb but reappears when the limb remains in a posture against gravity or "resets" to another resting position. In contrast, postural and action tremors (from essential tremor or cerebellar disease) appear only when the limb is being used.

The absence of a rest tremor often raises the possibility of other parkinsonian syndromes. Rest tremor is estimated to occur in only 75% of patients with Parkinson disease. Furthermore, this tremor can occur in other syndromes, including multiple system atrophy, progressive supranuclear palsy, and dementia with Lewy bodies. The presence of an action tremor in a patient with Parkinson disease complicates the diagnosis. Be aware that a patient can have both types of tremor.

Patients with rest tremor often hold their hands or an object to minimize the tremor. The tremor can be demonstrated by having patients place their hands on their legs during the interview. The tremor may also become apparent while gait is being assessed. In Parkinson disease, tremor of the head usually involves the lips, chin, or tongue. Although head (neck) tremor can occur in Parkinson disease, it is more common in essential tremor, cerebellar disease, or dystonic tremor.

Bradykinesia

Bradykinesia is best demonstrated when the patient initiates movement, as in getting up from a chair, or makes a turn while walking. Turning often requires several steps, and the patient turns en bloc. Reduced facial movement, decreased frequency of blinking, impaired upgaze and eye convergence, hypophonic speech with loss of inflection, drooling of saliva from decreased spontaneous swallowing, and micrographia are all examples of bradykinesia. Voluntary movement is slow and shows a decrease in amplitude. This decrease in amplitude can be demonstrated by having the patient perform repetitive finger or toe tapping during rapid alternate motion testing. The range of movement is reduced and the rate appears faster. Bradykinesia can be a feature in other parkinsonian syndromes and in Alzheimer disease, depression, and normal aging.

Rigidity

Rigidity is an increase in muscle tone or resistance to motion. Muscle tone is tested by moving a patient's extremity through its range of movement. Rigidity of the proximal joints can be elicited by swinging the patient's shoulders or rotating the hips. Rigidity can be differentiated from spasticity by the resistance that is present equally in all directions of passive movement in both flexor and extensor muscles. The rigidity in Parkinson disease is often called *cogwheel rigidity* because of the jerky nature of the resistance, which is due to the superimposed tremor. Rigidity can be painful, and it is not uncommon for shoulder pain to be an initial symptom of Parkinson disease. Rigidity is often associated with the change that occurs in the patient's posture, with flexion of the neck, trunk, elbows, and knees becoming more prominent as the disease progresses.

Rigidity is a feature of many movement disorders and lesions of the central nervous system, including neuroleptic malignant syndrome, tetanus, and decorticate and decerebrate posturing. Cogwheel rigidity may occur also in essential tremor.

Postural Instability

Postural instability is a late manifestation of Parkinson disease. The pull test is a useful office procedure to test for postural instability. Stand behind the patient and pull the patient by the shoulders toward you. Carefully explain how the test is performed, and tell the patient to try to maintain his or her balance by taking a step backward. Be prepared to catch the patient if he or she cannot maintain balance. If the patient is large, stand next to a wall for support. Normally, a person maintains balance by taking one step back.

Two features that contribute to the high rate of fall-related injuries in patients with parkinsonism are the loss of postural reflexes and the freezing phenomenon. Postural instability and flexed truncal posture often cause festination, in which patients walk progressively faster to catch up with their center of gravity to avoid falling. The combination of postural instability, bradykinesia, and axial rigidity causes patients to collapse when they attempt to sit down.

Postural instability is not unique to Parkinson disease. If it occurs early in a patient with parkinsonism, the diagnostic possibility of progressive supranuclear palsy should be considered. Postural instability and falls are the common initial symptoms of this disorder. Postural instability is also seen in many neurologic disorders associated with sensory loss or muscle weakness and in nonneurologic disorders such as severe arthritis.

Other Manifestations

Parkinson disease has many manifestations in addition to rest tremor, bradykinesia, rigidity, and postural instability. *Dystonia*, or sustained muscle contractions, can be either a symptom of Parkinson disease or a complication of drug therapy. It can result in abnormal posture or painful spasms. The most common types of dystonia in Parkinson disease are morning foot inversion dystonia, blepharospasm, and other focal dystonias.

With the *freezing phenomenon* (another motor manifestation of Parkinson disease), the patient's gait is affected initially by start hesitation. Before starting, the patient takes small shuffling steps. As the freezing phenomenon progresses, it seems as though the patient's feet are "glued" to the floor. This may be aggravated in situations such as going through a revolving door or crossing the street. The phenomenon can affect the arms and speech and is usually a late manifestation of the disease. The presence of the freezing phenomenon early in the course of the disease should raise the possibility of a parkinsonian syndrome.

Behavioral signs that may be found in patients with Parkinson disease include bradyphrenia, depression, and dementia. Bradyphrenia is mental slowness that may be reflected by slow thinking and a slow response to answering questions. Depression is estimated to occur in 30% to 50% of patients with Parkinson disease and is considered a biologic association of the disease and not a reaction to it. The prevalence of dementia among patients with Parkinson disease is about 40%, but it increases with age. The dementia can be due to the neuropathologic changes that occur either in the disease itself or in a coexisting condition such as Alzheimer disease or cerebrovascular infarcts.

Sleep disturbance is common in Parkinson disease and includes fragmentation of sleep, restless legs, periodic leg movements of sleep, and rapid eye movement (REM) sleep behavior disorder. Dysautonomia (including orthostatic hypotension), sphincter dysfunction, and erectile dysfunction are often late findings in the disease. Constipation and dysphagia are common gastrointestinal symptoms, and seborrhea is a common dermatologic feature. Other manifestations of Parkinson disease include paresthesias, akathisia, and oral and genital pain. It is important to recognize these symptoms as part of the disorder to avoid unnecessary diagnostic evaluation. These nonmotor manifestations of the disease often respond to dopaminergic therapy.

Differential Diagnosis

Several diagnostic features are useful in differentiating Parkinson disease from the other parkinsonian disorders. Features of parkinsonian disorders include little or no tremor, early gait trouble, postural instability, upper motor neuron signs, and poor response to levodopa. If dementia occurs before the onset of motor symptoms, the patient probably does not have Parkinson disease but another parkinsonian disorder. Prominent postural instability, freezing phenomenon, and hallucinations unrelated to medications should suggest an alternative diagnosis, such as multiple system atrophy. Combinations of parkinsonism, cerebellar dysfunction, autonomic failure, and corticospinal signs characterize multiple system atrophy. The clinical features of some parkinsonian disorders are summarized in Table 12.4.

Secondary parkinsonism should be considered if the patient has a known cause of parkinsonism, for example, exposure to dopamine receptor blocking agents. Medications that can induce parkinsonism are listed in Table 12.5. The first line of treatment is to discontinue the medication. Infectious causes of parkinsonism include acquired immunodeficiency syndrome and Creutzfeldt-Jakob disease and other prion diseases. Encephalitis can result in parkinsonism, as it did following the influenza pandemic at the end of World War I. Toxins that cause parkinsonism include carbon monoxide, manganese, mercury, cyanide, methanol, and ethanol. MPTP, a byproduct of meperidine synthesis, caused an outbreak of parkinsonism among drug abusers in northern California in the 1980s. Parathyroid abnormalities and hypothyroidism can cause parkinsonism, as can cerebral infarcts, trauma, brain tumors, paraneoplastic syndrome, and normal-pressure hydrocephalus.

Medical Treatment of Parkinson Disease

The goal of treating Parkinson disease is to keep the patient functioning independently as long as possible. Nonpharmacologic treatment includes exercise, education, peer and group support, and professional, legal, financial, and occupational counseling. Encourage the patient to remain active and mobile. Exercise is important in slowing the effects of the disease that limit the patient's functional activity. The exercise program should include aerobic, strengthening, and stretching activities. Formal physical therapy can be beneficial.

Therapy should be individualized and based on the patient's social, occupational, and emotional issues. For example, it may be more important to treat a mild tremor in a patient who is still working than in one who is retired. For younger Parkinson patients, who are more likely to develop motor fluctuations and dyskinesias, consider a dopamine agonist. The medication regimen should be simplified for older patients, who are more likely to experience the adverse effects of confusion, hallucinations, and sleep-wake alterations. Discuss the specific symptoms that bother a patient, the degree of functional impairment, and the risks and benefits of therapy. Medical therapy, physical therapy, speech therapy, and mental health treatment can be valuable. Surgical treatments are also available.

Table 12.4. Parkinsonian Disorders

Disorder	Clinical features
Parkinson disease	Resting tremor, bradykinesia, rigidity, asymmetrical onset, good response to levodopa
Cortical-basal ganglionic degeneration	Marked asymmetry, focal rigidity and dystonia, apraxia, tremor, myoclonus, cortical sensory deficit, alien limb phenomenon
Dementia with Lewy bodies	Early-onset dementia, gait impairment, rigidity, hallucinations, poor tolerance of neuroleptic agents, fluctuating cognitive status
Olivopontocerebellar atrophy*	Cerebellar ataxia
Progressive supranuclear palsy	Vertical gaze palsy, oculomotor problems, early postural instability, axial rigidity, neck extension
Shy-Drager syndrome*	Dysautonomia, gait disturbance, mild tremor, dysarthria, inspiratory stridor
Striatonigral degeneration*	Early falls, poor response to levodopa, dysarthria, respiratory stridor, upper motor neuron signs
Vascular parkinsonsim	Gait disturbance of legs more than arms, "lower-half" parkinsonism, upper motor neuron signs, pseudobulbar palsy, cerebrovascular risk factors

*Multiple system atrophy.

From Adams, AC: Neurology in Primary Care. FA Davis, Philadelphia, 2000, p 210. Used with permission of Mayo Foundation for Medical Education and Research.

Table 12.5. Drugs Capable of Inducing Parkinsonism

Amiodarone (Cordarone)
Amoxapine (Asendin)
Chlorpromazine (Thorazine)
Cytarabine (cytosine arabinoside, Cytosar-U)
Fluphenazinen (Prolixin)
Haloperidol (Haldol)
Lovastatin (Mevacor)
Methyldopa (Aldomet)
Metoclopramide (Reglan)
Olanzapine (Zyprexa)
Perphenazine (Trilafon), perphenazine/
  amitriptyline (Triavil, Etrafon)
Prochlorperazine (Compazine)
Quetiapine (Seroquel)
Reserpine (Serpasil)
Risperidone (Risperdal)
Thioridazine (Mellaril)
Thiothixene (Navane)
Trifluoperazine (Stelazine)
Verapamil (Calan)

Modified from Adams, AC: Neurology in Primary Care. FA Davis, Philadelphia, 2000, p 211. Used with permission of Mayo Foundation for Medical Education and Research.

The most effective medicine for symptomatic treatment of Parkinson disease is levodopa, usually given in combination with carbidopa. A favorable response to levodopa supports the diagnosis of Parkinson disease. Levodopa is converted to dopamine by dopa decarboxylase and acts on postsynaptic dopamine receptors. Carbidopa inhibits peripheral dopa decarboxylase and allows more levodopa to enter the central nervous system. The carbidopa/levodopa combination (Sinemet) reduces nausea and orthostatism (Sinemet = "without emesis"). Carbidopa/levodopa is available in a standard and controlled-release formulation. The standard, or immediate release, formulation provides more rapid onset of action, with a shorter half-life, whereas the controlled-release formulation has delayed onset but a longer half-life. Levodopa is absorbed in the small intestine, and the full amount of the controlled-release formulation may not be absorbed ($2/3$-$3/4$) by the time it reaches the large intestine.

Despite the effectiveness of levodopa, it is not free from controversy. Most patients who take levodopa develop serious complications that include motor fluctuations, dyskinesias, toxicity at therapeutic and subtherapeutic dosages, and loss of efficacy. Dopamine increases oxidative stress and, theoretically, may accelerate disease progression. Some neurologists argue that levodopa therapy should be delayed to avoid the neurotoxic effects of dopamine and to delay the onset of complications.

Dopamine agonists do not generate oxidative metabolites and may have potential neuroprotective benefits (Table 12.6). Advocates for delaying the use of levodopa favor the early use of dopamine agonists, especially in younger patients (younger than 60 years). The major disadvantages of dopamine agonists are their limited effectiveness and the frequency of adverse neuropsychiatric effects.

Carbidopa/levodopa is recommended for the initial treatment of symptomatic Parkinson disease. The starting dose is $1/2$ tablet 1 hour before meals, three times daily. Instruct the patient to take the medicine on an empty stomach. Emphasize this point, because dietary protein can compete with levodopa for facilitated transport into the bloodstream of the small intestine, and the delay in gastric emptying has the potential for aggravating motor fluctuations. The dose should be increased by $1/2$ tablet three times a day weekly ($1/2$ tablet three times daily for the first week, 1 tablet three times daily for the second week, $1 1/2$ tablets

Table 12.6. Drugs for Parkinson Disease

Drug, intial dose	Mechanism of action	Clinical advantages	Clinical disadvantages
Dopaminergic			
Carbidopa/levodopa (Sinemet) 25/100 mg ½ tablet 1 hour before meals, increase ½ tablet tid weekly to 3½ tablets tid (Parcopa, orally disintegrating tablet)	Decarboxylase inhibitor/dopamine precursor	Most effective symptomatic treatment, may improve mortality rate	Nausea, orthostatic hypotension, dyskinesias, motor fluctuations, confusion
Dopamine agonist		Reduced incidence of levodopa-related adverse events, levodopa-sparing effect	Nausea, hypotension, neuropsychiatric adverse effects, sleep attacks, leg edema
Apomorphine (Apokyn) 0.2-0.6 mL (2-6 mg) subcutaneous as needed for "off" episodes		Acute, intermittent treatment of hypomobility "off" episodes	Must determine initial dose, serious cardiovascular side effects, orthostatic hypotension
Bromocriptine (Parlodel) 1.25 mg bid			Weakest dopamine agonist
Cabergoline (Dostinex) 0.5-1 mg *orally* daily in morning		Longest acting, may prevent or reduce "wearing-off"	
Pergolide mesylate (Permax) 0.05 mg for first 2 days; increase dose by 0.1 or 0.15 mg/day every third day over the next 12 days of therapy			Association with valvular fibrotic heart disease
Pramipexole (Mirapex) 0.125 mg tid			
Ropinirole (Requip) 0.25 mg tid			

Table 12.6 (continued)

Drug, intial dose	Mechanism of action	Clinical advantages	Clinical disadvantages
Rotigotine (Neupro) 2 mg/24 hours (a single 10-cm² patch)		Transdermal delivery	Prolongs QT interval, sleep attack
COMT inhibitor Carbidopa/entacapone/ levodopa (Stalevo) Entacapone (Comtan) Adjunct: 200 mg *orally* with each dose of levodopa/carbidopa; *maximum*, 1,600 mg/day		Increases levodopa availability to brain, decreases "off" time in patients with fluctuations	Dyskinesias, hallucinations
Tolcapone (Tasmar) 100 mg tid			Must monitor for liver failure, explosive diarrhea
Dopamine releaser and antiglutamatergic Amantadine (Symmetrel) 100 mg bid		Reduces motor fluctuations, mild symptomatic effect	May contribute to confusion and hallucinations, livedo reticularis, ankle edema
MAO type B inhibitor Rasagiline (Azilect) 1 mg once daily Selegiline Eldepryl—5 mg bid Zelapar—1.25 mg dissolved on the tongue once daily		Mild symptomatic benefit, questionable neuroprotective effect	Nausea, arthralgia

bid, twice daily; COMT, catechol-O-methyltransferase; MAO, monoamine oxidase; tid, three times daily.

three times daily for the third week, and so forth), as tolerated and needed, to the initial maximal dose of 3½ tablets three times daily. The majority of patients should have marked improvement with this dose. A lack of response to levodopa therapy suggests that the patient has a parkinsonian syndrome instead of Parkinson disease.

Nausea is one of the most common side effects of levodopa therapy and may be avoided if the patient eats a soda cracker 30 minutes after each dose. Additional carbidopa (Lodosyn) taken 1 hour before each dose may also circumvent the problem. Trimethobenzamide (Tigan) may be effective for nausea and is not associated with drug-induced parkinsonism, as are metoclopramide (Reglan) and prochlorperazine (Compazine). Another strategy to combat nausea is to prescribe a controlled-release carbidopa/levodopa preparation. The controlled-release preparation is difficult to titrate, and the onset of the therapeutic effect is slow.

Orthostatic hypotension is a serious complication of levodopa therapy. Before getting up, patients should sit on the side of the bed for several minutes. They should drink six to eight glasses of water daily, use salt liberally, and drink a caffeinated beverage with each meal. The problem of hypotension can be minimized by elevating the head of the bed. Support or pressure stockings are useful, but, practically, they are difficult for hypokinetic patients to put on and wear. Medications that may be helpful include additional carbidopa, nonsteroidal anti-inflammatory drugs, fludrocortisone (Florinef), and midodrine (ProAmatine).

Hallucinations can be a complication of levodopa therapy and are more prominent in demented patients. Clozapine (Clozaril), an antipsychotic agent, can be used to treat levodopa-induced psychosis without worsening the parkinsonism. With clozapine therapy, the patient's leukocyte count has to be monitored weekly. If the number of leukocytes decreases, the agent has to be discontinued to avoid irreversible agranulocytosis. One-half of a 25-mg tablet can be taken at bedtime and increased to 1 tablet in 1 week if needed. Atypical antipsychotics such as risperidone, olanzapine, and quetiapine do not require hematologic monitoring. Although they can aggravate parkinsonism, they may reduce psychotic symptoms without causing a significant change in Parkinson disease if used at a low dose.

The dopaminergic medications prescribed to treat Parkinson disease are listed in Table 12.6. These agents are used early in the treatment of Parkinson disease when a dopa-sparing strategy is selected to reduce dyskinesias and motor fluctuations. Bromocriptine (Parlodel) and pergolide (Permax) are ergot dopa agonists. They have the potential to induce fibrosis, and pergolide has been associated with valvular heart disease. The non-ergot dopamine agonists (pramipexole [Mirapex] and ropinirole [Requip]) are prescribed to avoid this problem. Common side effects include nausea, hypotension, drowsiness, hallucinations, and leg edema. Sudden sleep attacks have been reported, and patients should be warned of this potential hazard.

The use of monoamine oxidase B inhibitors such as selegiline (Eldepryl) has fluctuated over the years. Initially it was thought to have some neuroprotective effect in Parkinson disease, and it was recommended as first-line therapy. Although further study has shown it to have mild symptomatic benefit, no neuroprotective benefit has been established. Serious drug interactions can occur with the concomitant use of selegiline and antidepressants or piperidine-containing agents such as thioridazine (Melleril). The combination of selegiline and antidepressants can cause a syndrome of hyperthermia, autonomic instability, and mental status changes.

Catechol-O-methyltransferase (COMT) inhibitors (tolcapone and entacapone) can extend the plasma half-life of levodopa without increasing the peak plasma concentration, prolonging the duration of action of each dose of levodopa. Explosive diarrhea is an adverse side effect that can occur 6 weeks after the patient starts taking the medication. Tolcapone has been associated with serious liver damage and, thus, requires monitoring with liver function tests. Because of this serious complication, entacapone (Comtan) is the preferred COMT inhibitor. A combination formulation of carbidopa, levodopa, and entacapone (Stalevo) is available.

Amantadine causes the release of dopamine from nerve terminals, blocks dopamine uptake, has antimuscarinic effects, and blocks glutamate receptors. It has limited antiparkinson effect but may be useful in reducing levodopa-induced dyskinesias. Its important adverse effects include livedo reticularis (reddish mottling of skin), edema, and hallucinations.

Parkinson disease is treated with several nondopaminergic agents. Because of the relative cholinergic sensitivity that results from dopamine depletion, the symptoms of Parkinson disease have been treated with anticholinergic agents. The anticholinergic agents trihexyphenidyl (Artane) and benztropine (Cogentin) are prescribed primarily for rest tremor in young patients who do not have dementia. Anticholinergic agents are limited by their side effects, including memory impairment, hallucinations, confusion, constipation, and urinary retention.

Managing Late Complications of Parkinson Disease

As Parkinson disease progresses, it becomes increasingly more difficult to treat. The pathogenesis for late complications is not fully known, but it involves altered dopaminergic mechanisms of the degenerating nigrostriatal system.

Motor Fluctuations

The most common complications include fluctuations, or *off states*, when parkinsonian symptoms predominate, and *on states*, when dyskinesias are prominent. The first complication that usually appears is a mild wearing-off, or end-of-dose failure. During the first few years of treatment, patients experience a long duration of response to levodopa therapy. Wearing-off occurs when the dose no longer lasts 4 hours. Initially, the off periods are short, but as the disease progresses, both the off and on periods shorten. In association with these fluctuations, dyskinesias (chorea and dystonia) develop in many patients.

The various strategies for managing motor fluctuations and dyskinesias are listed in Table 12.7. Small changes in the dose of levodopa may be necessary to treat motor fluctuations: liquefied carbidopa/levodopa can be used for this. To make liquefied carbidopa/levodopa, dissolve ten 25/100-mg tablets in 1 L of an acidified solution (diet soda, carbonated water, or ascorbic acid solution); 1 mL of solution = 1 mg of levodopa. Because the solution oxidizes easily, it should be prepared daily and stored in the refrigerator. Motor fluctuations can be lessened if gastrointestinal motility is improved. Cisapride (Propulsid) increases gastrointestinal motility and can reduce the motor fluctuations caused by poor gastric emptying.

When motor fluctuations develop, it is essential to establish the timing of the problem and the relation to the dose, dosage schedule, meals, and sleep. One way to do this is to have the patient keep a diary. This will help in determining whether the complication is related to being parkinsonian ("off") or "on." Wearing-off, or end-of-dose failure, is apparent when an increase in parkinsonian symptoms occurs before the next dose. Decreasing the dose interval will solve the problem. The distinction between off and on states for other fluctuations may be difficult. Types of fluctuations include sudden off, random off, yo-yoing, episodic failure to respond, delayed on, weak end-of-day response, response variability in relation to meals, and sudden transient freezing. In yo-yoing, the patient responds to levodopa rapidly, with a peak-dose dyskinesia followed by the wearing-off.

Dyskinesias

Dyskinesias are frequently a late complication of Parkinson disease and usually consist of chorea or dystonia (or both). The types of dyskinesia include peak-dose dyskinesias, diphasic dyskinesias, and off dystonia. Peak-dose dyskinesias represent an excessive level of levodopa. A patient with diphasic dyskinesia may

Table 12.7. Strategies for Managing Motor Fluctuations and Dyskinesias

Complication	Management options
Wearing-off	Decrease dose interval, add MAO B inhibitor, change to controlled-release form, add COMT inhibitor, add dopamine agonist
Sudden "off" or random "off"	Dissolve carbidopa/levodopa in carbonated water before ingestion, change to dopamine agonist
"Yo-yoing"	Liquid carbidopa/levodopa tiration, dopamine agonist
Dose failures	Liquid carbidopa/levodopa
Delayed "on"	Increase morning dose, add cisapride
Weak response at end of day	Increase evening dose
Freezing	Increase dose for "off" freezing, decrease dose for "on" freezing
Peak-dose dyskinesia	Decrease dose, decrease dose interval, decrease levodopa, dopamine agonists, controlled-release levodopa, amantadine
Diphasic dyskinesia	Dopamine agonists
Off dystonia	Dopamine agonists, controlled-release levodopa

COMT, catechhol-O-methyltransferase; MAO, monoamine oxidase.
From Adams, AC: Neurology in Primary Care. FA Davis, Philadelphia, 2000, p 214. Used with permission of Mayo Foundation for Medical Education and Research.

have dystonia followed by improvement and then the return of dystonia. This is thought to be the result of increasing and decreasing levels of levodopa. Off dystonia occurs when the level of levodopa is low; painful sustained muscle contractions can develop.

Other Late Complications

Other frequently encountered late complications include falling, sleep difficulty, autonomic dysfunction, psychiatric problems, and cognitive difficulty. Any complication that develops suddenly should prompt an investigation for a medical illness such as pneumonia or urinary tract infection. Scrutinize the patient's medications to determine if they are responsible for any complications.

Falling

Falling is a dangerous complication and the cause of significant morbidity and mortality. The twofold increase in the risk of death in parkinsonism is related directly to the presence of a gait disturbance and falling. The risk factors for falling include older age, advanced stages of disease, gait disturbance, freezing, and postural instability. Mental status changes, dyskinesias, orthostatic hypotension, arthritis, visual impairment, vestibular dysfunction, and sensory loss also contribute to the problem of falling. If a patient has a positive pull test or a gait disturbance with freezing, he or she is at risk for falling. Prescribe preventative measures for these patients, for example, the use of a cane or walker and home safety devices. Gait freezing that occurs with the initiation of walking is sometimes improved with visual cues such as stepping over the handle of an inverted cane or placing lines on the floor.

Sleep Disturbance

Sleep disorders are common in Parkinson disease. Sleep disturbance can result from the effects of medications, restless legs syndrome, sleep apnea, REM sleep behavior disorder, depression, anxiety, and circadian rhythm disorders. The management of these disorders is discussed in Chapter 9 and summarized in Table 12.8.

Cognitive Difficulty

Cognitive difficulty is common in Parkinson disease and becomes more pronounced as the disease progresses. The prevalence of dementia in Parkinson disease increases with age and severity of disease. The relationship of dementia in Parkinson disease, dementia with Lewy bodies, and Alzheimer dementia has not been delineated completely. Management of dementia is discussed in Chapter 8.

Psychiatric Complications

The psychiatric complications of Parkinson disease include hallucinations, psychoses, depression, and anxiety. Most psychiatric problems are treated in the same way they would be if Parkinson disease were not present, except that antipsychotic medications that can aggravate the disease are contraindicated. Psychiatric consultation is useful for managing these complications.

Surgical Therapy for Parkinson Disease

Several surgical options can be considered when Parkinson disease becomes refractory to medical therapy, including thalamotomy, pallidotomy, deep brain stimulation or neuromodulation, and cellular transplant. Surgery for the treatment of movement disorders has been enhanced by improved surgical technique, stereotactic imaging techniques, and microelectrode cell recording.

Deep Brain Stimulation

Deep brain stimulation (DBS) has replaced ablative surgery for Parkinson disease because of potential reversibility and lower risk of complications. A neurostimulator that is surgically implanted subcutaneously, similar to a cardiac pacemaker, delivers electrical stimulation to specific brain targets (Fig. 12.2). Stimulation parameters are programmed with noninvasive radiotelemetry.

The mechanism of DBS is not known, but there is evidence of increased transmitter release by neurons adjacent to the DBS electrode. DBS of the subthalamic nucleus (STN) (STN DBS) and the globus pallidus interna has been shown to be effective in reducing the motor signs of Parkinson disease, including tremor, bradykinesia, rigidity, and dyskinesias. The benefits of surgery include reduced motor fluctuations and, often, a reduction in the amount of antiparkinsonian medications. Follow-up studies have shown that patients have sustained benefit from DBS and improved quality-of-life measures. Bilateral STN DBS has become the preferred surgical treatment of Parkinson disease.

It is important to emphasize to patients who are considering DBS that it is not a cure for degenerative disease. It never improves symptoms that are unresponsive to medication or the patients' best "on." Any signs or symptoms that do not respond to medication are unlikely to improve with DBS.

The timing of DBS in Parkinson disease is still being defined. DBS should be considered if the patient has disabling symptoms despite optimal medical therapy. In selecting patients for DBS, it is important that they have idiopathic Parkinson disease and not parkinsonism. Features of Parkinson disease include

Table 12.8. Treatment of Sleep Disturbance in Parkinson Disease

Sleep hygiene
 Regular bedtime and waking time
 Appropriate amount of time in bed
 Bright light exposure
 Maximize daytime activity
 Reduce nap frequency and duration
 Avoid caffeinated products
Evaluate and treat sleep disorders
 Obstructive sleep apnea syndrome: CPAP, weight reduction
 Restless legs syndrome: adjust dopaminergic medications, anticonvulsants
 Periodic limb movement disorder: adjust dopaminergic medications
 REM sleep behavior disorder: clonazepam, melatonin
 Insomnia: sleep hygiene, hypnotics, sedative antidepressants, melatonin
 Circadian rhythm sleep disorders: melatonin, light exposure, daytime activity
Parkinson disease-related disorders
 Depression: antidepressants
 Psychosis: clozapine, low-dose atypical antipsychotics
 Dementia: cholinesterase inhibitors
Nightmares
 Reduce medications that affect REM sleep, including anticholinergics, antidepressants, and dopaminergic agents
Pain
 Analgesics: acetaminophen, NSAIDs, or opioid derivatives

CPAP, continuous positive airway pressure: NSAID, nonsteroidal antiinflammatory drug; REM, rapid eye movement.
Modified from Adler, CH, and Thorpy, MJ: Sleep issues in Parkinson's disease. Neurology 64 Suppl 3:S12-S20, 2005. Used with permission.

asymmetrical onset, robust response to levodopa, slowly progressive course, lack of early dysautonomia, lack of early cognitive dysfunction, normal eye movement, and lack of cerebellar or corticospinal tract involvement. Good candidates for bilateral STN DBS are patients who are still ambulatory during the "on" and have a continued response to levodopa. Dementia, severe depression, uncontrolled hypertension, and bleeding diatheses are contraindications to DBS.

The complication rate of DBS is low. Side effects can often be eliminated with programming adjustment of the neurostimulator and manipulating the patient's medication. Postoperative problems reported with STN DBS include weight gain, dyskinesias, hypophonia or dysarthria, depression, and other behavioral and cognitive problems.

TREMOR

Definition

Tremor, the most common form of involuntary movement disorder, is a rhythmic oscillation of agonist and antagonist muscles. It can be classified as either a *rest tremor* or *action*

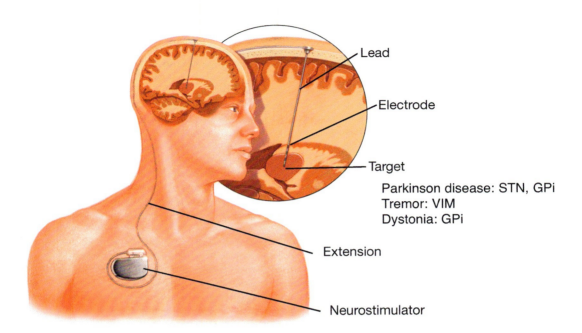

Fig. 12.2. Deep brain stimulation. The neurostimulator is placed under the skin and delivers electrical stimulation to a specific brain target. GPi, internal segment of globus pallidus; STN, subthalamic nucleus; VIM, ventral intermediate thalamic nucleus. (From Deep brain stimulation: program expansion. Neurosciences Update, 2007;4[2]:1-3. Used with permission of Mayo Foundation for Medical Education and Research.)

tremor (Table 12.9). Rest tremor is the tremor characteristic of parkinsonism. It occurs when the affected body part is supported against gravity and the muscles are not actively contracting. Rest tremor is absent or diminished during muscle contraction or movement. Most tremors are action tremors that become more prominent with voluntary movement, such as writing, eating, or drinking. Action tremors include postural, kinetic, task- or position-specific, and iometric tremors.

Types

Postural tremors occur when an antigravity posture is maintained, for example, holding the arms in front of the body. Kinetic tremors are seen with voluntary movement. Initial tremor,

dynamic tremor, and terminal tremor describe, respectively, kinetic tremor, tremor at the beginning of a movement, and tremor when the affected body part approaches the target. A *task-specific tremor* occurs with a specific activity, for example, a voice tremor that occurs with singing and a hand tremor that occurs only with writing. *Position-specific tremors* occur only when a specific posture is maintained, for example, holding a cup to the mouth. An *isometric tremor* occurs during voluntary muscle contraction not accompanied by a change in position of the body part. An example is orthostatic tremor, in which a fine, fast tremor occurs in the legs with standing.

A postural tremor that everyone has is *physiologic tremor*. It can be enhanced by several

Table 12.9. Classification of Tremor

Rest tremor	Action tremor
Parkinson disease	Postural
Multisystem degeneration	Physiologic tremor
Multiple system atrophy	Enhanced physiologic tremor
Progressive supranuclear palsy	Stress-induced, endocrine, drugs, toxins
Cortical-basal ganglionic degeneration	Essential tremor
Diffuse Lewy body disease	Autosomal dominant, sporadic
Heredodegenerative disorders	Parkinsonism
Huntington disease	Tardive tremor
Wilson disease	Midbrain (rubral) tremor
Neuroacanthocytosis	Cerebellar
Ceroid lipofuscinosis	Neuropathic
Secondary parkinsonism	Kinetic (intention, termination)
Drug-induced	Cerebellar disorders
Toxic	Midbrain lesions
Vascular	Task- or position-specific tremors
Trauma	Handwriting
Infectious	Occupational task-specific
Tardive tremor	Isometric
Severe essential tremor	Orthostatic
Midbrain (rubral) tremor	

From Adams, AC: Neurology in Primary Care. FA Davis, Philadelphia, 2000, p 217. Used with permission of Mayo Foundation for Medical Education and Research.

things, including emotion, exercise, fatigue, anxiety, and fever and by any condition that increases peripheral β-adrenergic activity. If a patient presents with an enhanced physiologic tremor, consider such endocrine disorders as thyrotoxicosis, hypoglycemia, and pheochromocytoma. Drugs that enhance physiologic tremor are listed in Table 12.10.

Essential Tremor

Essential tremor is the most common movement disorder and occurs equally in both sexes. The age at onset has a bimodal distribution, with peaks in the second and sixth decades. This tremor is most likely to involve the hands, but it can involve, in decreasing order, the head, voice, leg, jaw, trunk, and tongue. Patients with essential tremor often have other associated movement disorders. According to one study, a large proportion of patients with essential tremor have dystonia and parkinsonian signs.

Essential tremor occurs sporadically and is inherited. Familial tremor has an autosomal dominant inheritance pattern with variable penetrance. An association between essential tremor and Parkinson disease has been suggested by several studies, but the exact relation has not been identified. Complicating the distinction between essential tremor and Parkinson disease is the presence of both conditions in one patient and an incorrect diagnosis, for

Table 12.10. Drugs Associated With Enhanced Physiologic Tremor

Albuterol (Proventil, Ventolin)
Bromocriptine (Parlodel)
Buproprion (Wellbutrin)
Carbidopa/levodopa (Sinemet)
Caffeine (coffee, tea)
Cimetidine (Tagamet)
Cyclobenzaprine (Flexeril)
Cyclosporine (Neoral)
Fluoxetine (Prozac)
Haloperidol (Haldol)
Lithium (Lithobid)
Methylphenidate (Ritalin)
Metoclopramide (Reglan)
Pergolide (Permax)
Phenylpropanolamine (nasal decongestant)
Pramipexole (Mirapex)
Pseudoephedrine (Sudafed)
Ropinirole (Requip)
Tacrolimus (Prograf)
Terbutaline (Brethine)
Theophylline (Theo-Dur)
Valproate (Depakote)
Venlafaxine (Effexor)

Modified from Adams, AC: Neurology in Primary Care. FA Davis, Philadelphia, 2000, p 217. Used with permission of Mayo Foundation for Medical Education and Research.

example, Parkinson disease being misdiagnosed in a patient with essential tremor. Patients with essential tremor often are concerned about the possibility of having Parkinson disease.

Essential tremor is a postural tremor that becomes more prominent with voluntary movement. Some patients with parkinsonism have a postural tremor (with arms outstretched in front of them) that develops after a latency of a few seconds. This probably represents a rest tremor that has been "reset" during posture holding, for which reason it is sometimes called a *repose tremor*. In essential tremor, the tremor does not occur when the hands and arms are relaxed. Hand tremor that occurs with the arms hanging at the sides is more likely a parkinsonian tremor. Alcohol frequently decreases essential tremor, but it has no effect on a parkinsonian tremor. The differences between essential tremor and the tremor of Parkinson disease are summarized in Table 12.11. It is important to keep in mind that these two types of tremor overlap.

The treatment of essential tremor depends on its severity and the patient's functional impairment. Some patients with extremely mild tremor may require only reassurance about the absence of a serious problem. Many patients drink alcohol to suppress the tremor. Although the information about alcoholism and essential tremor is contradictory, drinking alcohol is not a recommended treatment.

Before drug therapy is initiated for the tremor, a sample of the patient's handwriting should be obtained. The handwriting or the patient's drawing of a spiral (Fig. 12.3) can be monitored to assess the response to treatment. Having patients maintain a daily sample of handwriting helps them visualize their response to treatment.

Propranolol (Inderal), a β-adrenergic-blocking drug, is effective for treating essential tremor. Other β-blockers, for example, atenolol (Tenormin) and sotalol (Betapace), are probably effective, and nadolol (Corgard) is possibly effective. A central mechanism of action has been suggested for these medications, but because some of these agents are not lipid soluble and do not cross the blood-brain barrier, the antitremor effect of β-blockers is mediated partly by peripheral mechanisms. The dose of propranolol ranges from 60 to 800 mg daily. These medications should not be taken by patients who have asthma, second-degree atrioventricular

Table 12.11. Comparison of Essential Tremor and Parkinson Tremor

Characteristic	Essential tremor	Parkinson tremor
Tremor type	Action	Rest
Anatomical distribution	Head and voice, not in leg	Limbs of the same side
Symmetry	Symmetrical	Asymmetrical
Effect of alcohol	Decreases	No effect
Other neurologic signs	None	Bradykinesia, rigidity, postural instability

From Adams, AC: Neurology in Primary Care. FA Davis, Philadelphia, 2000, p 218. Used with permission of Mayo Foundation for Medical Education and Research.

block, or insulin-dependent diabetes mellitus. Extra care should be extended to patients with any cardiopulmonary disease. Frequent side effects include fatigue, sedation, and depression. However, according to a review of clinical trials of β-blockers, the data do not support that these agents are associated with a risk of depressive symptoms, fatigue, or sexual dysfunction.

Primidone (Mysoline) is also effective in treating essential tremor. Its tremor-suppressant effect is due primarily to the parent compound rather than the metabolites (phenobarbital or phenylethylmalonamide). Treatment should be started at a very low dose (25 mg at bedtime) to prevent the common side effects of sedation, confusion, and ataxia. The daily dose

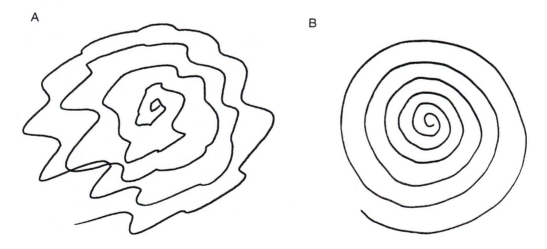

Fig. 12.3. Spirals, as drawn by a person with essential tremor (*A*) and a person without tremor (*B*). (From Adams, AC: Neurology in Primary Care. FA Davis, Philadelphia, 2000, p 219. Used with permission of Mayo Foundation for Medical Education and Research.)

should be increased gradually to achieve the optimal therapeutic response. The combination of propranolol and primidone may provide greater benefit if monotherapy with either drug is not sufficient. Other anticonvulsants that have been shown to probably be effective in treating essential tremor are gabapentin (Neurontin) and topiramate (Topamax).

The benzodiazepines have shown efficacy in the treatment of essential tremor. Alprazolam (Xanax) is considered probably effective and clonazepam (Klonopin) as possibly effective. Caution should be used with these medications because of the potential for abuse and dependency.

An option for medically refractory essential tremor is the injection of botulinum toxin (Botox) into muscles that produce the oscillatory movement. This intervention is limited because of dose-dependent weakness.

DBS has become the surgical treatment of choice for medically refractory tremor. The DBS electrode is placed in the ventralis intermedius (VIM) nucleus of the thalamus, also known as the ventral lateral nucleus. After the perioperative complications of surgery, the most common adverse effects of bilateral VIM DBS are dysarthria, paresthesias, and disequilibrium. Many of these effects can be eliminated with appropriate programming of the neurostimulator. The interventions available for treating tremor are summarized in Table 12.12.

DYSTONIA

Dystonia is a heterogeneous movement disorder of sustained muscle contractions that frequently cause twisting and repetitive movements or abnormal postures. Dystonias have been classified by distribution. Focal dystonias include cervical (torticollis), hand or writer's cramp, voice or spasmodic dysphonia, and blepharospasm. Classification of dystonia by distribution also includes segmental (contiguous regions), multifocal, and generalized. Dystonias are also classified by cause, including primary dystonias, secondary dystonias (dystonia-plus, heredodegenerative, and acquired), and dystonias of unknown cause.

Currently, 15 subtypes of dystonia have been identified (designated DYT1-15). The dystonia-plus syndromes include dopa-responsive dystonia, rapid-onset dystonia, and myoclonus-dystonia. The heredodegenerative dystonias include Huntington disease, spinocerebellar ataxia, dentatorubral pallidoluysian atrophy, Wilson disease, GM_1 and GM_2 gangliosidosis, metachromatic leukodystrophy, and homocystinuria. The most common cause of acquired dystonia is drug-induced (tardive dystonia). Any injury to the basal ganglia circuitry (especially the putamen), such as stroke, tumor, or demyelination, can also cause acquired dystonia.

The clinical presentation of dystonia can be as varied as its different types. A unique feature of dystonic movement is a reduction in movement caused by a tactile or sensory stimulus (sensory trick, or *geste antagoniste*). Examples of this include a patient who has cervical dystonia touching his or her face or a patient who has oromandibular dystonia placing something in the mouth. Pain is uncommon in most forms of dystonia, although most patients with cervical dystonia experience neck pain.

Treatment of Dystonia

Dopa-responsive dystonia and Wilson disease are examples of the few dystonic syndromes that have specific treatment. Because the syndrome of dopa-responsive dystonia tends to occur in young people, a trial of levodopa is reasonable for a child or adolescent who presents with generalized or segmental dystonia. The classic features of dopa-responsive dystonia include lower limb dystonia, diurnal variation,

Table 12.12. Treatments for Tremor

Intervention	Efficacy	Dose	Adverse effects
Propranolol (Inderal)	Effective	60-800 mg/day	Hypotension, fatigue, sedation, depression
Primidone (Mysoline)	Effective	25-750 mg/day	Sedation, confusion, ataxia
Alprazolam (Xanax)	Probably effective	0.125-3 mg/day	Fatigue, sedation, abuse
Atenolol (Tenormin)	Probably effective	50-150 mg/day	Dizziness, fatigue
Gabapentin (Neurontin)	Probably effective	1,200-1,800 mg/day	Somnolence, peripheral edema
Sotalol (Betapace)	Probably effective	75-200 mg/day	Chest pain, light-headedness
Topiramate (Topamax)	Probably effective	50-400 mg/day	Weight loss, concentration difficulty
Clonazepam (Klonopin)	Possibly effective	0.5-6 mg/day	Sedation, depression
Clozapine (Clozaril)	Possibly effective	6-75 mg/day	Sedation, agranulo-cytosis, requires monitoring
Nadolol (Corgard)	Possibly effective	120-240 mg/day	Fatigue, dizziness
Nimodipine (Nimotop)	Possibly effective	120 mg/day	Diarrhea, nausea
Botulinum toxin (Botox)	Possibly effective		Hand weakness, hoarseness, dysarthria for voice tremor
Deep brain stimulation	Effective		Dysarthria, paresthesias, dysequilibrium (programming adjustment may eliminate)

parkinsonian features, and a sustained and dramatic response to levodopa. Patients with dopa-responsive dystonia typically have a response in the first few months to a low dose of levodopa (< 600 mg daily).

Anticholinergic medications such as trihexyphenidyl (Artane) and benztropine mesylate (Cogentin) have been used to treat dystonia, as have baclofen (Lioresal), clonazepam (Klonopin), carbamazepine (Tegretol), and tizanidine (Zanaflex). Botulinum toxin is the treatment of choice for focal dystonia. Intrathecal baclofen has been used to treat generalized dystonia. DBS, with the globus pallidus interna as the target site, has been shown to be effective in selected cases of dystonia.

TICS AND TOURETTE SYNDROME

Definition and Types

Tics are brief and intermittent movements (motor) or sounds (phonic) that can be classified as either simple or complex. Simple motor tics involve only one group of muscles and cause a brief jerklike movement. Phonic, or vocal, tics are essentially motor tics that involve the respiratory, pharyngeal, laryngeal, oral, and nasal musculature. Simple phonic tics consist of grunting, throat-clearing, sniffing, coughing, or blowing sounds. Examples of complex vocal tics include using obscenities and profanities (coprolalia), repeating what is said by others (echolalia), or repeating oneself (palilalia). Complex motor tics consist of coordinated sequenced movements that are inappropriately timed and intense, for example, making obscene gestures (copropraxia) and imitating gestures (echopraxia).

Tics are paroxysmal and occur abruptly for brief moments from a background of normal motor activity. They are frequently diagnosed as habits, allergies, or hyperactivity. Distinguishing a simple motor tic from myoclonus or chorea may be difficult in isolation. The patient is aware that the tic is going to happen. Many times the tic can be provoked by suggestion. Compared with other hyperkinetic movement disorders, tics tend to be repetitive and the patient is more likely to have other complex motor tics. Eye movement abnormalities are frequent in tics but infrequent in other hyperkinetic movement disorders. Tics are usually induced by an inner sensory stimulus that is relieved by the movement. This premonitory sensation is compared with the urge to "scratch an itch." Tics are suppressible and frequently vary in severity over time. Remissions and exacerbations are common, with worsening in late adolescence and improvement in later adulthood. Tics are often associated with obsessive-compulsive disorder and attention-deficit/hyperactivity disorder.

The combination of chronic simple and complex motor and vocal tics is characteristic of Tourette syndrome. This syndrome usually begins in childhood and has been associated with attention-deficit disorder, lack of impulse control, and obsessive-compulsive disorder. Genetic and autoimmune mechanisms have been implicated in the pathophysiology of the syndrome. Neuroimaging has identified involvement of the basal ganglia and frontal lobes. Functional studies of Tourette syndrome have also demonstrated alterations in dopaminergic activity.

Treatment

The treatment of tics and Tourette syndrome begins with educating the patient, family, and those who interact with the patient about the disorder. National and local support groups are an invaluable resource for support and education. Many patients do not require pharmacologic therapy. Often, tic triggers can be identified and modified. Psychiatric assessment may be important, and cognitive-behavioral therapy may be beneficial for selected patients.

Medication should be considered when the symptoms interfere with academic or job performance, social interactions, or activities of daily living. Many medications can be used to treat the symptoms of Tourette syndrome, but therapy should be individualized and tailored to the specific needs of the patient. It is important to give the medication a trial of adequate dose and time to avoid unnecessary changes in response to the normal variations in symptoms that occur during the natural course of the disease. Clonidine (Catapres), guanfacine (Tenex), and clonazepam are three of the medications prescribed to treat Tourette syndrome. Many neuroleptics have been used, including pimozide (Orap), fluphenazine (Prolixin), risperidone (Risperdal), olanzapine (Zyprexa), quetiapine

(Seroquel), ziprasidone (Geodon), aripiprazole (Abilify), and haloperidol (Haldol). The neuroleptics are effective but have the risk of causing tardive dyskinesias. Other medications that have been used are modafinil (Provigil), topiramate, baclofen, levetiracetam (Keppra), pergolide mesylate, ropinirole, nicotine patch, and atomoxetine (Strattera). Botulinum toxin may be useful if a small number of trigger muscles are identified. DBS may be a consideration for the treatment of medically refractory Tourette syndrome. The targets that have been used in Tourette include the globus pallidus interna and the medial part of the thalamus (centromedian nucleus, the substantia periventricularis, and the nucleus ventro-oralis internus).

TARDIVE SYNDROMES

Tardive dyskinesia is an iatrogenic syndrome of persistent abnormal involuntary movements that occurs as a complication of drugs that block dopamine receptors (Table 12.13). The diagnosis of a tardive syndrome is based on exposure of the patient to a dopamine receptor-blocking agent within 6 months before the onset of the movement and the persistence of the movement for 1 month after the patient stops taking the offending drug.

The most common tardive syndrome is *oral-buccal-lingual dyskinesia*. This movement involves rapid, repetitive, and stereotypic movements of the oral, buccal, and lingual areas. *Akathisia* can occur as a tardive syndrome. It is described as an inner restlessness of the whole body, but it can involve an uncomfortable sensation in a specific part of the body. Focal akathisias are often described as a burning pain, commonly in the mouth and genital areas. A patient with generalized akathisia has rhythmical, repetitive, stereotypic movements like body rocking, crossing and uncrossing the

legs, and moaning. Dystonia can be part of a tardive syndrome. It is not uncommon for patients to have both dystonia and oral-buccal-lingual dyskinesia. Both akathisia and dystonia can occur acutely after exposure to dopamine receptor-blocking drugs. Acute dystonia that affects the ocular muscles is called an *oculogyric crisis*. The acute reactions can be treated with parenteral anticholinergic and antihistamine agents such as diphenhydramine and benztropine mesylate.

Table 12.13. Drugs That Can Cause Tardive Syndromes

Amoxapine (Asendin)
Aripiprazole (Abilify)
Chlorpromazine (Thorazine)
Clozapine (Clozaril)
Droperidol (Inapsine)
Fluphenazine (Prolixin)
Haloperidol (Haldol)
Loxapine (Loxitane)
Mesoridazine (Serentil)
Metoclopramide (Reglan)
Molindone (Moban)
Olanzapine (Zyprexa)
Perphenazine (Trilafon)
Pimozide (Orap)
Prochlorperazine (Compazine)
Promethazine (Phenergan)
Quetiapine (Seroquel)
Risperidone (Risperdal)
Thioridazine (Mellaril)
Thiothixene (Navane)
Trifluoperazine (Stelazine)
Ziprasidone (Geodon)

From Adams, AC: Neurology in Primary Care. FA Davis, Philadelphia, 2000, p 222. Used with permission of Mayo Foundation for Medical Education and Research.

Unlike drug-induced parkinsonism, in which the symptoms disappear when the drug is withdrawn, tardive dyskinesia can persist and be permanent. This emphasizes the importance of avoiding dopamine receptor-blocking drugs unless absolutely necessary. The patient should be informed about the potential complication of these agents, and this should be documented in the medical record. Patients at risk for tardive dyskinesia are older, female, and those exposed to higher daily doses and greater cumulative amounts of dopamine receptor-blocking drugs.

Treatment

The first step in treating tardive syndromes is to remove the offending drug. Gradual withdrawal is recommended to avoid an exaggeration of the movement (withdrawal emergent syndrome). If the drug can be avoided, the tardive symptoms may resolve. If it is necessary to treat the symptoms, dopamine receptor-depleting drugs (reserpine [Resa] and tetrabenazine [available in Europe]) can be prescribed. Other useful drugs are clonazepam, alprazolam (Xanax), baclofen, and anticholinergic agents (for dystonia). If continued treatment with an antipsychotic medication is needed, the atypical or second-generation antipsychotic agents may be preferred. The results of a pilot study of bilateral DBS of the globus pallidus are encouraging.

SUGGESTED READING

Adler, CH, and Thorpy, MJ: Sleep issues in Parkinson's disease. Neurology 64 Suppl 3:S12-S20, 2005.

Bhidayasiri, R: Dystonia: Genetics and treatment update. Neurologist 12:774-785, 2006.

Bonuccelli, U, and Del Dotto, P: New pharmacologic horizons in the treatment of Parkinson disease. Neurology 67 Suppl 2:S30-S38, 2007.

Damier, P, et al, French Stimulation for Tardive Dyskinesia (STARDYS) Study Group: Bilteral deep brain stimulation of the globus pallidus to treat tardive dyskinesia. Arch Gen Psychiatry 64:170-176, 2007.

Diamond, A, and Jankovic, J: The effect of deep brain stimulation on quality of life in movement disorders. J Neurol Neurosurg Psychiatry 76:1188-1193, 2005.

Fahn, S, et al, Parkinson Study Group: Levodopa and the progression of Parkinson's disease. N Engl J Med 351:2498-2508, 2004.

Ferreri, F, Agbokou, C, and Gauthier, S: Recognition and management of neuropsychiatric complications in Parkinson's disease. CMAJ 175:1545-1552, 2006.

Galvin, JE: Cognitive change in Parkinson disease. Alzheimer Dis Assoc Disord 20:302-310, 2006.

Halpern, C, et al: Deep brain stimulation in neurologic disorders. Parkinsonism Relat Disord 13:1-16, 2007. Epub 2006 Dec 1.

Holloway, RG, et al, Parkinson Study Group: Pramipexole vs levodopa as initial treatment for Parkinson disease: A 4-year randomized controlled trial. Arch Neurol 61:1044-1053, 2004. Erratum in: Arch Neurol 62:430, 2005.

Jankovic, J: Botulinum toxin in clinical practice. J Neurol Neurosurg Psychiatry 75:951-957, 2004.

Jenner, P: Preclinical evidence for neuroprotection with monoamine oxidase-B inhibitors in Parkinson's disease. Neurology 63 Suppl 2:S13-S22, 2004.

Ko, DT, et al: Beta-blocker therapy and symptoms of depression, fatigue, and sexual dysfunction. JAMA 288:351-357, 2002.

Lester, J, and Otero-Siliceo, E: Parkinson's disease and genetics. Neurologist 12:240-244, 2006.

Lippa, CF, et al, DLB/PDD Working Group: DLB and PDD boundary issues: Diagnosis, treatment, molecular pathology, and biomarkers. Neurology 68:812-819, 2007.

Louis, ED, et al: Neuropathologic findings in essential tremor. Neurology 66:1756-1759, 2006.

Mink, JW, et al, Tourette Syndrome Association, Inc: Patient selection and assessment recommendations for deep brain stimulation in Tourette syndrome. Mov Disord 21:1831-1838, 2006.

Ondo, WG, et al, Topiramate Essential Tremor Study Investigators: Topiramate in essential tremor: A double-blind, placebo-controlled trial. Neurology 66:672-677, 2006. Epub 2006 Jan 25.

Pahwa, R, et al, Quality Standards Subcommittee of the American Academy of Neurology. Practice parameter: Treatment of Parkinson disease with motor fluctuations and dyskinesia (an evidence-based review): Report of the Quality Standards Subcommittee of the American Academy of Neurology. Neurology 66:983-995, 2006.

Pringsheim, T, Davenport, WJ, and Lang, A: Tics. Curr Opin Neurol 16:523-527, 2003.

Shahed, J, et al: GPi deep brain stimulation for Tourette syndrome improves tics and psychiatric comorbidities. Neurology 68:159-160, 2007.

Waller, EA, Kaplan, J, and Heckman, MG: Valvular heart disease in patients taking pergolide. Mayo Clin Proc 80:1016-1020, 2005.

Watts, RL, et al: Randomized, blind, controlled trial of transdermal rotigotine in early Parkinson disease. Neurology 68:272-276, 2007. Epub 2007 Jan 3. Erratum in: Neurology 69:617, 2007.

Zesiewicz, TA, et al, Quality Standards Subcommittee of the American Academy of Neurology: Practice parameter: Therapies for essential tremor: Report of the Quality Standards Subcommittee of the American Academy of Neurology. Neurology 64:2008-2020, 2005. Epub 2005 Jun 22.

CHAPTER 13

Immune and Infectious Diseases

Many immune-mediated diseases and infections affect the central and peripheral nervous systems. The common feature that characterizes both immune-mediated diseases and infections is a subacute temporal profile. Immune-mediated disease can affect only the nervous system or involve the nervous system as part of a systemic illness, as in vasculitis and connective tissue disease (Table 13.1). Multiple sclerosis, the most common disabling neurologic illness of young people, is the prototypical immune-mediated disease of the central nervous system. The availability of disease-modifying treatments for multiple sclerosis emphasizes the importance of accurate diagnosis and therapeutic intervention.

IMMUNE DISEASE OF THE NERVOUS SYSTEM

Multiple Sclerosis

Features and Types

Multiple sclerosis is a relapsing or progressive immune-mediated disorder of the central nervous system. It is characterized by recurrent patches of inflammation, with damage to myelin (demyelination) and axons of the brain, spinal cord, and optic nerves. Multiple sclerosis is not a single disease but several idiopathic inflammatory demyelinating syndromes (Table 13.2). The demyelinating syndromes are described by their course (monophasic, relapsing-remitting, progressive) and the site of nervous system involvement.

The most common clinical category of multiple sclerosis is *relapsing-remitting*. Approximately 80% of patients present with this type of multiple sclerosis. Episodes (relapses, attacks, or exacerbations) of neurologic dysfunction are followed by recovery and a stable phase between relapses (remission). The length of time for most relapses, or attacks of neurologic deficit, is 4 to 16 weeks.

More than 50% of patients with relapsing-remitting multiple sclerosis develop the secondary progressive stage of the disease. Patients with secondary progressive multiple sclerosis have progressive neurologic deterioration with or without superimposed acute relapses. Patients whose condition deteriorates continuously from the onset of symptoms have *primary progressive multiple sclerosis*.

Table 13.1. Immune-Mediated Disorders of the Neuromuscular System

Muscle
  Polymyositis
  Dermatomyositis
  Inclusion body myositis
Neuromuscular junction
  Myasthenia gravis
  Lambert-Eaton myasthenic syndrome
Peripheral nerve
  Acute inflammatory demyelinating polyneuropathy (AIDP, or Guillain-Barré syndrome)
  Chronic inflammatory demyelinating polyneuropathy (CIDP)
  Monoclonal gammopathy of undetermined significance (MGUS)
Central nervous system
  Acute disseminated encephalomyelitis (postviral demyelination)
  Multiple sclerosis
  Optic neuritis
  Transverse myelitis
  Central nervous system vasculitis
Systemic
  Vasculitis: polyarteritis nodosa, Wegener granulomatosis, Churg-Strauss syndrome,
    Kawasaki disease, hypersensitivity vasculitis, giant cell arteritis (temporal arteritis)
  Connective tissue disease: systemic lupus erythematosus, rheumatoid arthritis, Sjögren
    syndrome, mixed connective tissue disease, scleroderma
  Sarcoidosis
  Behçet disease
  Cogan syndrome
  Hypersensitivity angiitis: drug-induced, serum sickness, cryoglobulinemia
  Infection-related vasculitis
  Malignancy-related: paraneoplastic, lymphoma, leukemia
  Vasculitis in substance abuse: amphetamines, cocaine, heroin

From Adams, AC: Neurology in Primary Care. FA Davis Company, Philadelphia, 2000, p 226. Used with permission of Mayo Foundation for Medical Education and Research.

Multiple sclerosis can present as a monosymptomatic illness. Optic neuritis is a common monosymptomatic demyelinating syndrome. The patient presents with unilateral loss of vision, and ophthalmoscopic examination may show a swollen optic nerve head (papillitis) or no abnormality (retrobulbar neuritis). Isolated brainstem and spinal cord (transverse myelitis) syndromes are included in this category.

Fulminant, or severe, demyelinating syndromes include acute disseminated encephalomyelitis, Baló concentric sclerosis, and Marburg variant. These disorders are associated with high morbidity and mortality. Neuromyelitis optica

Table 13.2. Idiopathic Inflammatory Demyelinating Diseases of the Central Nervous System

Clinical category	Description
Relapsing-remitting multiple sclerosis	Episodic neurologic deficits with stable phase between attacks
Secondary progressive multiple sclerosis	Gradual neurologic deterioration from relapsing-remitting course, with or without superimposed acute attacks
Primary progressive multiple sclerosis	Gradual, continuous neurologic deterioration from onset of symptoms
Monosymptomatic demyelinating disease	Single episode of neurologic deficit
Optic neuritis	Loss of vision
Transverse myelitis	Bilateral lower extemity motor and sensory deficit, bladder difficulty
Isolated brainstem syndrome	Cranial nerve, motor and sensory deficits
Fulminant demyelinating disease	
Acute disseminated encephalomyelitis	Postinfectious, monophasic, diffuse white matter encephalopathy
Marburg variant	Fatal multifocal cerebral involvement
Baló concentric sclerosis	Rapidly progressive demyelination presenting as solitary mass lesion
Restricted distribution demyelinating disease	
Neuromyelitis optica (Devic disease)	Relapsing bilateral optic neuritis and transverse myelitis
Benign multiple sclerosis	Minimal neurologic disability at 10 years after onset of symptoms

From Adams, AC: Neurology in Primary Care. FA Davis Company, Philadelphia, 2000, p 227. Used with permission of Mayo Foundation for Medical Education and Research.

(Devic disease) is a demyelinating syndrome of restricted distribution, affecting only the optic nerves and spinal cord.

Patients whose disease has a mild course and minimal neurologic disability have *benign multiple sclerosis*. There is no consensus on the definition of benign multiple sclerosis, but prolonged (10-25 years) clinical observation is needed for the diagnosis. Patients with this type of multiple sclerosis tend to have the relapsing subtype and have prolonged remission after their first attack, mild and infrequent relapses, and little neurologic deficit or disability after an extended period.

Diagnostic Approach

The diagnosis of multiple sclerosis is a clinical diagnosis that can be supported by findings obtained with magnetic resonance imaging (MRI), cerebrospinal fluid (CSF) analysis, and visual evoked potentials. The central criterion for the diagnosis of multiple sclerosis is the presence of central nervous system lesions disseminated in time and space. Using both clinical and paraclinical investigations, an international panel on the diagnosis of multiple sclerosis established recommended diagnostic criteria (Tables 13.3 and 13.4). The diagnosis of multiple sclerosis can be made if the patient has two or more attacks (an episode of neurologic disturbance [subjective report or objective observation] of at least 24 hours) and objective clinical evidence of two or more lesions. In this clinical setting, no additional testing is needed; however, if the MRI and CSF findings are negative, alternative diagnoses need to be considered.

Although any neurologic symptom can occur in multiple sclerosis, the most frequent initial symptoms are sensory disturbances, motor dysfunction, and monocular visual impairment. Initial somatosensory disturbances may include complaints of tingling, burning, tightness, or numbness. The sensory symptoms often do not correlate with a recognizable anatomical pattern. Balance and gait difficulty are common complaints. Bladder disturbance is one of the most disabling symptoms of multiple sclerosis and occurs most often with advanced disease; however, symptoms of urgency and frequency and frequent urinary tract infections may be present early in the disease. In the case of a young man who presents with acute urinary retention, demyelinating disease is one of the first diagnostic considerations. Other signs and symptoms that should raise suspicion of multiple sclerosis include double vision, a "useless hand," trigeminal neuralgia in a person younger than 50 years, and symptoms induced by heat or exercise (Uhthoff phenomenon). Postpartum onset of symptoms and a diurnal fatigue pattern are also important findings. An electric-like sensation that radiates down the spine with flexion of the neck (Lhermitte sign) is also a characteristic symptom in multiple sclerosis.

When performing a neurologic examination on a patient with suspected multiple sclerosis, it is important to check the uninvolved, or "good," side and to attend to subtle asymmetries. The most frequent neurologic deficits found on examination involve the optic nerves, ocular motility, corticospinal pathway, and somatosensory pathways. Cerebellar findings of ataxia, dysmetria, and intention tremor usually occur later in the course of the disease. Cortical (or gray matter) signs such as early cognitive dysfunction, language disturbance, and extrapyramidal features do not suggest multiple sclerosis.

Findings of optic nerve dysfunction include diminished visual acuity, central scotoma, and, on ophthalmoscopic examination, optic nerve pallor (optic atrophy) (Fig. 13.1). Impaired color vision can be detected with the use of Ishihara plates. An afferent pupillary defect (also called a *Marcus Gunn pupil*) can be demonstrated with the swinging flashlight test. When a light source is moved back and forth between the eyes, the eye with the afferent defect appears to dilate when stimulated by the light. Because of the lesion, the direct response is slow in the affected eye and the dilatation that is seen with the swinging flashlight test is from the consensual response (Fig. 13.2).

Ocular motility problems such as nystagmus and ophthalmoparesis are frequently found on examination and indicate brainstem and cerebellar involvement. An early manifestation of multiple sclerosis is often *internuclear ophthalmoplegia*. It is the result of a lesion of the medial longitudinal fasciculus, the tract that connects the nucleus abducens (origin of cranial nerve VI) and the oculomotor nucleus (origin of cranial nerve III), which produce conjugate lateral eye movements (Fig. 13.3). The eye ipsilateral to the lesion cannot adduct on lateral gaze, but the contralateral eye can abduct and has horizontal nystagmus.

Table 13.3. Diagnostic Criteria for Multiple Sclerosis (MS)

Clinical presentation	Additional data needed for diagnosis
Two or more attacks; objective clinical evidence of two or more lesions	None*
Two or more attacks; objective clinical evidence of one lesion	Dissemination in space demonstrated by: • MRI,[†] *or* • Two or more MRI lesions consistent with MS plus positive CSF,[‡] *or* • Await further clinical attack implicating a different site
One attack; objective clinical evidence of two or more lesions	Dissemination in time demonstrated by: • MRI,[†] *or* • Second clinical attack
One attack; objective clinical evidence of one lesion (clinically isolated syndrome)	Dissemination in space demonstrated by: • MRI,[†] *or* • Two or more MRI lesions consistent with MS plus positive CSF[‡] And dissemination in time, demonstrated by: • MRI,[†] *or* • Second clinical attack
Insidious neurologic progression suggestive of MS	Positive CSF,[‡] and dissemination in space, demonstrated by: • 1) Nine or more T2 lesions in brain, *or* 2) Two or more lesions in spinal cord, *or* 3) Four to eight brain lesions plus one spinal cord lesion; *or* • Abnormal visual evoked potentials with MRI demonstrating four to eight brain lesions, or fewer than four brain lesions plus one spinal cord lesion; *and* • Dissemination in time demonstrated by MRI,[†] *or* • Continued progression for 1 year

CSF, cerebrospinal fluid; MRI, magnetic resonance imaging.
Brain MRI is recommended to exclude other causes.
[†]*MRI criteria for dissemination in space or time are described in Table 13.4.*
[‡]*"Positive CSF" is defined as oligoclonal bands differerent from those in serum, or elevated IgG index.*
Modified from McDonald, WI, et al: Recommended diagnostic criteria for multiple sclerosis: Guidelines from the International Panel on the Diagnosis of Multiple Sclerosis. Ann Neurol 50:121-127, 2001. Used with permission.

Table 13.4. Magnetic Resonance Imaging (MRI) Criteria for Dissemination of Lesions in Space and Time

MRI lesions disseminated in space:
At least three of the following criteria must be met:
1. One gadolinium-enhancing lesion or nine T2 hyperintense lesions if there is no gadolinium-enhancing lesion
2. At least one infratentorial lesion
3. At least one juxtacortical lesion
4. At least three periventricular lesions

MRI lesions disseminated in time:
At least one criterion must be met:
1. If MRI is more than 3 months after clinical event, then a gadolinium-enhancing lesion at a site different from the original clinical event is sufficient; if there is no gadolinium enhancement, then a follow-up scan is required (usually >3 months later). A new T2 or gadolinium-enhancing lesion on this second or subsequent MRI fulfills the requirement.
2. If first MRI scan is less than 3 months after the onset of the clinical event, then a second scan more than 3 months later showing a new gadolinium-enhancing lesion fulfills the requirement. If no gadolinium enhancement is seen on this second scan, a further scan not less than 3 months after the first scan that shows a new T2 lesion or an enhancing lesion will suffice.

Modified from McDonald, WI, et al: Recommended diagnostic criteria for multiple sclerosis: Guidelines from the International Panel on the Diagnosis of Multiple Sclerosis. Ann Neurol 50:121-127, 2001. Used with permission.

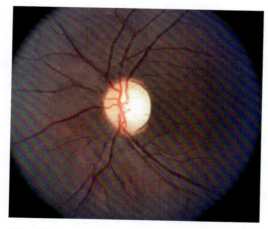

Fig. 13.1. Optic atrophy. Note that the optic disc is pale and small.

However, the eye ipsilateral to the lesion is able to adduct on accommodation because convergence does not require the medial longitudinal fasciculus.

Corticospinal tract (upper motor neuron) abnormalities are frequently elicited on examination. These include hyperactive reflexes, spasticity, extensor plantar reflexes, clonus, and loss of superficial reflexes. The absence or asymmetry of abdominal or cremasteric reflexes is useful when evaluating a person with suspected demyelinating disease, because the loss or asymmetry of these reflexes indicates upper motor neuron involvement. The sensory examination often shows reduced vibratory

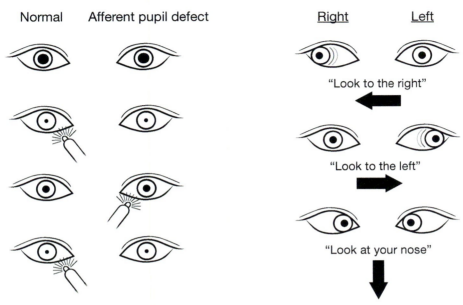

Normal   Afferent pupil defect   Right   Left

"Look to the right"

"Look to the left"

"Look at your nose"

Fig. 13.2. Afferent pupil defect. When a light source is moved back and forth between the eyes, the eye with the afferent defect appears to dilate when stimulated by the light. Because of the lesion, the direct response is slow in the affected eye and the dilatation that is seen with the swinging-flashlight test is from the consensual response.

Fig. 13.3. Bilateral internuclear ophthalmoplegia. This diagram represents what is seen when a lesion affects the medial longitudinal fasciculus bilaterally. Conjugate eye movement is affected by the inability to adduct the eye when looking to the left or right. Compensatory nystagmus occurs in the abducting eye. Convergence is normal.

sensation, which precedes any detectable loss in joint position sense.

Diagnostic Laboratory Support

The clinical diagnosis of multiple sclerosis is made on the basis of the history and examination findings of neurologic lesions disseminated in space and time. MRI, CSF analysis, and visual evoked potentials can support the diagnosis and may be essential in making the diagnosis when the clinical presentation alone is not sufficient. MRI is the most sensitive supportive test for the diagnosis of multiple sclerosis. CSF analyses can provide inflammatory and immunologic information. Visual evoked potentials are particularly useful when MRI findings are nonspecific or minimal. Somatosensory and

brainstem auditory evoked potentials are thought to contribute little to the diagnosis.

MRI

MRI has been invaluable in the diagnosis of multiple sclerosis and is included in the diagnostic criteria (Fig. 13.4). In patients with established disease, MRI is used to monitor disease activity and progression. The lesions of multiple sclerosis are of high intensity on T2-weighted images and of isointensity to low intensity on T1-weighted images. Fluid-attenuated inversion-recovery images are useful for showing juxtacortical and periventricular lesions because of the suppression of CSF intensity. It is important to remember that white matter abnormalities are nonspecific and can be

1. One gadolinium-enhancing lesion (*arrow*) *or*

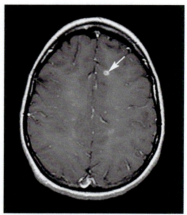

Nine T2 hyperintense lesions (*arrows* indicate three lesions) if no gadolinium-enhancing lesion

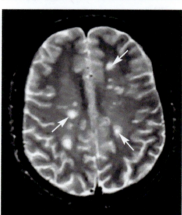

2. At least one infratentorial lesion (*arrow*)

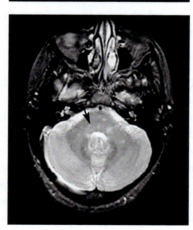

Fig. 13.4. MRI criteria for multiple sclerosis.

3. At least one juxtacortical lesion (*arrow*)

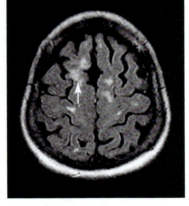

4. At least three periventricular lesions (*arrows*)

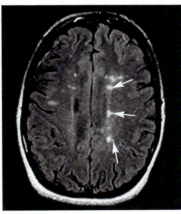

Fig. 13.4 (continued)

seen in ischemic and degenerative disorders (Fig. 13.5). In multiple sclerosis, white matter lesions are characteristically found in the periventricular white matter, on the inner surface of the corpus callosum, at the juxtacortical gray-white matter junction, and in the brainstem and cerebellum.

The low-intensity lesions seen on T1-weighted images are often referred to as black holes. Black holes that persist for several months represent areas of axon loss. Measurement of T1-lesion load correlates better with clinical disability than does T2-lesion load. Gadolinium-enhanced lesions are seen when the blood-brain barrier is disrupted; they represent active inflammation. Lesion enhancement can last for approximately 3 weeks and can be useful in monitoring active disease. Central nervous system atrophy can also be seen with MRI.

MRI has a pivotal role in the evaluation of patients who initially present with what is called a clinically isolated syndrome, such as optic neuritis or transverse myelitis. MRI findings can be used to predict in which patients clinically definite multiple sclerosis will develop. This is important when discussing disease-modifying therapy.

After the history and neurologic examination, the next diagnostic test should be cranial MRI. Although the diagnosis of multiple sclerosis can be made on clinical grounds alone

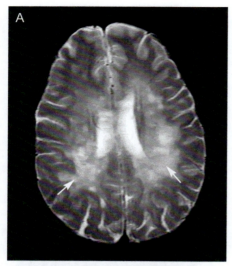

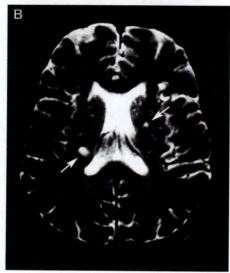

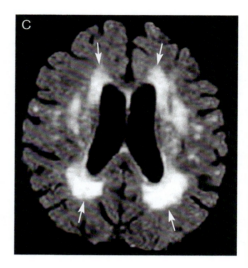

Fig. 13.5. Appearance of white matter abnormalities on MRI. *A*, Multiple sclerosis plaques (*arrows*); *B*, multiple lacunar infarcts (*arrows*); *C*, leukoaraiosis (*arrows*) in Alzheimer disease.

(two or more attacks; objective clinical evidence of two or more lesions), MRI can exclude other diagnoses in the differential diagnosis (Table 13.5). MRI of the spine should be performed if the patient presents with a myelopathy.

Cerebrospinal Fluid Analysis

CSF analysis can be useful in supporting the diagnosis of multiple sclerosis by providing evidence of immune and inflammatory disease. This is important if patients have an atypical clinical presentation and inconclusive imaging results. CSF immunoglobulin levels, especially immunoglobulin G (IgG), are increased in most patients with multiple sclerosis, presumably because of immune activation. CSF abnormalities supportive of the diagnosis of multiple sclerosis include the presence of oligoclonal IgG bands (not present in the serum) or elevated IgG index or both. Oligoclonal bands are not specific for multiple sclerosis and can occur with several infectious and inflammatory diseases, including Lyme disease, syphilis, human T-lymphotropic virus myelopathy, sarcoidosis, vasculitis, and chronic meningitis. Rarely, oligoclonal bands have been reported in healthy persons. The CSF of patients with multiple sclerosis may show a mild leukocytic (lymphocytes) pleocytosis (should be <50/mm^3 [0.05×10^9/L]) and increased concentration of protein. Infection

Table 13.5. Differential Diagnosis of Multiple Sclerosis

Disease	Distinguishing clinical or paraclinical features
Infectious	
Lyme	Rash, arthralgias, Lyme serology
Syphilis	Positive results: RPR, VDRL, FTA-ABS
HTLV-1 (myelopathy)	HTLV-1 detected
HIV infection	HIV detected
Inflammatory	
Sarcoidosis	ACE increased, meningeal enhancement at base of brain on MRI
Systemic lupus erythematosus	Other organ involvement, MRI abnormalities more subcortical than periventricular, autoantibodies
Sjögren syndrome	Sicca complex antibodies SS-A and SS-B, MRI lesion may involve gray matter
Behçet syndrome	Mucocutaneous lesions
Degenerative	
Cervical spondylosis (myelopathy)	Abnormal cervical spine MRI findings
Spinocerebellar or olivoponto-cerebellar degeneration	Family history, normal CSF, pes cavus
Leukodystrophies	Peripheral nerve involvement, increased levels of long-chain fatty acids
Hereditary spastic paraplegia (myelopathy)	Family history
Nutritional	
Vitamin B_{12} deficiency	Serum vitamin B_{12} level decreased
Neoplastic	
Sphenoid wing meningioma (optic neuritis)	Abnormal MRI findings
Optic nerve tumors (optic neuritis)	Abnormal MRI findings
Primary CNS lymphoma	Abnormal MRI findings
Paraneoplastic syndromes	Paraneoplastic antibodies, other evidence of malignancy
Psychogenic	Absence of objective neurologic signs; inconsistent weakness or sensory loss; normal MRI, CSF, evoked potentials; disability out of proportion to neurologic examination findings

ACE, angiotensin-converting enzyme; CNS, central nervous system; CSF, cerebrospinal fluid; FTA-ABS, fluorescent treponemal antibody absorption test; HIV, human immunodeficiency virus; HTLV-1, human T-lymphotropic virus type 1; MRI, magnetic resonance imaging; RPR, rapid plasma reagin test; SS, Sjögren syndrome; VDRL, Venereal Disease Research Laboratory test.
From Adams, AC: Neurology in Primary Care. FA Davis Company, Philadelphia, 2000, p 232. Used with permission of Mayo Foundation for Medical Education and Research.

or malignancy should be investigated if these values are high. CSF is valuable in excluding other infectious diseases (eg, neuroborreliosis [Lyme disease] and neurosyphilis) and malignancy.

Visual Evoked Potentials

Visual evoked potentials may be valuable in making the diagnosis of multiple sclerosis by establishing the presence of a lesion disseminated in space. This may be particularly useful when the patient presents with minimal or nonspecific MRI findings, for example, a patient with primary progressive multiple sclerosis and a progressive myelopathy or an older patient who has ischemic and degenerative changes visible on MRI. The usual finding in multiple sclerosis is a delayed visual evoked potential with a well-preserved wave form (Fig. 13.6).

Differential Diagnosis

Many infectious, inflammatory, degenerative, and neoplastic diseases of the nervous system need to be considered in the differential diagnosis of multiple sclerosis (Table 13.5). If the clinical presentation or MRI findings are atypical for multiple sclerosis, further laboratory evaluation is needed to investigate another possible diagnosis. It is important to consider these other diagnoses when patients have progressive deterioration from the onset of symptoms. Evaluation for systemic disease, MRI of the spine, CSF analysis, evoked potentials, and infectious and inflammatory serologic testing may be needed for accurate diagnosis.

Epidemiology

Patients often ask what causes multiple sclerosis and if it can be passed on to their children. Currently, multiple sclerosis is considered an autoimmune disease of the central nervous system that is initiated by an undefined environmental trigger in a genetically susceptible person. Environmental factors are suggested by the geographic distribution of multiple sclerosis. Its prevalence increases the greater the distance from the equator. High-risk areas are within the temperate zones in the northern and southern hemispheres. This

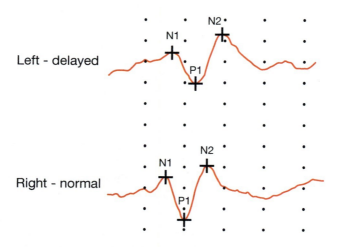

Fig. 13.6. Visual evoked potential in patient with left eye optic neuritis. (Modified from Mancall, EL, general editor: Continuum: Lifelong Learning in Neurology. Part A: Clinical Neurophysiology 4:58, October 1998. Used with permission.)

risk can be affected by migration if the person migrates before puberty. If the person moves before puberty, the prevalence rate will be that of the new residence; however, if he or she moves after puberty, the prevalence rate will be that of the previous location. Epidemics of multiple sclerosis have been reported and support an environmental cause for the disease. Viruses have been thought to trigger autoimmune demyelination in susceptible persons. Epstein-Barr virus, human herpesvirus 6, and many other pathogens have been suggested as a cause, but currently, no evidence shows direct involvement of a virus as a cause of multiple sclerosis.

Ample evidence supports a genetic component to disease susceptibility. Of patients with multiple sclerosis, 15% have a first-degree relative with the disease. The incidence of the disease in studies of twins supports both environmental and genetic factors. The concordance rate of monozygotic twins is 6 to 10 times that of dizygotic twins, but not the 100% that would be expected for a purely genetic disease. Although the lifetime risk that a child of an affected parent will develop multiple sclerosis is low (3%-5%), it is still 20 to 50 times that of the general population. The risk is increased for children, particularly daughters, of mothers with multiple sclerosis. Multiple sclerosis has been associated with certain human leukocyte antigen genotypes, and a consistent relation has been reported with the class II region of the major histocompatibility complex gene on chromosome 6. Genetic susceptibility to multiple sclerosis is complex, and additional investigation is needed to define the relation between genetic and environmental factors.

Prognosis

Multiple sclerosis is a disorder that evolves over decades. The clinical course is often unpredictable, and the individual variation is considerable, making a discussion about prognosis difficult. Most patients have relapsing-remitting multiple sclerosis, and 50% of these develop secondary progressive multiple sclerosis. This transition occurs gradually over 10 to 20 years, when clinical relapses become less distinct and recovery is less vigorous. Patients with primary progressive multiple sclerosis (10%-15% of those with multiple sclerosis) have continuous clinical deterioration from the onset of symptoms.

Because multiple sclerosis is seldom fatal, survival is an insensitive measure of disease outcome. More than one-half of the deaths of multiple sclerosis patients are not related to the disease. Expected survival is approximately 80% that of an age- and sex-matched population. Prognosis is better discussed in terms of disability and quality-of-life issues. Most patients will be ambulatory 15 years after the onset of disease (50% may depend on a walking aid), but 15% will require a wheelchair.

Several clinical features provide prognostic information. Indicators for a favorable prognosis include sensory symptoms or optic neuritis at the onset, infrequent attacks during the first few years, and good recovery from the attacks. Poor prognostic indicators include age at onset older than 40 years; male sex; progressive disease from onset; early motor, cerebellar, and sphincter signs; more than four attacks in the first 2 years; short intervals between attacks; and permanent disability within 3 years from the onset of symptoms.

Pregnancy

Multiple sclerosis is twice as common in women as in men, and the majority of patients are of childbearing age. Many patients are concerned about the effect of pregnancy on multiple sclerosis and about the effect of the disease on pregnancy. Multiple sclerosis has no adverse effect on pregnancy, labor, or delivery. However, an increased risk of relapse has been shown during the six-month postpartum period for women with relapsing-remitting multiple sclerosis. However, this increased risk does not appear to have a detrimental effect on the rate of developing sustained disability. The patient's current level of disability may be the most significant factor to consider in family planning. Therapies with disease-modifying medications and many symptom-relieving drugs need to be considered for women anticipating pregnancy.

Disease-Modifying Therapy

The medical treatment of multiple sclerosis has changed remarkably since the approval of interferon β-1b (Betaseron), interferon β-1a (Avonex, Rebif), and glatiramer acetate (Copaxone). Interferon β-1b and β-1a are recombinant interferon β preparations that have multiple immunomodulatory actions and inhibit cell-mediated inflammation. Glatiramer acetate is a random polymer of basic amino acids that inhibits T-cell recognition of myelin antigens. All three drugs reduce the relapse rate by one-third in patients who have relapsing-remitting multiple sclerosis. Some evidence suggests that interferons may reduce long-term disability. All three drugs have shown a reduction in MRI-visualized lesion activity, but the clinical significance of this is not known.

When therapy should be initiated and how long it should be maintained are not known and are matters of controversy. Advocates for starting therapy early, including the time of the first clinically isolated demyelinating event, believe that early treatment will prevent or delay immune-mediated axonal injury and reduce long-term disability. Before initiating therapy, other neurologists favor further clinical observation to determine if the patient has mild disease with infrequent relapses. They cite the modest efficacy of the drugs and their unknown long-term benefits and risks, adverse effects, and high cost. Also, patients who receive interferon therapy can develop neutralizing

antibodies that are associated with reduced clinical and radiographic evidence of effectiveness. Neutralizing antibodies may reduce the likelihood of long-term benefit. Because studies have shown return of disease activity after discontinuation of drug treatment, therapy should be continued indefinitely. The patient's clinical status and MRI findings are followed to determine disease activity and the effectiveness of treatment.

Interferons β-1a (Rebif and Avonex) and β-1b and glatiramer acetate are considered first-line disease-modifying therapy for relapsing-remitting multiple sclerosis. The decision about which of the four drugs to be used may be based on clinician and patient preference, dosage schedule, and adverse effects. No study has directly compared the four medications. Evidence suggests that higher dose interferon therapy may be more effective, as indicated clinically and radiographically, but the adverse effects are more prominent. During the first few months of treatment with interferon, flulike symptoms are common. Interferon therapy can cause depression and should not be given to a patient who has severe depression. Also, it should not be administered to women who are pregnant or anticipate becoming pregnant. Glatiramer acetate is not recommended for pregnant women (class B pregnancy drug), but the risk may be less than it is with interferon treatment.

Natalizumab (Tysabri) was approved by the US Food and Drug Administration in 2004 to treat relapsing-remitting multiple sclerosis after studies showed it could possibly reduce the rate of relapse and the risk of sustained disability. This monoclonal antibody, thought to reduce inflammation, was withdrawn 3 months after it was introduced because of the rare association with progressive multifocal leukoencephalopathy. However, in 2006, the drug was reintroduced and is available under a restricted distribution system. Other monoclonal antibodies for the treatment of multiple sclerosis are being investigated.

Mitoxantrone (Novantrone), an antineoplastic drug, has been approved for the treatment of aggressive relapsing-remitting and secondary progressive multiple sclerosis. This drug has been shown to slow progression of the disease. The most serious concerns about this agent are the development of cardiotoxicity and secondary acute myelogenous leukemia. The disease-modifying drugs available for treating multiple sclerosis are summarized in Table 13.6.

Symptomatic Therapy

Despite the advances in disease-modifying therapy, symptomatic treatment of multiple sclerosis is essential to help maintain function and to improve quality of life (Table 13.7). Before a specific medical therapy is initiated, the patient needs to be evaluated for factors that may contribute to the symptoms, such as infections or medication side effects. Patients should maintain a well-balanced diet, not smoke, and avoid excessive alcohol consumption. Currently, there is little evidence to recommend a specific diet rather than a well-balanced one. Patient education, rehabilitation (eg, supervised fitness program for fatigue), and counseling (eg, for depression) are important nonpharmacologic management measures that may be preferable to drug therapy for some patients. Many of the symptoms of patients with multiple sclerosis, for example, pain and depression, are treated in the same way as they are in patients who do not have multiple sclerosis.

Acute attacks or relapses of the disease in patients with marked disability (eg, loss of vision or paraplegia) are frequently treated with corticosteroids. Methylprednisolone given intravenously has a rapid onset of action, produces consistent results, has few adverse effects, and can be administered on an outpatient basis. The recommended therapy is 3 to 5 days of 1,000 mg given intravenously over 2 to 3 hours. An oral prednisone taper (60 mg/day, decreasing by 10 mg every 2-3 days) is optional after intravenous therapy. Corticosteroid treatment accelerates recovery and shortens the duration of the disability. However, no evidence suggests that it alters the outcome.

Occasional adverse effects of intravenous methylprednisolone include flushing, fluid retention, hyperglycemia, depression, and insomnia. The fasting serum glucose level and electrolyte levels may need to be monitored. Oral corticosteroids generally have not been prescribed since the optic neuritis trial demonstrated an increased risk of subsequent clinical relapse in patients treated with prednisone.

Depression is relatively common in patients with multiple sclerosis and needs to be considered seriously by the physician. Suicide is a leading cause of death among those who are mildly to moderately disabled. Many medications prescribed for multiple sclerosis (interferon, baclofen, and benzodiazepines) can aggravate depression. Psychiatric consultation can be useful. Depression in multiple sclerosis is treated with the same medications used to treat depression in the general population. Emotional lability (pathologic crying and laughing) can be socially disabling. Low-dose amitriptyline or nortriptyline is effective in reducing this problem.

Fatigue is the most common symptom in multiple sclerosis and can be extremely disabling. Nonpharmacologic measures that can reduce fatigue include sleep hygiene measures, a supervised fitness program, the use of air conditioners or fans for cooling, and improved nutrition. Other diagnoses such as sleep disorders or depression should be considered. Medication options include amantadine, selective serotonin reuptake inhibitors, and modafinil.

Spasticity is also a common symptom in multiple sclerosis and can be worsened by

Table 13.6. Disease-Modifying Drugs for Multiple Sclerosis

Drug	Adverse effects	Safety monitoring
Glatiramer acetate (Copaxone) 20 mg SQ daily	Transient flushing, chest tightness, palpitations, anxiety, injection site reaction	None
Interferon	Myalgias, fever, malaise, depression, local rejection reaction	CBC with differential and platelet counts and liver function tests: at 1, 3, and 6 months after initiation of therapy and periodically thereafter Thyroid function: periodically
Interferon β-1a (Avonex) 30 μg IM once weekly Interferon β-1a (Rebif) 22 or 44 μg SQ 3 times weekly Interferon β-1b (Betaseron) 0.25 mg SQ every other day		
Mitoxantrone (Novantrone) 5 or 12 mg/m² IV every 12 weeks for 2 or 3 years	Alopecia, diarrhea, amenorrhea, cardiotoxicity	Echocardiography with each dose, discontinue if ejection fraction decreases
Natalizumab (Tysabri) 300 mg IV infused over approximately 1 hour given at 28-day intervals	Headache, fatigue, arthralgias	Available only through a restricted distribution program because of increased risk of PML

CBC, complete blood count; IM, intramuscularly; IV, intravenous; PML, progressive multifocal leukoencephalopathy; SQ, subcutaneously.

bladder or bowel distention or by any infection. Regular stretching and exercise can reduce the discomfort and improve function. Many medications are available to treat spasticity, including baclofen, tizanidine, dantrolene, diazepam, and clonazepam. For all these agents, treatment should be started at the lowest dose and increased gradually. The most common adverse effects are increasing weakness, sedation, and hypotension. Dantrolene (Dantrium) is given primarily to nonambulatory patients. Botulinum toxin (Botox) may be useful if focal control of spasticity is needed. The muscle spasms that frequently accompany spasticity can be treated with many of the anticonvulsant medications. For these, too, treatment should be started at a low

Table 13.7. Symptomatic Therapy for Multiple Sclerosis

Symptom	Treatment options
Acute attack	Methylprednisolone (Solu-Medrol), 1,000 mg intravenously daily for 3-5 days
	Seven courses of plasma exchange on alternate days
Depression	All antidepressants
Emotional lability	Amitriptyline (Elavil), 10-25 mg before bedtime
Erectile dysfunction	Sildenafil (Viagra), 25-100 mg 1 hour before sexual activity
Fatigue	Amantadine (Symmetrel), 100 mg twice daily
	Fluoxetine (Prozac) 20 mg in morning, other SSRIs
	Modafinil (Provigil), 200 mg in morning
Muscle spasms	Carbamazepine (Tegretol), titrate dose
	Phenytoin (Dilantin), titrate dose
	Gabapentin (Neurontin), titrate dose
	Baclofen (Lioresal), 5 mg 3 times daily (maximum 80 mg/day)
Neurogenic bladder	Oxybutynin (Ditropan), 2.5-5 mg 3-4 times daily
	Tolterodine (Detrol), 1-2 mg twice daily
Spasticity	Baclofen (Lioresal), 5 mg 3 times daily (maximum 80 mg/day), baclofen pump for intrathecal administration
	Tizanidine (Zanaflex), 2 mg daily–12 mg 3 times daily
	Clonazepam (Klonopin), titrate dose
	Botulinum toxin (Botox)

SSRI, selective serotonin reuptake inhibitor.
Modified from Adams, AC: Neurology in Primary Care. FA Davis Company, Philadelphia, 2000, p 236.
Used with permission of Mayo Foundation for Medical Education and Research.

dose and increased until the desired therapeutic effect is achieved or toxicity occurs. If an oral medication is not effective in treating spasticity, consider intrathecal baclofen.

Bladder dysfunction, like fatigue, is an extremely disabling symptom. Urgency, frequency, and incontinence are the most frequent symptoms. Many patients attribute bladder difficulty to the effects of aging. Estrogen deficiency and prostatic hypertrophy can be contributing factors, but check for other causes of neurogenic bladder. If the urinary residual volume is less than 100 mL, suspect a spastic bladder. Recommend that the patient avoid alcohol and caffeine, which stimulate the bladder, drink plenty of fluid to prevent concentrated urine, perform pelvic floor strengthening exercises, and have frequent voiding times throughout the day. Anticholinergic agents help. Patients who have a large postvoid residual volume may need intermittent catheterization. Whenever patients have symptoms of bladder dysfunction, they should be evaluated for a urinary tract infection. Urologic consultation may be necessary.

Optic Neuritis

Optic neuritis, a syndrome caused by inflammation of the optic nerve, is characterized by painful loss of vision in one eye. The patient usually reports subacute (hours to days) loss of vision and pain with eye movement. Impaired visual acuity and color vision and an afferent pupillary defect are the common findings on physical examination. Central scotomas are the usual visual field findings. The optic disc can appear normal (retrobulbar neuritis) or show swelling without hemorrhages (Fig. 13.7). As mentioned above, multiple sclerosis is a frequent cause of optic neuritis. It is the first symptom in 20% of patients with multiple sclerosis and occurs in 70% of patients sometime during the course of the illness. Optic neuritis can also be caused by viral, bacterial (syphilis, Lyme disease, or tuberculosis), and fungal (cryptococcosis or histoplasmosis) infections and by such inflammatory disorders as sarcoidosis and systemic lupus erythematosus.

MRI is usually part of the diagnostic evaluation of a patient who has optic neuritis (Fig. 13.8). Evidence of other inflammatory lesions provides prognostic information about demyelinating disease and may lead to more aggressive treatment. Other tests that might be considered for a patient who presents with optic neuritis are antinuclear antibodies for connective tissue disease, fluorescent treponemal antibody absorption for syphilis, and chest radiography for sarcoidosis.

Intravenous methylprednisolone followed by optional oral prednisone speeds the recovery of the loss of vision from optic neuritis. Oral prednisone is ineffective and increases the risk of new episodes. Also, intravenous methylprednisolone was shown over a 2-year period to decrease the rate of development of multiple sclerosis. If MRI of the head shows that the patient is at risk for the development of multiple sclerosis (two or more white matter lesions that are 3 mm or more in diameter, ovoid, and periventricular in location), disease-modifying therapy should be considered.

Neuromyelitis Optica

Neuromyelitis optica, also know as *Devic disease*, is a demyelinating disorder that involves predominantly the spinal cord and optic nerves. In 2006, specific diagnostic criteria were developed to distinguish neuromyelitis optica from multiple sclerosis. The criteria include optic neuritis, acute myelitis, and at least two or three supportive criteria. Supportive criteria include

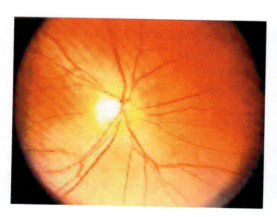

Fig. 13.7. Optic neuritis. The funduscopic examination shows papilledema due to the swelling of the myelin sheaths of optic nerve axons.

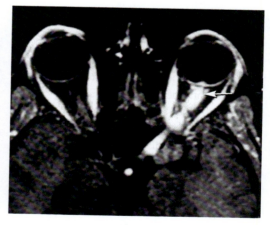

Fig. 13.8. Optic neuritis. MRI of the head showing increased signal in the left optic nerve (*arrow*) in optic neuritis.

a continuous spinal cord MRI lesion extending over three or more contiguous vertebral segments (Fig. 13.9), MRI findings at onset not meeting the diagnostic criteria for multiple sclerosis, and the presence of the serum autoantibody, neuromyelitis optica (NMO)-IgG.

No definitive treatment protocol has been published for neuromyelitis optica. Acute attacks are often treated with corticosteroids. Various immune therapies have been used for preventive treatment, including the disease-modifying therapies for multiple sclerosis, azathioprine, methotrexate, and mycophenolate mofetil. Research findings involving mono-clonal antibodies are encouraging.

Connective Tissue Diseases and the Vasculitides

The systemic inflammatory diseases that affect the neuromuscular system are listed in Table 13.1. Several potential pathogenic mechanisms can explain how connective tissue diseases and vasculitides affect the nervous system, including direct immune-mediated effects (immune complex, autoantibodies, or cytokine-mediated effects) and indirect effects (vasculopathy, coagulopathy, or cardiac emboli). Injury to the nervous system may be due to toxic effects, including the effects of medications. It is important to know how these disorders affect the nervous system because the patient may present initially with a neurologic problem. The neurologic, systemic, and diagnostic features of several of these disorders are highlighted in Table 13.8.

INFECTIOUS DISEASE OF THE NERVOUS SYSTEM

Meningitis

The clinical features of meningitis include headache, stiff neck (nuchal rigidity), and mental status changes. Nuchal rigidity indicates irritation of the meninges. The diagnosis of meningitis is confirmed by an infectious CSF profile (ie, leukocytosis, increased protein concentration, and decreased glucose level). Acute meningitis can develop over hours to days and is usually caused by a viral or bacterial infection in a patient with normal immune status. The most common cause of bacterial meningitis in adults is infection with *Streptococcus pneumoniae* or *Neisseria meningitidis*. In neonates, the elderly, alcoholics, and immunosuppressed patients, *Listeria monocytogenes* is a likely organism. Chronic meningitis, usually caused by granulomatous disease, tumor, or syphilis, can be associated with encephalitis. Cortical dysfunction and cranial nerve palsies may occur in chronic meningitis. *Cryptococcus neoformans* is the most common opportunistic organism that causes meningitis in a patient

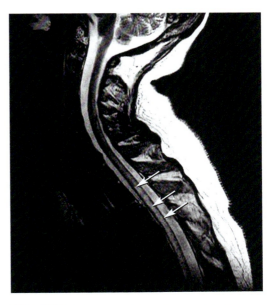

Fig. 13.9. MRI of the spine in neuromyelitis optica. MRI shows a continuous lesion (*arrows*) in the spinal cord extending over three contiguous vertebral segments.

with human immunodeficiency virus (HIV) infection. The CSF findings may be only mildly abnormal (mild pleocytosis and increased protein concentration), so it is important to test for *Cryptococcus* with the India ink preparation, the antigen assay, and fungal culture. Because *Cryptococcus* and other fungal pathogens may be present in low concentrations, it is important to provide the laboratory with several milliliters of CSF for these studies. In a patient with HIV infection, tuberculous meningitis or aseptic meningitis (thought to be secondary to the virus itself) can occur. The pathogens associated with meningitis, the common risk factors, and treatment are summarized in Table 13.9. Infectious disease consultation is recommended when treating these serious infections.

CSF analysis is essential in the diagnostic evaluation of a patient with an infection of the nervous system (Table 13.10). Infections of the central nervous system cause an increase in the leukocyte count (pleocytosis) and protein level and a decrease in the glucose level, depending on the infectious organism. The CSF leukocyte count and differential need to be interpreted carefully. Generally, bacterial infections cause a neutrophilic pleocytosis, but this may be altered if the infection has been partially treated. Some viral infections such as mumps can produce a

Table 13.8. Neurologic, Systemic, and Diagnostic Features of Connective Tissue Disease and Vasculitis

Disease	Neurologic feature	Systemic feature	Diagnostic feature
Systemic lupus erythematosus	Encephalopathy, seizures, behavioral change	Butterfly rash, pleuritic pain, proteinuria	Anti-Sm and anti-DNA antibodies
Sjögren syndrome	Trigeminal sensory neuropathy, autonomic neuropathy	Sicca complex	Anti-SSA
Wegener granulomatosis	Cranial mononeuropathy	Hemoptysis	cANCA, pANCA
Rheumatoid arthritis	Cervical myelopathy, compression neuropathies, peripheral neuropathies	Erosive inflammation of joints	Rheumatoid factor
Polyarteritis nodosa	Mononeuropathy multiplex, polyneuropathy, brachial plexopathy	Renal disease	Angiography, sural nerve biopsy, ANA
Temporal arteritis	Headache, visual impairment, cranial neuropathies	Anemia, weight loss, jaw claudication	Increased ESR, temporal artery biopsy

ANA, antinuclear antibody; ANCA, antineutrophil cytoplasmic antibody (c, classic; p, peripheral); ESR, erythrocyte sedimentation rate; SSA, soluble substance A antigen.
Modified from Adams, AC: Neurology in Primary Care. FA Davis Company, Philadelphia, 2000, p 239. Used with permission of Mayo Foundation for Medical Education and Research.

neutrophilic pleocytosis during the first few days of infection. Eosinophils occur in allergic and parasitic diseases but can also be present in fungal infections, tuberculosis, and lymphoma. Diagnostic possibilities for the presence of erythrocytes in the CSF include traumatic tap, subarachnoid hemorrhage, and herpes encephalitis. An increased concentration of protein in the CSF occurs in most infections and tends to be greater in bacterial than viral infections. Neoplasm should be considered if the protein concentration is more than 400 mg/dL. The CSF glucose level usually is low in bacterial infections, but there are exceptions.

Computed tomography (CT) or MRI should be performed before lumbar puncture. If imaging or examination findings provide any evidence of a space-occupying lesion, initiate empirical therapy without delay. Although treatment may impair CSF culture results, the etiologic agent often can be found with blood cultures or by a positive result on the CSF antigen test. Other diagnostic measures include Gram stain, culture, serology, antigen detection, polymerase chain reaction, and brain biopsy.

Human Immunodeficiency Virus Infection

Infectious diseases of the nervous system are well illustrated by considering a patient who has HIV infection. The neurologic complications of this infection involve every level of the central and peripheral nervous systems (Table 13.11). Because of the compromised immune status of these patients, every infectious agent needs to be considered in the diagnostic evaluation.

Focal findings in a patient with HIV infection suggest the possibility of a mass lesion. The three major diagnostic considerations include cerebral toxoplasmosis, progressive multifocal leukoencephalopathy, and primary central nervous system lymphoma (Fig. 13.10). Tuberculous and other fungal brain abscesses can occur. In persons who are not immunosuppressed, brain abscesses can result from such underlying infections as otitis, mastoiditis, sinusitis, head wounds, endocarditis, and pulmonary infections. Brain abscesses cause focal syndromes such as hemiparesis, aphasia, or focal seizures. Neurosurgical and infectious disease consultation is valuable in the diagnosis and treatment of brain abscesses.

Headache in a patient with HIV infection should always prompt an evaluation for an underlying mass lesion. When no other cause of the headache can be identified, the diagnosis is *HIV headache*. Its cause is not known, but it may be related to the release of vasoactive cytokines.

The most common neurologic complication of HIV-1 is *acquired immunodeficiency syndrome dementia complex*. Other terms used to describe this disorder are *HIV encephalopathy* and *HIV-1–associated cognitive/motor complex*. The clinical features include cognitive, motor, and behavioral abnormalities. Early in the course of the disorder, the patient may complain of impaired memory and concentration. Apathy and withdrawal are the usual early behavioral disturbances. Motor features can include ataxia, leg weakness, tremor, and loss of fine motor coordination. The disorder is progressive and, when advanced, can include severe dementia, mutism, paraplegia, and incontinence. Antiretroviral agents are used for treatment.

HIV infection has numerous neuromuscular complications (Table 13.11). The pathogenesis of many of these disorders is autoimmune, as in chronic inflammatory demyelinating neuropathy. Treatment includes corticosteroids, plasma exchange, and intravenous immunoglobulin. An important opportunistic infection of the peripheral nervous system can occur with cytomegalovirus, which can cause a subacute progressive polyradiculoneuropathy. CSF analysis shows pleocytosis with neutrophil predominance. Ganciclovir is used to treat this disorder.

Table 13.9.   Pathogens Associated With Meningitis, Risk Factors, and Treatment

Pathogen	Risk factors	Treatment
Bacterial		
Neisseria meningitidis	Childhood to early adulthood	Penicillin G or ampicillin Ceftriaxone or cefotaxime plus vancomycin
Streptococcus pneumoniae	All ages Otitis, sinusitis, head injury, CSF leak	Penicillin G (plus vancomycin) or ampicillin or third-generation cephalosporin
Haemophilus influenzae type b	Infants and children Otitis, sinusitis	Ceftriaxone or cefotaxime plus vancomycin
Listeria monocytogenes	Neonate and elderly, diabetes, immunocompromised	Ceftazidime plus ampicillin
Group B streptococcus	Neonate	Ampicillin plus cefotaxime or aminoglycoside
Klebsiella-Enterobacter species	Neonate	Ampicillin plus cefotaxime or aminoglycoside
Escherichia coli	Neonate	Ampicillin plus cefotaxime or aminoglycoside
Staphylococcus aureus	Penetrating head trauma	Vancomycin plus ceftazidime
Viral		Supportive
Herpes simplex	Cutaneous herpes lesions	
Varicella-zoster	Shingles or chickenpox	
Enterovirus	Contact with small children, diarrhea	
Mumps	Parotitis, not vaccinated	
HIV	Primary infection, advanced immunodeficiency	
Mycobacterial		
Tuberculous	Tuberculous exposure, associated with HIV	Isoniazid plus rifamprin plus pyrazinamide plus ethambutol
Fungal		
Cryptococcus neoformans	Immunosuppression, especially HIV	Amphotericin B

CSF, cerebrospinal fluid; HIV, human immunodeficiency virus.

Table 13.10. Cerebrospinal Fluid Findings in Infectious Meningitis

Condition	Opening pressure	Protein	Glucose	Cell count	Other studies
Normal	50-200 mm H_2O	15-45 mg/dL	45-80 mg/mL (2/3 of serum)	No RBCs WBCs 0-5/mm³ ($0-0.005\times10^9$/L) (lymphocytes or monocytes)	
Bacterial meningitis	Increased	Increased Usually >100 mg/dL	Decreased Usually <50% of blood glucose	Increased >100/mm³ ($>0.1\times10^9$/L), often >1,000/ mm³ ($>1\times10^9$/L) WBCs (PMNs)	Positive Gram stain Positive culture (reduced if patient partially treated)
Viral meningitis	Normal or increased	Normal or increased	Normal or decreased	Increased WBCs (lymphocytes)	Negative Gram stain Negative culture PCR sensitive for enterovirus, herpesvirus, and some arboviruses
Tuberculous meningitis	Increased	Increased, 60-500 mg/dL	Decreased	Increased WBC 30->1,000/mm³ ($0.03->1\times10^9$/L) lymphocytes (PMNs can occur)	Positive acid-fast smear in 25% Positive culture in 33% PCR is specific, not sensitive
Fungal meningitis	Normal or increased	Increased, 50-1,000 mg/dL	Normal or decreased	Increased WBC 20-1,000/mm³ ($0.02-1\times10^9$/L) lymphocytes (PMNs can occur)	Culture usually negative except for *Cryptococcus* Antigen and antibody testing

PCR, polymerase chain reaction; PMN, polymorphonuclear neutrophil; RBC, erythrocytes; WBC, leukocyte.

Focal CNS disorder	Time course (onset to presentation)	Associated symptoms	MRI focal lesion	
Cerebral toxoplasmosis	Few days	Altered consciousness, fever, headache, constitutional symptoms	Mass effect with surrounding edema; ring-like contrast enhancement; located in gray matter of diencephalon and cerebral cortex	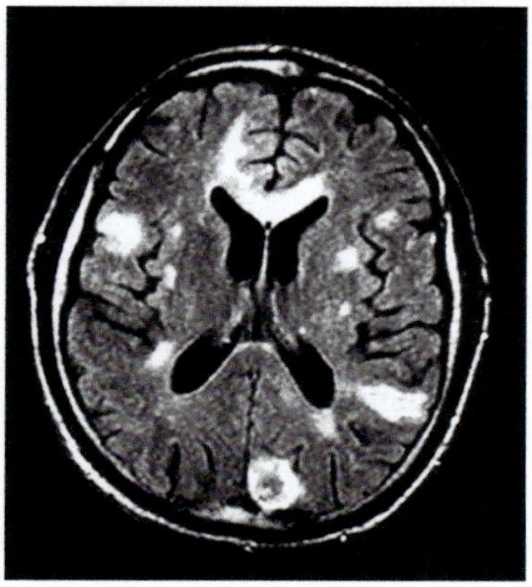
Progressive multifocal leukoencephalopathy	Weeks	Progressive focal syndrome, cognitive dysfunction	No mass effect or edema; lesions confined to white matter	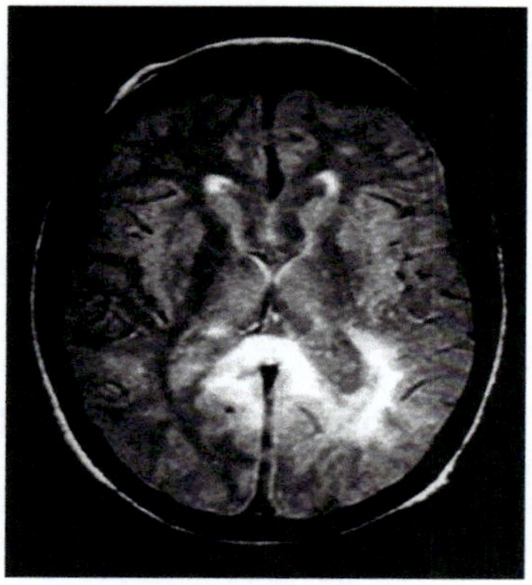
Primary CNS lymphoma	1-2 weeks	Focal syndrome, headache, confusion, seizures, cranial nerve deficits	Mass effect with surrounding edema; diffuse contrast enhancement, involvement of white matter adjacent to ventricles	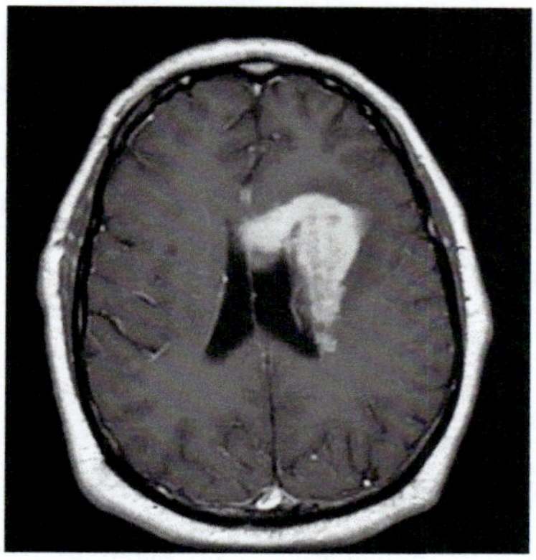

Fig. 13.10. Major focal central nervous system (CNS) disorders in human immunodeficiency virus infection. MRI, magnetic resonance imaging.

The most frequent neuropathy in patients with HIV infection is a distal sensory polyneuropathy. Management of the painful dysesthesias includes many of the medications used to treat other painful disorders, such as painful diabetic neuropathy (see Table 10.2). Many of the antiretroviral agents can cause peripheral neuropathies and myopathies.

Lyme Disease

Lyme disease is a bacterial infection caused by *Borrelia burgdorferi*, a tick-transmitted spirochete that occurs along the U.S. Atlantic coast and in parts of the U.S. West and Midwest and in Western Europe. Peripheral nervous system manifestations of the infection include multifocal axonal neuropathy, painful radiculitis, mononeuritis multiplex, sensorimotor neuropathy, facial nerve palsy, and myositis. Central nervous system manifestations include lymphocytic meningitis, focal and diffuse encephalitis, encephalomyelitis, and encephalopathy.

The illness begins (stage 1) with flulike symptoms and may be associated with an expanding ringlike skin rash that has a clear center (erythema migrans). After several weeks or months (stage 2), the patient may experience meningeal and radicular symptoms, with headache, stiff neck, or cranial nerve (facial nerve) or spinal root involvement. Arthritis is typical at this stage. Late central nervous system complications (stage 3) can include encephalopathy, seizures, and dementia. The late syndrome may resemble multiple sclerosis.

The results of laboratory tests to detect Lyme disease can be difficult to interpret, and it is most important to interpret the results in relation to clinical findings. Currently, serologic tests are the best measure of infection. Most laboratories use enzyme-linked immunosorbent assays to measure specific antibodies. The most helpful way to confirm CNS infection is to demonstrate the specific antibody in the CSF.

Table 13.11. Neurologic Complications of Human Immunodeficiency Virus Infection

Muscle
  Inflammatory myopathy
  Noninflammatory myopathy
  Zidovudine (AZT) myopathy

Peripheral nerve
  Focal neuropathy
  Mononeuritis multiplex
  Polyneuropathy
  Acute and chronic demyelinating
   polyneuropathy
  Distal sensory polyneuropathy
  CMV polyneuropathy
  Nucleoside polyneuropathy
  Brachial plexitis
  Autonomic neuropathy

Spinal cord
  Vacuolar myelopathy

Meninges
  Aseptic meningitis
  Cryptococcal meningitis
  Tuberculous meningitis

Brain
  Postinfectious encephalomyelitis
  CMV encephalitis
  AIDS dementia complex
  Cerebral toxoplasmosis
  Progressive multifocal leukoencephalopathy
  Primary CNS lymphoma

AIDS, acquired immunodeficiency syndrome; CMV, cytomegalovirus; CNS, central nervous system.
From Adams, AC: Neurology in Primary Care. FA Davis Company, Philadelphia, 2000, p 239. Used with permission of Mayo Foundation for Medical Education and Research.

Parenteral ceftriaxone (2 g intravenously every 24 hours for 10-30 days) is recommended for meningitis, radiculoneuritis, encephalomyelitis, peripheral neuropathy, and encephalopathy. Oral doxycycline (100 mg orally twice daily for 10-30 days) is used to treat cranial neuritis or facial palsy if the results of the CSF analysis are normal.

West Nile Virus

West Nile virus infection is a mosquito-borne disease. The infection is usually asymptomatic, and involvement of the nervous system is rare. However, it is important to know that the infection can cause a meningoencephalitis and acute flaccid paralysis similar to poliomyelitis. The acute flaccid paralysis can involve only one limb or be more diffuse. Autonomic and cranial nerve involvement has been reported. The CSF findings are consistent with a viral infection, and electromyography shows decreased amplitude of compound muscle action potentials in the affected limbs, with intact nerve conduction velocities. Detection of the IgM antibody in the CSF is consistent with the diagnosis. Treatment is supportive.

Prion Diseases

Prion diseases include a group of transmissible sporadic, familial, and acquired neurodegenerative disorders. These diseases are the result of an abnormally folded isoform of the prion protein, a normal constituent of the neuronal cell membrane. Prion diseases include Creutzfeldt-Jakob disease, Gerstmann-Sträussler-Scheinker syndrome, fatal insomnia, new variant Creutzfeldt-Jakob disease, and kuru (Table 13.12). Prion diseases are rare, but with the association of new variant Creutzfeldt-Jakob disease and bovine spongiform encephalopathy, or "mad-cow disease," they have received considerable publicity. Currently, no specific treatment is known for these disorders.

Table 13.12. Summary of Prion Diseases

Disease	Clinical presentation	Diagnostic tests	Cause
Creutzfeldt-Jakob disease			
Sporadic	Cognitive disburbance, ataxia, myoclonus Rapid course (months)	Periodic EEG Increased 14-3-3 protein in CSF	
Familial	Same as above	Same as above	Mutations of the *PRNP* gene
New variant	Personality changes, sensory symptoms, cerebellar dysfunction	Normal or slow EEG	Associated with consumption of beef with bovine spongiform encephalopathy
Iatrogenic	Cerebellar dysfunction more prominent than dementia	Slow EEG	From growth hormone, dura mater, corneal implants, human chorionic gonadotropin
Gerstmann-Sträussler-Scheinker syndrome	Cerebellar dysfunction more prominent than cognitive disturbance	Slow EEG	Mutations of *PRNP* gene
Fatal insomnia			
Sporadic	Insomnia, autonomic dysfunction, minimal dementia	Normal or slow EEG	
Familial	Same as above	Same as above	Mutations of *PRNP* gene
Kuru	Cerebellar dysfunction	Normal or slow EEG	From ritualistic consumption of brain by Fore people of Papua, New Guinea

CSF, cerebrospinal fluid; EEG, electroencephalogram; PRNP, prion protein.

SUGGESTED READING

Bakshi, R, et al: The use of magnetic resonance imaging in the diagnosis and long-term management of multiple sclerosis. Neurology 63 Suppl 5:S3-S11, 2004.

Balcer, LJ: Clinical practice: Optic neuritis. N Engl J Med 354:1273-1280, 2006.

Beck, RW, et al, The Optic Neuritis Study Group: A randomized, controlled trial of corticosteroids in the treatment of acute optic neuritis. N Engl J Med 326:581-588, 1992.

Bennett, KA: Pregnancy and multiple sclerosis. Clin Obstet Gynecol 48:38-47, 2005.

Collinge, J: Molecular neurology of prion disease. J Neurol Neurosurg Psychiatry 76:906-919, 2005.

Crayton, H, Heyman, RA, and Rossman, HS: A multimodal approach to managing the symptoms of multiple sclerosis. Neurology 63 Suppl 5:S12-S18, 2004.

Cree, B: Emerging monoclonal antibody therapies for multiple sclerosis. Neurologist 12:171-178, 2006.

Frohman, EM, et al: Most patients with multiple sclerosis or a clinically isolated demyelinating syndrome should be treated at the time of diagnosis. Arch Neurol 63:614-619, 2006.

Frohman, EM, Racke, MK, and Raine, CS: Multiple sclerosis: The plaque and its pathogenesis. N Engl J Med 354:942-955, 2006.

Goodin, DS, et al, Therapeutics and Technology Assessment Subcommittee of the American Academy of Neurology: The use of mitoxantrone (Novantrone) for the treatment of multiple sclerosis: Report of the Therapeutics and Technology Assessment Subcommittee of the American Academy of Neurology. Neurology 61:1332-1338, 2003.

Kantarci, O, and Wingerchuk, D: Epidemiology and natural history of multiple sclerosis: New insights. Curr Opin Neurol 19:248-254, 2006.

Kappos, L, et al: Treatment with interferon beta-1b delays conversion to clinically definite and McDonald MS in patients with clinically isolated syndromes. Neurology 67:1242-1249, 2006. Epub 2006 Aug 16.

Marra, CM: Infections of the central nervous system in patients infected with human immunodeficiency virus in infectious disease. Continuum: Lifelong Learning in Neurology 12:111-132, June 2006.

McDonald, WI, et al: Recommended diagnostic criteria for multiple sclerosis: Guidelines from the International Panel on the Diagnosis of Multiple Sclerosis. Ann Neurol 50:121-127, 2001.

Nath, A, and Sacktor, N: Influence of highly active antiretroviral therapy on persistence of HIV in the central nervous system. Curr Opin Neurol 19:358-361, 2006.

Noseworthy, JH, and Hartung, H-P: Multiple sclerosis and related conditions. In Noseworthy, JH (ed): Neurological Therapeutics: Principles and Practice. Vol 1. Martin Dunitz, London, 2003, pp 1107-1131.

Noseworthy, JH, et al: Multple sclerosis. N Engl J Med 343:938-952, 2000.

Pirko, I, et al: Gray matter involvement in multiple sclerosis. Neurology 68:634-642, 2007.

Rizvi, SA, and Agius, MA: Current approved options for treating patients with multiple sclerosis. Neurology 63 Suppl 6:S8-S14, 2004.

Roos, KL: Acute meningitis in infectious disease. Continuum: Lifelong Learning in Neurology 12:13-26, June 2006.

Schwid, SR, et al, EVIDENCE (Evidence of Interferon Dose-Response: European North American Comparative Efficacy) Study Group; University of British Columbia MS/MRI Research Group. Enhanced benefit of increasing interferon beta-1a dose and frequency in relapsing multiple sclerosis: the EVIDENCE Study. Arch Neurol 62:785-792, 2005.

Sorensen, PS, et al: Neutralizing antibodies hamper IFNβ bioactivity and treatment effect on MRI in patients with MS. Neurology 67:1681-1683, 2006.

Torno, M, Vollmer, M, and Beck, CK: West Nile virus infection presenting as acute flaccid paralysis in an HIV-infected patient: A case report and review of the literature. Neurology 68:E5-E7, 2007.

Tunbridge, A, and Read, RC: Management of meningitis. Clin Med 4:499-505, 2004.

Whiting, P, et al: Accuracy of magnetic resonance imaging for the diagnosis of multiple sclerosis: Systematic review. BMJ 332:875-884, 2006. Epub 2006 Mar 24.

Wingerchuk, DM: Diagnosis and treatment of neuromyelitis optica. Neurologist 13:2-11, 2007.

Wingerchuk, DM, et al: Revised diagnostic criteria for neuromyelitis optica. Neurology 66:1485-1489, 2006.

CHAPTER 14

Neuro-oncology

Neuro-oncology is a rapidly evolving specialty involving the study of cancer and the nervous system. The nervous system can be affected by cancer directly, indirectly, or as a result of treatment-related side effects. The diagnosis and treatment of cancer of the nervous system require the skills of several medical disciplines to help patients who have one of the most frightening medical problems.

INTRACRANIAL NEOPLASMS

A modified version of the World Health Organization's classification of tumors of the central nervous system is provided in Table 14.1. Tumors of neuroepithelial tissue (glial tumors or gliomas) include the most common primary brain tumor, astrocytoma. Other major types of tumors are tumors of cranial and spinal nerves (schwannomas) and the meninges (meningiomas), lymphomas and hematopoietic neoplasms, germ cell tumors, tumors of the sellar region (pituitary), and metastatic tumors.

To determine prognosis and the most appropriate treatment, the tumor needs to be classified. Certain types of tumors have a predilection for specific locations in the brain. Gliomas (astrocytoma, glioblastoma multiforme, oligodendroglioma), meningiomas, and metastatic tumors usually occur in the cerebral hemispheres. Pituitary adenomas and pineal tumors are midline tumors. In adults, the most common infratentorial tumors are acoustic schwannomas, metastases, and meningiomas. Primary brain tumors in children are usually infratentorial and include cerebellar astrocytomas, medulloblastomas, ependymomas, and brainstem gliomas.

The histologic grade of a brain tumor is important for classification. The four astrocytoma grades correlate directly with mortality rate. Grade 1 astrocytomas (pilocytic astrocytoma) can be cured with surgical removal. Grade 2, or low-grade, astrocytoma is an infiltrating lesion with nuclear atypia but little or no mitotic activity. Grade 2 tumors can progress to higher grades of malignancy. Grade 3, or anaplastic, astrocytoma has mitoses. Grade 4, glioblastoma multiforme, has nuclear atypia, mitoses, necrosis, and endothelial proliferation.

Table 14.1. World Health Organization Classification of Tumors of the Central Nervous System

Neuroepithelial tumors

Astrocytic tumors

Pilocytic astrocytoma, diffuse astrocytoma (fibrillary, gemistocytic, proptoplasmatic), anaplastic astrocytoma, glioblastoma (giant cell glioblastoma, gliosarcoma), pleomorphic xanthoastrocytoma, subependymal giant cell astrocytoma, gliomatosis cerebri

Oligodendroglial tumors

Oligodendroglioma, anaplastic oligodendroglioma

Oligoastrocytic tumors

Oligoastrocytoma, anaplastic oligoastrocytoma

Ependymal tumors

Ependymoma (cellular, papillary, clear cell, tanycytic), anaplastic ependymoma, myxopapillary ependymoma, subependymoma

Choroid plexus tumors

Choroid plexus papilloma, atypical choroid plexus papilloma, choroid plexus carcinoma

Other neuroepithelial tumors

Astroblastoma, choroid glioma of the third ventricle, angiocentric glioma

Neuronal and mixed neuronal-glial tumors

Gangliocytoma, dysembryoplastic neuroepithelial tumor, ganglioglioma, anaplastic ganglioglioma, central neurocytoma, dysplastic gangliocytoma of the cerebellum, desmoplastic infantile astrocytoma/ganglioglioma, extraventricular neurocytoma, cerebellar liponeuronal tumor, rosette-forming glioneuronal tumor of the fourth ventricle, paraganglioma

Tumors of the pineal region

Pineocytoma, pineoblastoma, pineal parenchymal tumor of intermediate differentiation, papillary tumor of the pineal region

Embryonal tumors

Medulloblastoma (desmoplastic/nodular medulloblastoma, medulloblastoma with extensive nodularity, anaplastic medulloblastoma, large cell medulloblastoma), primitive neuroectodermal tumor (PNET) (CNS neuroblastoma, CNS ganglioneuroblastoma, medulloepithelioma, ependymoblastoma), atypical teratoid/rhabdoid tumor

Tumors of cranial and paraspinal nerves

Schwannoma

Cellular, plexiform, melanotic

Neurofibroma

Plexiform

Perineurioma

Perineurioma (not otherwise specified), malignant perineurioma

Malignant peripheral nerve sheath tumor (MPNST)

Epithelioid MPNST, MPNST with mesenchymal differentiation, melanotic MPNST, MPNST with glandular differentiation

Table 14.1 (continued)

Tumors of the meninges
Meningioma
Meningothelial, fibrous, transitional, psammomatous, angiomatous, microcystic, secretory, lymphoplasmacyte-rich, metaplastic choroid, clear cell, atypical, papillary, rhabdoid, anaplastic
Mesenchymal tumors
Lipoma, angiolipoma, hibernoma, liposarcoma, solitary fibrous tumor, fibrosarcoma, malignant fibrous histiocytoma, leiomyosarcoma, rhabdomyosarcoma, chondroma, chondrosarcoma, osteoma, osteosarcoma, osteochondroma, hemangioma, epithelioid hemangioendothelioma, hemangiopericytoma, angiosarcoma, Kaposi sarcoma, Ewing sarcoma
Primary melanocytic lesions
Diffuse melanocytosis, melanocytoma, malignant melanoma, meningeal melanomatosis
Lymphomas and hematopoietic neoplasms
Malignant lymphomas
Plasmacytoma
Granulocytic sarcoma
Germ cell tumors
Germinoma
Embryonal carcinoma
Yolk sac tumor
Choriocarcinoma
Teratoma
Mature, immature, teratoma with malignant transformation
Mixed germ cell tumors
Tumors of the sellar region
Craniopharyngioma
Adamantinomatous, papillary
Granular cell tumor
Pituicytoma
Spindle cell oncocytoma of the adenohypophysis
Metastatic tumors

CNS, central nervous system.
Modified from Louis DN, Ohgaki H, Wiestler OD, Cavenee WK, editors. WHO Classification of Tumours of the Central Nervous System. Lyon (FR), International Agency for Research in Cancer, 2007. Used with permission.

DIAGNOSTIC APPROACH

The most common symptoms of brain tumors are headache and personality changes, and the temporal profile is chronic and progressive. Headache is the initial symptom in more than one-third of patients with brain tumors, and more than two-thirds will experience headache in the course of the illness. The headache can be mild and intermittent, characteristics of a tension-type headache. Symptoms of increased intracranial pressure or focal findings, or both, are more indicative of a brain tumor than headache. With increased intracranial pressure, headache can be worse in the morning (it can even awaken the patient) and improve in the afternoon. Also, it can worsen with a change in position, cough, or exercise.

Seizures, both focal and generalized, can be the first sign of a brain tumor. Slower growing tumors, such as low-grade astrocytomas or oligodendrogliomas, are more likely to cause seizures than rapidly growing ones. Seizures are more likely to occur when the tumor is in the cerebral cortex. Subcortical or infratentorial tumors are rarely epileptogenic.

Changes in mental status may also be the first symptom of a brain tumor. Patients may complain of problems with concentration or memory, and family members may note a change in personality. In a study of patients older than 65 years who had brain tumors, the most frequent presenting symptoms were confusion, aphasia, and memory loss.

You should focus the neurologic examination on the presence of focal findings that suggest localization of the problem (Table 14.2). All tumors can cause an increase in intracranial pressure. Infratentorial tumors and tumors of the third ventricle frequently obstruct the ventricular system and cause hydrocephalus. Papilledema is a nonlocalizing sign of increased intracranial pressure and is a late finding. It is important to remember two false-localizing features of increased intracranial pressure: compression of the abducens nerve (cranial nerve VI) where it passes over the petrous ligament and compression of the cerebral peduncle by the free edge of the tentorium cerebelli that causes ipsilateral hemiparesis.

Computed tomography (CT) and magnetic resonance imaging (MRI) have been indispensable in evaluating intracranial neoplasms. These diagnostic studies provide information about size, location, midline shift, mass effect, ventricular compression, and obstructive hydrocephalus. The imaging characteristics of the lesion, such as location, amount of edema, and type of enhancement, can suggest the diagnosis (Fig. 14.1). The use of an intravenous contrast agent improves the sensitivity of CT in detecting brain tumors. However, CT is not as good as MRI for the evaluation of posterior fossa tumors, isodense infiltrating gliomas, and leptomeningeal metastases (meningeal carcinoma). MRI with gadolinium enhancement is the preferred imaging technique for the evaluation of intracranial malignancies.

Several other diagnostic tests may aid in the diagnosis and management of brain tumors. Audiometry and brainstem auditory evoked potentials are useful in the evaluation of acoustic neuromas. Visual field testing is valuable for indicating the presence of tumors in the sellar region (pituitary adenomas or craniopharyngiomas). The presence of bitemporal hemianopia indicates that a tumor is present in the sellar region and is affecting the optic chiasm. Determining hormonal levels in the blood and urine is helpful in identifying pituitary and hypothalamic tumors. Electroencephalography (EEG) should be performed if the patient has seizures. Focal tumors can cause focal slowing or epileptogenic activity (spikes) seen on EEG.

Table 14.2. Clinical Features of Brain Tumors Based on Location

Location	Clinical features
Frontal cortex	Personality change: disinhibition, abulia
	Seizures
	Hemiparesis
	Urinary urgency and frequency
	Gait ataxia
	Aphasia (dominant hemisphere)
	Gaze preference
Temporal cortex	Seizures
	Memory disturbance
	Superior quadrantanopia
Parietal cortex	Hemianesthesia
	Aphasia (dominant hemisphere)
	Neglect (nondominant hemisphere)
	Constructional apraxia
	Seizures
Occipital cortex	Hemianopia
	Visual agnosia
	Seizures
Thalamus	Hemianesthesia
	Cognitive impairment
Brainstem	Cranial neuropathies
	Ataxia
	Limb weakness
	Nystagmus
Pineal region	Parinaud syndrome (impaired upward gaze and dissociation of pupillary light reflex and near reflex)
Third ventricle	Hydrocephalus
	Hypothalamic dysfunction
	Autonomic dysfunction
Cerebellum	Headache
	Ataxia
	Hydrocephalus

From Adams, AC: Neurology in Primary Care. FA Davis, Philadelphia, 2000, p 247. Used with permission of Mayo Foundation for Medical Education and Research.

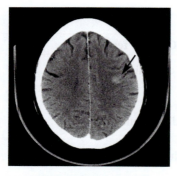

Low-grade astrocytoma (*arrow*)

Location: cerebral hemisphere
NECT: hypodense
MRI: hyperintense
Enhancement: 0/+
Edema: rare
Hemorrhage: rare
Calcification: 10%-20% of cases

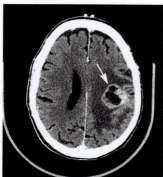

Anaplastic astrocytoma (*arrow*)

Location: cerebral white matter
NECT: inhomogeneous
MRI: heterogeneous signal
Enhancement: ++ inhomogeneous
Edema: common
Hemorrhage: occasional
Calcification: uncommon

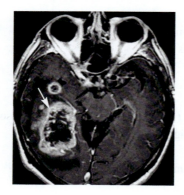

Glioblastoma multiforme (*arrow*)

Location: cerebral hemisphere
NECT: heterogeneous
MRI: heterogeneous
Enhancement: +++ inhomogeneous
Edema: common
Hemorrhage: common
Calcification: rare

Fig. 14.1. Imaging characteristics of intracranial tumors. CT, computed tomography; MRI, magnetic resonance imaging; NECT, nonenhanced computed tomography. (Images continued on next 2 pages).

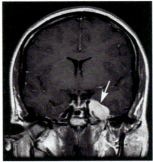

Meningioma (*arrow*)

Location: extra-axial dural based
NECT: hyperdense
MRI: isodense
Enhancement: +++ homogeneous on CT, het-
  erogeneous
Edema: present
Hemorrhage: rare
Calcification: 20%-25% of cases

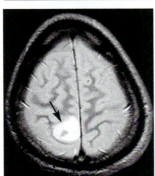

Oligodendroglioma (*arrow*)

Location: frontal lobe, cortex
NECT: calcified mixed density
MRI: mixed hypo- and isodense
Enhancement: +/++ inhomogeneous
Edema: rare
Hemorrhage: rare
Calcification: 70%-90% of cases

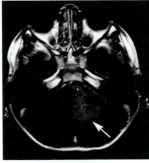

Ependymoma (*arrow*)

Location: Fourth ventricle
NECT: isodense
MRI: hypo-/isodense on T1
Enhancement: +/++ variable
Edema: hydrocephalus
Hemorrhage: can occur
Calcification: 1%-8% of cases

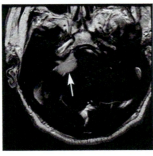

Acoustic neuroma (schwannoma) (*arrow*)

Location: cerebellopontine angle
NECT: hypo-/isodense
MRI: hypodense on T1
Enhancement: +++ homogeneous, inhomoge-
  neous, heterogeneous
Edema: rare
Hemorrhage: can occur
Calcification: rare

Fig. 14.1 (continued).

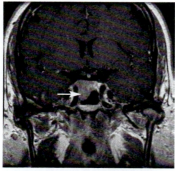

Pituitary adenoma (*arrow*)

Location: sellar region
NECT: isodense
MRI: hypodense, mixed intensity
Enhancement: +++
Edema: can occur
Hemorrhage: can occur
Calcification: 1%-8% of cases

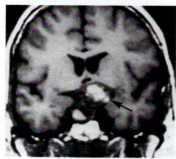

Craniopharyngioma (*arrow*)

Location: sellar region
NECT: calcification
MRI: hyperdense on T2, heterogeneous
Enhancement: ++ heterogeneous
Edema: rare
Hemorrhage: rare
Calcification: 90% of cases

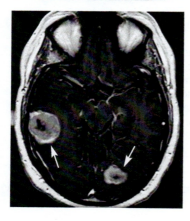

Metastasis (*arrows*)

Location: all areas, corticomedullary junction
NECT: iso-/hyperdense
MRI: hypodense on T1, hyperdense on T2
Enhancement: +++ ring
Edema: present
Hemorrhage: common
Calcification: rare

Fig. 14.1 (continued).

Cerebrospinal fluid (CSF) abnormalities (eg, pleocytosis) may provide important diagnostic information about leptomeningeal disease. CSF cytology is useful in the diagnosis of pineal tumors and leptomeningeal metastases (meningeal carcinoma). Biologic markers of germ cell tumors (alpha fetoprotein, β-subunit of human chorionic gonadotropin, and placental alkaline phosphatase) can be detected in the CSF. Remember, lumbar puncture should not be performed in a patient with increased intracranial pressure who is at risk for herniation.

MANAGEMENT

The management of a brain tumor is facilitated by the involvement of several medical specialties, including primary care, neurology, neurosurgery, oncology, radiation oncology, and psychiatry. Most brain tumors require the combination of surgery, radiotherapy, and chemotherapy. Some slow-growing tumors require only continued neurologic surveillance and serial imaging studies. An example is a small meningioma on the convexity of the brain that is often asymptomatic and requires only observation and reassurance of the patient.

For most brain tumors, surgery is the first step in management. It is curative for many tumors, including meningiomas, pituitary adenomas, pilocytic astrocytomas, and acoustic neuromas. The additional advantages of surgery are that it provides histologic diagnosis and improves the effectiveness of radiotherapy and chemotherapy.

Radiotherapy is essential in the treatment of all malignant gliomas, low-grade gliomas, and inoperable or recurrent benign tumors. Radiation of the whole brain, involved-field radiotherapy, stereotactic placement of radioactive isotopes directly into the tumor (brachytherapy), stereotactic radiosurgery (gamma knife), and stereotactic radiotherapy are techniques used to deliver cytotoxic ionizing radiation to tumor cells. Elderly patients and those with a very poor prognosis (poor performance status or high-grade malignancy) may be considered for an abbreviated course of radiotherapy or supportive care without radiotherapy. Fatigue, alopecia, headache, nausea, and scalp irritation are the common side effects of radiotherapy.

Many chemotherapeutic agents are used to treat brain tumors. Chemotherapy is complicated by the blood-brain barrier, which limits the distribution of water-soluble drugs into the brain. Various strategies have been used to bypass the blood-brain barrier to deliver the medication to the intended target, for example, intrathecal administration and implantation of chemotherapy-impregnated polymer wafers in the surgical cavity after resection.

Common chemotherapeutic regimens to treat patients with gliomas included BCNU (carmustine) or PCV (combination procarbazine, lomustine [CCNU], and vincristine). Since 2005, temozolomide has become the preferred chemotherapeutic agent for treating gliomas. Novel treatment strategies being developed for brain tumors include gene therapy, antiangiogenesis, immunotherapy, and targeting of tumor cells. Specialty consultation will provide the most up-to-date treatment recommendations.

Several medical issues are common to patients with intracranial tumors and include seizures, cerebral edema, fatigue, gastrointestinal dysfunction (anorexia, constipation, nausea, and vomiting), cognitive dysfunction, depression, and venous thromboembolism. Seizures are common in patients with brain tumors, and the usual antiepileptic medications are prescribed (see Table 9.5). Enzyme-inducing anticonvulsants (phenobarbital, phenytoin, and carbamazepine) should be avoided because of the interactions between these drugs and antineoplastic agents. Also, the enzyme-inducing antiepileptic drugs can cause an accelerated metabolism of chemotherapeutic drugs and, thus, reduce their plasma concentrations and anticancer effect. Furthermore, chemotherapeutic drugs can alter the metabolism of these antileptic drugs and either increase the likelihood of toxicity or diminish the anticonvulsant effect. Levetiracetam (Keppra) and lamotrigine (Lamictal) have been recommended as first-line agents for the treatment of patients who have brain tumors and seizures. Gabapentin (Neurontin) may be a reasonable add-on agent. Prophylactic anticonvulsant therapy is not recommended for patients with brain tumors.

Cerebral edema associated with a brain tumor is treated with corticosteroids. The dose of dexamethasone often ranges from 16 mg/day to 100 mg/day. This is effective in reducing the headache and may lessen the neurologic deficits. Common complications of corticosteroid therapy include behavioral changes, fragile skin, osteoporosis, gastrointestinal tract bleeding, visual blurring, hypertension, hyperglycemia, and opportunistic infections. Steroid myopathy occurs after prolonged treatment (in the 9th to 12th week of treatment). Proximal muscle weakness and wasting develops. The medication should be discontinued, if possible, or given at the lowest effective dose.

Venous thromboembolic disease is a frequent complication of intracranial malignancy. The risk of brain hemorrhage from anticoagulation may not be significantly increased beyond the immediate postoperative period, but some physicians have used inferior vena cava filtration devices to avoid anticoagulation and the risk of hemorrhage into the brain. The supportive treatment that can be used for the medical issues common to patients with brain tumors is summarized in Table 14.3.

SPINAL CORD TUMORS

Spinal cord tumors can cause myelopathy, with bilateral lower extremity weakness, spasticity, sensory level, spastic bladder, and extensor plantar reflexes. Involvement of the cauda equina causes lower motor neuron weakness, sensory loss, flaccid bladder, and decreased muscle reflexes (Fig. 14.2). MRI is the primary diagnostic imaging method (Fig. 14.3).

The three types of spinal cord tumors are distinguished by their anatomical location. Extradural tumors are external to the dura mater. Extramedullary tumors (meningiomas and neurofibromas) and intramedullary tumors

Table 14.3. Medical Management of Common Problems of Patients With Intracranial Tumors

Symptom	Management options
Seizures	Levetiracetam (Keppra), lamotrigine (Lamictal)
	Avoid enzyme-inducing anticonvulsants
Cerebral edema	Dexamethasone (Decadron)
Complications of corticosteroid therapy	
Osteoporosis	Calcium, vitamin D, bisphosphonates
Gastrointestinal tract bleeding	Proton pump inhibitors
Myopathy	Dose reduction, physical therapy
Fatigue	Modafinil (Provigil), other stimulants
Depression	Antidepressants
Venous thromboembolism	Anticoagulants, inferior vena cava filters
Nausea, vomiting	Antiemetics
Anorexia	Dronabinol (Marinol), megestrol (Megace)
Pneumocystis pneumonia	Trimethoprim-sulfamethoxazole (Bactrim)

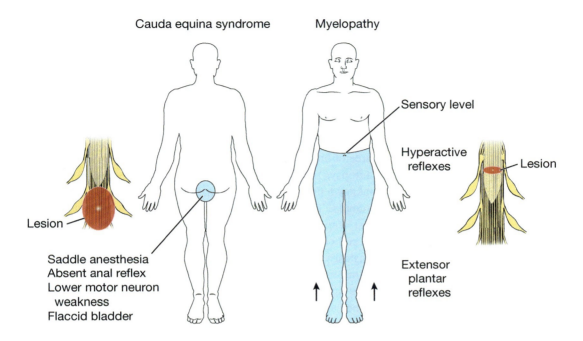

Fig. 14.2. Comparison of deficits associated with cauda equina syndrome and myelopathy. (From Adams, AC: Neurology in Primary Care. FA Davis, Philadelphia, 2000, p 73. Used with permission of Mayo Foundation for Medical Education and Research.)

(ependymomas, astrocytomas, oligodendro-gliomas, hemangioblastomas, and metastatic tumors) are internal to the dura mater.

The treatment of choice for spinal cord tumors is surgical removal. Radiotherapy is used if surgical excision is incomplete. High-grade gliomas of the spinal cord tend to undergo leptomeningeal spread. Specialty consultation is recommended for further management advice.

NEUROLOGIC COMPLICATIONS OF SYSTEMIC DISEASE

Brain Metastases

Brain metastases are neoplasms that originate outside the nervous system. The incidence is not known exactly, but evidence suggests

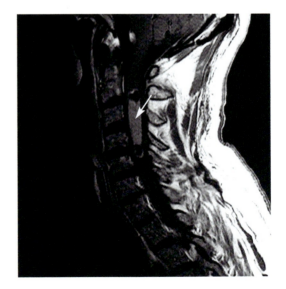

Fig. 14.3. MRI of the cervical spine showing an ependymoma (*arrow*).

that intracranial metastases equal, if not exceed, the incidence of primary brain tumors. Brain metastases occur in 20% to 40% of cancer patients, and an increased incidence is anticipated with improved neuroimaging techniques and the extended survival of cancer patients.

Metastases can occur in the parenchyma of the brain, in the leptomeninges, or in the dura mater. The most common source of brain metastases is lung cancer. On autopsy, the majority of "brain metastases of unknown primary" are found to be from lung tumors. The second leading source is breast cancer. Melanoma, colon cancer, and renal cell carcinoma can also cause brain metastases. In patients younger than 21 years, brain metastases are often from sarcomas and germ cell tumors.

Tumor cells spread to the brain hematogenously. Metastases are usually located in the cerebral hemispheres at the junction of the gray and white matter (the corticomedullary junction). The reduced size of blood vessels at this junction is thought to serve as a trap for metastatic cells, as for emboli. Metastases are also located at the border zones of the major blood vessels (the watershed areas). They can occur anywhere intracranially, with their distribution reflecting the relative volume of blood flow: 80% cerebral hemispheres, 15% cerebellum, and 5% brainstem.

Most brain metastases are diagnosed after the systemic cancer has been identified. The neurologic symptoms reflect the location of the tumors. Contrast-enhanced MRI is the preferred diagnostic test. Metastases are round, well-circumscribed lesions that may be surrounded by edema and enhance with contrast agent. The number of metastases, whether single or multiple, has important treatment implications. Also, a single metastasis needs to be distinguished from a primary brain tumor, abscess, cerebral infarct, and hemorrhage. Surgical resection or biopsy may be needed to establish the diagnosis.

Treatment options for brain metastases include corticosteroids, surgery, radiotherapy, stereotactic radiosurgery, interstitial brachytherapy, and chemotherapy. Whole brain radiation is used for disseminated or uncontrolled systemic cancer and multiple metastases. If there is a single, surgically accessible metastasis in a patient with limited or no systemic cancer, surgical removal followed by radiotherapy is recommended. For a patient with multiple metastases and a single, surgically accessible, life-threatening lesion, the lesion should be removed surgically, followed by radiotherapy. Specialty consultation will provide the most up-to-date treatment options.

Epidural Spinal Cord Compression

Spinal cord compression is a medical emergency and requires immediate treatment if the patient is to maintain neurologic function. The patient may have a known cancer and complain of back pain or trouble urinating. Examination findings are consistent with a myelopathy or cauda equina syndrome. Emergency MRI of the spine should be performed to confirm the diagnosis. Give a high dose of corticosteroids (intravenous administration of 100 mg of dexamethasone followed by 24 mg four times daily) to reduce spinal cord edema. Initiate radiotherapy immediately. Surgical evaluation should be considered for spinal instability, for known radioresistant tumors such as renal carcinoma, or for acute deterioration of neurologic function.

Meningeal Carcinoma

Meningeal carcinoma, also known as leptomeningeal metastases, neoplastic meningitis, or carcinomatous meningitis, is the result of disseminated and multifocal seeding of the leptomeninges by malignant cells in the subarachnoid space. The tumors that most commonly metastasize to the meninges are breast and lung tumors and melanoma. It is important that meningeal carcinoma be recognized because of the associated high morbidity and mortality.

The clinical features of meningeal carcinoma are numerous because the disorder can involve all or several levels of the neuraxis. Leptomeningeal metastases can invade the brain and spinal cord parenchyma, cranial nerves, nerve roots, and blood vessels supplying the nervous system. Neck or back pain is a common initial complaint, and lower motor neuron weakness and hyporeflexia are the most common signs. Headache, cognitive changes, gait difficulty, cranial nerve palsies, and radicular symptoms are all possible clinical features. Meningeal carcinoma should be considered in a cancer patient who has evidence of multifocal neurologic involvement. However, single-level neurologic involvement occurs in a large percentage of patients. Like other neurologic complications of systemic cancer, meningeal carcinoma can be the initial presentation of the cancer.

The diagnosis of meningeal carcinoma is made on the basis of positive cytologic findings on CSF analysis. MRI identifies most intraparenchymal lesions and provides information about the risk of herniation with lumbar puncture. Multiple subarachnoid mass lesions and hydrocephalus without an identifiable mass lesion are consistent with the diagnosis. Meningeal enhancement, beading, and root clumping are also suggestive findings.

CSF findings include an increased opening pressure, increased protein concentration, decreased glucose level, and positive cytologic findings. Repeated lumbar punctures may be needed to demonstrate malignant cells in the CSF. Biochemical markers such as carcinoembryonic antigen and β-glucuronidase have been used as an aid in diagnosis but are limited by poor sensitivity and specificity.

Treatment for meningeal carcinoma includes radiotherapy directed at symptomatic sites of the neuraxis and intrathecal chemotherapy. Without treatment, the median survival of patients is 4 to 6 weeks from the time of diagnosis.

Neurologic Complications of Therapy

The neurologic complications of cancer therapy are extensive. Chemotherapeutic agents can affect any level of the central or peripheral nervous system (Table 14.4). It is important to recognize these complications in order to modify treatment and to avoid confusion with the direct and indirect effects of cancer.

Radiotherapy can also damage the central and peripheral nervous systems. Brain injury from radiation is classified by the time of onset. *Acute encephalopathy* can occur during the first few days of therapy. *Early delayed encephalopathy*, including headaches and somnolence, can occur from 1 to 4 months after the completion of therapy, and *delayed radiotherapy neurotoxicity* can occur from several months to 10 or more years after therapy. Other adverse effects of radiation include cranial neuropathy, myelopathy, peripheral neuropathy, cerebrovascular damage, and radiation-induced tumors. A multidisciplinary approach may be needed to distinguish recurrent cancer from the complications of treatment.

Paraneoplastic Syndromes

The term *paraneoplastic syndrome* is used to describe the clinical features of the remote effects of cancer on the nervous system. Paraneoplastic syndromes are rare disorders that can affect both the central and peripheral nervous systems (Table 14.5). They can be specific for one cell type (eg, lower motor neuron axonal ending [cholinergic synapse] in Lambert-Eaton myasthenic syndrome and Purkinje cells in paraneoplastic cerebellar degeneration). Multiple levels of the nervous system may be affected, as in encephalomyelitis, which is a paraneoplastic syndrome that affects the cerebral

Table 14.4. Neurologic Complications of Cancer Therapy

Acute cerebellar syndrome: cytosine arabinoside, 5-fluorouracil, hexamethylmelamine, procarbazine, vinca alkaloids

Acute encephalopathy: asparaginase, 5-azacytidine, carmustine, cisplatin, cytosine arabinoside, etoposide, fludarabine, 5-fluorouracil, glucocorticoids, hexamethylmelamine, ifosfamide, inteferons, interleukin-2, methotrexate, procarbazine, tamoxifen, thiotepa, vinca alkaloids

Aseptic meningitis: cytosine arabinoside, methotrexate, levamisole

Cranial neuropathies: carmustine, cisplatin, vincristine

Dementia: carmustine, carmofur, cytosine arabinoside, fludarabine, 5-fluorouracil, interferon α, levamisole, methotrexate

Headache: asparaginase, cytosine arabinoside, etoposide, fludarabine, glucocorticoids, hexamethylmelamine, interferons, interleukin-2, mechlorethamine, methotrexate, retinoic acid, tamoxifen, temozolomide, thiotepa

Myelopathy: methotrexate, cytosine arabinoside, thiotepa

Neuropathy: 5-azacytidine, carboplatin, cisplatin, cytosine arabinoside, etoposide, 5-fluorouracil, gemcitabine, hexamethylmelamine, ifosfamide, interferon α, oxaliplatin, procarbazine, purine analogues, suramin, paclitaxel, docetaxel, vinca alkaloids

Seizures: asparaginase, busulfan, carmustine, cisplatin, dacarbazine, etoposide, 5-fluorouracil, ifosfamide, interferons, interleukin-2, methotrexate, nitrogen mustard, pentostatin, teniposide, vinca alkaloids

Vasculopathy and stroke: asparaginase, carmustine, cisplatin, doxorubicin, estramustine, methotrexate

Visual loss: carmustine, cisplatin, fludarabine, tamoxifen, taxanes

From Wen, PY: Neurologic complications of chemotherapy. In Samuels, MA, and Feske, S (eds): Office Practice of Neurology. ed 2. Churchill Livingstone, Philadelphia, 2003, pp 1134-1140. Used with permission.

hemispheres, brainstem, spinal cord, dorsal root ganglia, and nerve roots.

The serum and CSF of patients with a paraneoplastic syndrome contain antibodies that are directed to neuronal proteins expressed by the associated tumor. The immune system recognizes these proteins as foreign and mounts an immune attack. This immune response partially controls tumor growth but also attacks the portion of the nervous system that expresses the antigen. The identification of these antibodies confirms the paraneoplastic origin of the neurologic dysfunction and helps direct the search for the underlying cancer. Several of the antibody-associated paraneoplastic disorders and their related cancers are summarized in Table 14.6.

Paraneoplastic syndromes are difficult to diagnose. The neurologic syndrome often occurs before the cancer is discovered. Also, many other inflammatory conditions can mimic these syndromes. Paraneoplastic syndromes have a subacute progressive temporal profile and should be suspected in a patient who has

Table 14.5. Paraneoplastic Syndromes and Clinical Features

Syndrome	Clinical features
Central nervous system syndromes	
Paraneoplastic encephalomyelitis	Combination of clinical features of limbic encephalitis, brainstem encephalitis, cerebellar degeneration, myelopathy, autonomic dysfunction
Limbic encephalitis	Behavioral and psychiatric symptoms, complex partial seizures, dementia
Brainstem encephalitis	Diplopia, dysarthria, dysphagia, spastic quadriparesis, ataxia, gaze palsies
Subacute cerebellar degeneration	Ataxia, dysarthria, limb ataxia, nystagmus
Opsoclonus-myoclonus	Abnormal ocular motility, quick muscle jerks
Retinopathy	Scotomas, blindness, visual hallucinations
Peripheral nervous system syndromes	
Motor neuronopathy	Predominant motor weakness
Sensory neuronopathy	Large-fiber sensory loss (joint position and vibration more than pain and temperature), sensory ataxia, dysesthesias, minimal motor involvement
Autonomic neuronopathy	Gastroparesis, orthostatic hypotension, impotence, reduced sweating, dry eyes and mouth
Length-dependent sensorimotor neuronopathy	Distal sensory loss, muscle weakness
Polyradiculoneuropathy	Proximal sensory loss and motor weakness, pain
Mononeuritis multiplex	Multiple mononeuropathies
Stiff person syndrome	Stiffness of axial muscles, painful tonic spasms, fixed lumbar lordosis
Neuromyotonia (Isaacs syndrome)	Muscle stiffness, myalgias, fasciculations, cramps, hyperhydrosis, tachycardia
Cramp-fasciculation syndrome	Cramps
Neuromuscular junction and muscle syndromes	
Myasthenia gravis	Fatigable weakness
Lambert-Eaton myasthenic syndrome	Fatigue, proximal muscle weakness, reduced or absent muscle stretch reflexes, dry mouth, impotence
Dermatomyositis	Proximal muscle weakness associated with rash
Necrotizing myopathy	Muscle weakness

From Adams, AC: Neurology in Primary Care. FA Davis, Philadelphia, 2000, p 255. Used with permission of Mayo Foundation for Medical Education and Research.

Table 14.6. Antibodies Found in Paraneoplastic Syndromes

Antibody	Associated tumor	Clinical syndrome
Acetylcholine receptor	Thymoma, SCLC	Myasthenia gravis
Amphiphysin	Breast, lung	Stiff person syndrome, encephalomyelitis, neuronopathy
ANNA 1 (anti-Hu)	SCLC, neuroblastoma	Sensory neuronopathy, encephalomyelitis
ANNA 2 (anti-Ri)	Breast, gynecologic, SCLC	Opsoclonus, cerebellar ataxia
ANNA 3	SCLC	Encephalomyelitis
Anti-glial nuclear	SCLC	Lambert-Eaton myasthenic syndrome
Anti-Ma	Lung, breast, testicular	Limbic and brainstem encephalitis, cerebellar degeneration
Anti-Tr	Hodgkin lymphoma	Cerebellar degeneration
Anti-Zic	SCLC	Cerebellar degeneration
CRMP-5	SCLC or thymoma	Encephalomyelitis, chorea, neuropathy, optic neuritis
Glutamate receptor antibody	Hodgkin lymphoma	Cerebellar degeneration
PCA 1 (anti-Yo)	Gynecologic, breast	Cerebellar degeneration
PCA 2	SCLC	Encephalomyelitis
Retinal	SCLC, melanoma, gynecologic	Cancer-associated retinopathy
Voltage-gated calcium channel (P/Q type)	SCLC	Lambert-Eaton myasthenic syndrome, cerebellar degeneration
Voltage-gated calcium channel (N type)	Lung or breast	Encephalomyelitis, neuropathy
Voltage-gated potassium channel	SCLC or thymoma	Neuromyotonia, limbic encephalitis

ANNA, antinuclear neuronal antibody; CRMP, collapsin response-mediator protein; PCA, Purkinje cell antibody; SCLC, small cell lung carcinoma.

cancer or risk factors for cancer. This diagnosis should also be considered if the patient's clinical features are consistent with one of the characteristic syndromes and no other cause is found on standard evaluation.

The diagnostic approach to the patient depends on whether the patient has a known cancer. If cancer has not been diagnosed, focus the evaluation on detecting the cancer. Some of the tests that may need to be performed are MRI or CT of the chest and abdomen, mammography and pelvic ultrasonography in women, testicular ultrasonography in men, lymph node examination, positron emission tomography, and serum tumor markers. If the patient has a peripheral neuropathy, include a bone survey and serum protein electrophoresis in the evaluation. Further diagnostic evaluation includes tests for paraneoplastic antibodies and CSF analysis for cells, immunoglobulin, oligoclonal bands, and cytology. Evaluate the CSF and serum for the presence of paraneoplastic antibodies. If no cancer is detected, follow the patient's condition. If paraneoplastic antibodies are present or CSF analysis results are positive for an immune reaction, repeat the diagnostic evaluation. If a paraneoplastic syndrome occurs in a patient with a known cancer, direct the evaluation at excluding metastatic complications, complications of therapy, or problems related to systemic disease.

The first line of treatment for paraneoplastic syndromes is to treat the underlying malignancy. However, many syndromes do not respond to treatment. Treatment with plasma exchange, intravenous immunoglobulin, and other immunosuppressive agents is being investigated.

SUGGESTED READING

Bloomer, CW, Ackerman, A, and Bhatia, RG: Imaging for spine tumors and new applications. Top Magn Reson Imaging 17:69-87, 2006.

Chamberlain, MC: Neoplastic meningitis. Neurologist 12:179-187, 2006.

Darnell, RB, and Posner, JB: Paraneoplastic syndromes involving the nervous system. N Engl J Med 349:1543-1554, 2003.

DeAngelis, LM: Brain tumors. N Engl J Med 344:114-123, 2001.

Ewend, MG, Elbabaa, S, and Carey, LA: Current treatment paradigms for the management of patients with brain metastases. Neurosurgery 57 Suppl:S66-S77, 2005.

Forsyth, PA, and Posner, JB: Headaches in patients with brain tumors: A study of 111 patients. Neurology 43:1678-1683, 1993.

Henson, JW: Spinal cord gliomas. Curr Opin Neurol 14:679-682, 2001.

Henson, JW: Treatment of glioblastoma multiforme: A new standard. Arch Neurol 63:337-341, 2006.

Kleihues, P, and Cavenee, WK (eds): Pathology and Genetics of Tumours of the Nervous System. International Agency for Research on Cancer, Lyon, France, 2000.

Loblaw, DA, et al: Systematic review of the diagnosis and management of malignant extradural spinal cord compression: The Cancer Care Ontario Practice Guidelines Initiative's Neuro-Oncology Disease Site Group. J Clin Oncol 23:2028-2037, 2005.

Newton, HB, Ray-Chaudhury, A, and Cavaliere, R: Brain tumor imaging and cancer management: The neuro-oncologists perspective. Top Magn Reson Imaging 17:127-136, 2006.

Norden, AD, and Wen, PY: Glioma therapy in adults. Neurologist 12:279-292, 2006.

Norden, AD, Wen, PY, and Kesari, S: Brain metastases. Curr Opin Neurol 18:654-661, 2005.

Plotkin, SR, and Wen, PY: Neurologic complications of cancer therapy. Neurol Clin 21:279-318, 2003.

Vecht, CJ, and van Breemen, M: Optimizing therapy of seizures in patients with brain tumors. Neurology 67 Suppl 4:S10-S13, 2006.

Vernino, S: Paraneoplastic neurologic syndromes. Curr Neurol Neurosci Rep 6:193-199, 2006.

Wen, PY: Neurologic complications of chemotherapy. In Samuels, MA, and Feske, SK (eds): Office Practice of Neurology. ed 2. Churchill Livingstone, Philadelphia, 2003, pp 1134-1140.

INDEX

*For Product Safety Concerns and Information please contact
our EU representative GPSR@taylorandfrancis.com Taylor & Francis
Verlag GmbH, Kaufingerstraße 24, 80331 München, Germany*

T - #0156 - 090625 - C408 - 254/178/19 - PB - 9781420079739 - Gloss Lamination